Editor's introduction

Horizons in medicine is a collation of reviews based on the annual Advanced Medicine conference held over four days at the Royal College of Physicians in London. The conference has a consistent reputation for extremely high quality presentations by speakers who are leaders in their fields. It has been a pleasure to organise the 2006 conference, not least because even the most distinguished speakers seemed genuinely delighted to be asked and clearly 'pulled out all the stops' to ensure a very high standard.

The Advanced Medicine conference is more than a collection of reviews across the range of internal medicine – it deliberately includes cutting-edge developments some of which may not yet be established in routine clinical practice. Arguably there is a growing and worrying division between clinical practice and academic medicine and one of the intentions in the programming was to reinforce the relevance of experimental medicine to the evolution of clinical practice. I was conscious, though, that most of the attendees (and readers of *Horizons*) are practising clinicians and we have tried to ensure a balance that includes practical guidance for the physician.

Whilst writing this several months after the event I challenged myself to remember what I had learnt without reference to notes or the manuscripts for this edition. I learnt that multi-organ failure was primarily mitochondrial failure, that heart valves could be replaced by a catheter-wielding physician, and I, at least temporarily, remembered a beautifully clear and scientific approach to the management of hypertension. We also had a stunning Croonian Lecture illustrating the surprisingly broad impact of the actions of the hypoxia response protein – HIF1, a superb bio-medical review lecture on inflammation and cancer, and excellent Linacre and William Withering lectures. I think I have sufficient insight to recognise that my recall may be very eccentric and incomplete (but it is not as incomplete as my recall of most other conferences I have attended) and I do remember that all the presentations, now presented here, were very high quality.

We also had good fun at the conference with some interactive case discussions, many of which were deliberately rather 'grey' and difficult. I am most grateful to our speakers for providing the cases and for joining in the panel discussions of these with such good spirit, and to my colleague from Liverpool, Dr Solomon Almond, for all the hard work he put into collating and chairing these cases. Increasing pressures on clinicians sometimes squeeze some of the fun out of clinical medicine and I hope the conference did a little to redress this. I am sorry that it was not possible to reproduce the cases in print here – this would have required a great deal of time and effort from all the speakers and we felt that was probably one demand too many. I can only suggest that you book early for next year's conference!

The conference as always has been enthusiastically supported and efficiently run by the College staff and I am most grateful to Anne McSweeney and her team in the Conference Department, Barry Lewis and the audiovisual team, and Hannah Thompson in the Publications Office.

JONATHAN RHODES
July 2006

Horizons in Medicine

Royal College
of Physicians

Acknowledgement

The Royal College of Physicians acknowledges with thanks a grant from the Haymills Trust and the contribution of The Lavenham Press towards the cost of printing this book.

The Royal College of Physicians of London

The Royal College of Physicians plays a leading role in the delivery of high quality patient care by setting standards of medical practice and promoting clinical excellence. We provide physicians in the UK and overseas with education, training and support throughout their careers. As an independent body representing over 20,000 Fellows and Members worldwide, we advise and work with government, the public, patients and other professions to improve health and healthcare.

Citation of this book: Royal College of Physicians. *Horizons in medicine*, volume 18. London: RCP, 2006.

Front cover photograph:
Ingram Publishing/SuperStock

Royal College of Physicians of London
11 St Andrews Place, London NW1 4LE

Registered Charity No. 210508

ISBN-13: 978-1-86016-292-3
ISBN-10: 1-86016-292-4

Typeset by Dan-Set Graphics, Telford, Shropshire
Printed in Great Britain by The Lavenham Press Ltd, Suffolk

British Library Cataloguing in Publication Data
A catalogue record of this book is available from the British Library

Contributors

QASIM AZIZ *Professor of Gastroenterology, Department of GI Sciences, University of Manchester, Clinical Sciences Building, Hope Hospital, Stott Lane, Salford M6 8HD*

SIMON V BAUDOUIN *Senior Lecturer in Critical Care Medicine, University of Newcastle upon Tyne, Department of Anaesthesia, Leazes Wing, Royal Victoria Infirmary, Newcastle upon Tyne NE1 4LP*

PHILIPP BONHOEFFER *Chief of Cardiology and Director of the Cardiac Catheterisation Laboratory, Cardiothoracic Unit, Great Ormond Street Hospital for Children, Great Ormond Street, London WC1N 3JH*

SIR ALASDAIR BRECKENRIDGE *Chair, Medicines and Healthcare products Regulatory Agency, Market Towers, 1 Nine Elms lane, London SW8 5NQ*

MORRIS J BROWN *Professor of Clinical Pharmacology, University of Cambridge and Honorary Consultant Physician, Addenbrooke's Hospital, Hills Road, Cambridge CB2 2QQ*

PATRICK F CHINNERY *Professor of Neurogenetics and Wellcome Trust Senior Fellow in Clinical Science, Department of Neurology, The Medical School, Framlington Place, Newcastle upon Tyne NE2 4HH*

LOUISE COATS *British Heart Foundation Junior Fellow, Cardiothoracic Unit, Great Ormond Street Hospital for Children, Great Ormond Street, London WC1N 3JH*

MICHAEL DOHERTY *Professor of Rheumatology, Academic Rheumatology, Clinical Sciences Building, Nottingham City Hospital, Nottingham NG5 1PB*

RACHELLE DONN *Senior Lecturer in Molecular Genetics, Centre for Molecular Medicine, Stopford Building, University of Manchester M13 9PT*

CHUNDAMANNIL E EAPEN *EASL Sheila Sherlock visiting fellow, Liver Unit, Queen Elizabeth Hospital, Birmingham B15 2TH*

ELWYN ELIAS *Consultant Hepatologist, Liver Unit, Queen Elizabeth Hospital, Birmingham B15 2TH*

EMAD M EL-OMAR *Professor of Gastroenterology/Honorary Consultant Physician, Department of Medicine & Therapeutics, Institute of Medical Sciences, Aberdeen University, Foresterhill, Aberdeen AB25 2ZD*

JOHN FEEHALLY *Professor of Renal Medicine, The John Walls Renal Unit, Leicester General Hospital, Gwendolen Road, Leicester LE5 4PW*

MICHAEL FISHER *Consultant Cardiologist and Honorary Lecturer, Cardiothoracic Centre Liverpool and Department of Cardiology, Royal Liverpool University Hospital, Prescot Street, Liverpool L7 8XP*

DANIEL R GAYA *Specialist Registrar and Research Fellow, Gastrointestinal Unit, Molecular Medicine Centre, Western General Hospital, University of Edinburgh, EH4 2XU*

TIMOTHY HJ GOODSHIP *Professor of Renal Medicine, The Institute of Human Genetics, University of Newcastle upon Tyne, The International Centre for Life, Central Parkway, Newcastle upon Tyne NE1 3BZ*

DAVID KAVANAGH *Kidney Research UK Training Fellow, Washington University School of Medicine, Campus Box 8045, 660 South Euclid, St Louis, MO 63110, USA*

MIDORI KAYAHARA *Research Associate, Centre for Molecular Medicine, Stopford Building, University of Manchester M13 9PT*

CHARLES W LEES *Clinical Lecturer in Gastroenterology, Gastrointestinal Unit Molecular Medicine Centre, University of Edinburgh, Western General Hospital, Crewe Road, Edinburgh EH4 2XU*

MAIRI MACARTHUR *Clinical Research Fellow, Department of Medicine & Therapeutics, Institute of Medical Sciences, Aberdeen University, Foresterhill, Aberdeen AB25 2ZD*

ISLA S MACKENZIE *Clinical Lecturer in Clinical Pharmacology, University of Cambridge and Honorary Specialist Registrar, Addenbrooke's Hospital, Hills Road, Cambridge CB2 2QQ*

MICHAEL S MARBER *Professor of Cardiology, Department of Cardiology, King's College London, The Rayne Institute, St Thomas' Hospital, London SE1 7EH*

JOHN MOXHAM *Professor of Respiratory Medicine, King's College London School of Medicine; Consultant Physician, King's College Hospital, Denmark Hill, London SE5 9PJ*

JOHN NEWELL-PRICE *Consultant Endocrinologist and Senior Lecturer, Academic Unit of Diabetes and Endocrinology, University of Sheffield, Room OU142, Floor O, Royal Hallamshire Hospital, Glossop Road, Sheffield S10 2JF*

JEREMY R PLAYFER *Consultant Physician in Geriatric Medicine, Royal Liverpool University Hospital, Prescot Street, Liverpool L7 8XP*

MICHAEL I POLKEY *Consultant Physician and Reader in Respiratory Medicine, Respiratory Muscle Laboratory, Royal Brompton Hospital and National Heart & Lung Institute, Fulham Road, London SW3 6NP*

D MARK PRITCHARD *Wellcome Trust Advanced Clinical Fellow and Senior Lecturer in Medicine, Division of Gastroenterology, School of Clinical Sciences, University of Liverpool, 5th Floor UCD Building, Daulby St, Liverpool L69 3GA*

PETER J RATCLIFFE *Nuffield Professor of Medicine, Nuffield Department of Medicine, John Radcliffe Hospital, Oxford OX3 9DU*

DAVID WILLIAM RAY *Professor of Medicine and Endocrinology, Centre for Molecular Medicine, Stopford Building, University of Manchester M13 9PT*

JONATHAN L REES *Grant Chair of Dermatology, Dermatology, Room 4.018, First Floor, The Lauriston Building, Lauriston Place, Edinburgh, EH3 9HA*

PETER SANDERCOCK *Professor of Medical Neurology, University of Edinburgh, Division of Clinical Neurosciences, Western General Hospital, Edinburgh EH4 2XU*

JACK SATSANGI *Professor of Gastroenterology and Consultant Physician, Gastrointestinal Unit, Molecular Medicine Centre, University of Edinburgh, Western General Hospital, Crewe Road, Edinburgh EH4 2XU*

ABHISHEK SHARMA *Clinical Research Fellow, Department of GI Sciences, University of Manchester, Clinical Sciences Building, Hope Hospital, Stott Lane, Salford M6 8HD*

MERVYN SINGER *Professor of Intensive Care Medicine, Bloomsbury Institute of Intensive Care Medicine, Department of Medicine and Wolfson Institute of Biomedical Research, University College London, Gower Street, London WC1E 6BT*

STEPHEN G SPIRO *Professor of Respiratory Medicine, Consultant Physician, Department of Thoracic Medicine, University College Hospital, UCLH NHS Foundation Trust, Grafton Way, London WC1E 6AU*

DEBORAH PM SYMMONS *arc Epidemiology Unit, University of Manchester, Stopford Building, Oxford Road, Manchester M13 9PT*

LYNNE TURNER-STOKES *Professor of Rehabilitation, Herbert Dunhill Chair of Rehabilitation, King's College, London, and Director, Regional Rehabilitation Unit, Northwick Park Hospital, Watford Road, Harrow HA1 3UJ*

JITEN VORA *Consultant Physician/Endocrinologist, Royal Liverpool University Hospital, Prescot Street, Liverpool L7 8XP*

JULIA WENDON *The Institute of Liver Studies, King's College Hospital, Denmark Hill, London SE5 9RS*

RAINER ZBINDEN *Honorary Consultant Cardiologist, Department of Cardiology, King's College London, The Rayne Institute, St Thomas' Hospital, London SE1 7EH*

Contents

Respiratory

Management of acute respiratory distress syndrome

Simon V Baudouin

☐ INTRODUCTION

Acute respiratory distress syndrome (ARDS) was first defined in detail only about 50 years ago and arose because of the success of modern critical care, anaesthesia, and surgery. It was first described in trauma and military casualties and later was extended to include patients after major surgery and those with a variety of clinical conditions, including sepsis, pancreatitis, and pneumonia.[1,2]

As the name suggests, ARDS is a symptom of acute respiratory failure that usually develops within 24–48 hours of the initiating insult and follows successful resuscitation. It is characterised by the radiological development of diffuse widespread alveolar shadowing on plain chest radiographs, which is caused by the presence of severe alveolar oedema. In theory, the absence of increased left atrial pressure distinguishes this from cardiogenic pulmonary oedema, but, in practice, complete separation of the two conditions may be difficult. Flooding and collapse of alveolar gas exchanging units produce marked ventilation–perfusion mismatching. The end result of this process is worsening, and ultimately intractable, hypoxaemia. Although the occasional patient may be managed successfully by non-invasive methods, almost all patients who develop ARDS will need intubation and often a prolonged period of mechanical ventilation.

Early descriptions of ARDS emphasised the important role of increased pulmonary vascular permeability in the pathophysiology of the condition. Radio-isotope studies confirmed the early appearance of a breakdown in the endothelial and epithelial barrier in the lung, which corresponds to the marked alveolar epithelial damage seen in histological sections of lung. Subsequent research has shown that an intense inflammatory process occurs at a very early stage; this is focused on the alveolar airspace and surrounding lung interstitium (Fig 1).[2] In a landmark study of patients at high risk of developing ARDS, the early appearance of proinflammatory cytokines in the alveolar space was shown to predict the subsequent development of acute lung injury.[3] These cytokines seem to amplify the initial insult by recruiting acute inflammatory cells, including neutrophils and mononuclear cells, to the lung. These innate immune cells became activated and release a complex mixture of proinflammatory mediators that contribute to further epithelial and endothelial damage. In patients who recover from ARDS, the inflammatory response ultimately resolves but frequently produces a stage of fibrosis and scarring that may result in irreversible destruction of pulmonary parenchyma.[4] In most survivors, however, lung

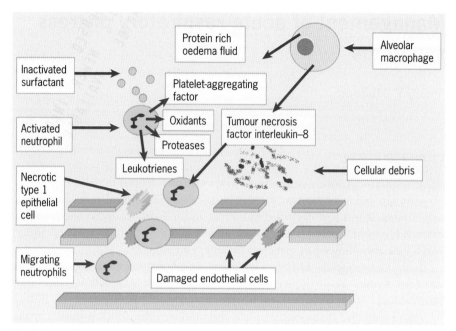

Fig 1 Acute inflammatory response in patients with acute respiratory distress syndrome. The airspaces of the lung are filled with acute inflammatory cells, as well as proteinaceous debris. Proinflammatory mediators are locally released from inflammatory cells and the damaged endothelial–epithelial barrier. Many of these mediators act as chemokine attractants to circulating inflammatory cells that amplify the injury process.

function ultimately recovers, although improvement of pulmonary gas exchange continues for a prolonged period.[5]

☐ EPIDEMIOLOGY OF ACUTE RESPIRATORY DISTRESS SYNDROME

Research into the epidemiology of ARDS has been facilitated by the international adoption of consensus definitions (Box 1). Even when these relatively straightforward definitions are used, however, the reported incidence of ARDS seems to have wide variation.[6] Most surveys have found ARDS to be a relatively uncommon condition, with a reported incidence of 1.5–8.3 cases per 100,000

Box 1 American–European consensus conference committee's definitions of acute respiratory distress syndrome and acute lung injury.

- Acute onset of respiratory failure
- Bilateral infiltrates in chest radiograph
- Pulmonary artery wedge pressure <18 mmHg (if obtained by pulmonary artery catheterisation)
- If the ratio of PaO_2 (mmHg) to FiO_2 is <300, acute lung injury is considered to be present
- If the ratio of PaO_2 (mmHg) to FiO_2 is <200, acute respiratory distress syndrome is considered to be present

person-years. A recent large and well conducted survey from North America, however, suggested that ARDS is much more common, with an incidence of 78.9 cases per 100,000 person-years.[7] A strong influence of patients' ages on incidence was also found, with the incidence increasing to 306 cases per 100,000 person-years for those older than 75 years. These findings are important in predicting the future incidence given the increasing age of patients on admission to critical care units.

Variation in outcome, as measured by hospital mortality, is also a feature of ARDS. A recent North American survey reported an in-hospital mortality of 38.5%, and previous surveys and trials have found that mortality varied from <30% to >80%.[6] Much of this variation can be explained by differing casemixes. Outcome from ARDS is determined mostly by the age of the patient and the cause and severity of the illness that induced the ARDS. In general critical care practice, severe sepsis is the most common underlying cause and is associated with a hospital mortality that often exceeds 50%. In contrast, patients who develop ARDS after trauma have a better outlook, with mortality <20%. Direct injury to the lung (for example, pneumonia and aspiration) also carries a higher mortality than indirect injury (for example, after major surgery). These differences are a consequence of the fact that ARDS is a clinical syndrome rather than a single distinct condition. Although the final common pathway of lung injury probably is similar, the impact of the illness on other vital organ systems is variable.

☐ ACUTE RESPIRATORY DISTRESS SYNDROME AND MULTIPLE ORGAN FAILURE

The importance of the severity of overall illness in determining outcome in ARDS has been confirmed in numerous surveys and clinical trials.[8] The initial severity of lung injury, as assessed indirectly by gas exchange criteria, has little or no predictive power in determining hospital outcome. In contrast, well established measures of the severity of critical illness and the degree of multiple organ failure have a much stronger relation with outcome. These factors underscore one of the most important aspects of the management of ARDS: most patients with ARDS will develop multiple organ failure and will require high quality support of several organ systems. Management of ventilation in ARDS has generated a huge and clinically useful literature. This is just one aspect of clinical care, however. A patient with ARDS presents the critical care team with one of their most challenging problems. A full range of skills thus are needed, including the use of inotropes, renal replacement therapy, fluid management, and nutritional support.

☐ MANAGEMENT OF VENTILATION

Patients with ARDS have characteristic changes in lung mechanics, with a marked alteration in pressure and volume relations. In simple terms, the lungs are stiff and need an increased inflation pressure to achieve any given tidal volume.[9] The aim of supportive treatment in critical care often is to normalise physiology. This approach to ventilation in ARDS was adopted in the 1970s and 1980s and led to the use of high tidal volumes and inflation pressures to achieve normocapnia. It also was established that a reasonably linear relation often exists between arterial oxygen pressure (PaO_2)

and mean airway pressure; again, this encouraged the use of relatively high inflation pressures.

Positive end expiratory pressure (PEEP) was also recognised to often improve oxygenation. Normally, at the end of expiration, alveolar pressure equilibrates with atmospheric pressure, which leads to what is sometimes described as 'zero end expiratory pressure'. By introducing resistance into the expiratory limb of the ventilator, alveolar pressure can be held at a set level above atmospheric pressure: commonly within a range of 5–15 cm water. Although widely used in critical care practice, PEEP was viewed as potentially harmful to the lung, and most practitioners would try to use the least PEEP possible.

Two decades of intense research – both experimental and clinical – have altered our approach to ventilation in ARDS.[9,10] This has been complemented by a new era of large multicentre clinical trials in critical care. A number of these have focused on the ventilatory management of ARDS, and the important input of a group of mostly North American and Canadian researchers – known as the ARDS Network – should be acknowledged.

The first important conceptual change came from cross sectional imaging and functional gas exchange studies in patients with ARDS. These techniques showed that lung injury is not a uniform process in the initial stages of ARDS.[9] In one popular model of this process, the lung can be divided into three compartments (Fig 2):

- □ normal gas exchanging units

- □ units that are completely collapsed, flooded, or destroyed

- □ units in which collapse is only partial.

This model has immediate practical implications for the ventilatory management of ARDS:

- □ the use of supranormal or even normal tidal volumes will eventually overdistend and stretch the normal lung units. This idea was popularised by one group of investigators under the name of 'baby lung' to emphasise the problem of ventilating a small effective lung

- □ the population of 'partly damaged' lung units indicates a potential for rapid improvement in gas exchange if these can be 'recruited' back into the normal population. This explains the apparent effectiveness of increasing airway pressure. Collapsed lung units would be recruited but at the cost of overdistension of existing units

- □ the model also provided an explanation for the effect of PEEP. Dynamic lung imaging showed that even during a single respiratory cycle, collapsed lung units could be recruited and subsequently derecruited. The addition of suitable levels of PEEP could stabilise the recruited lung units, thereby improving gas exchange.

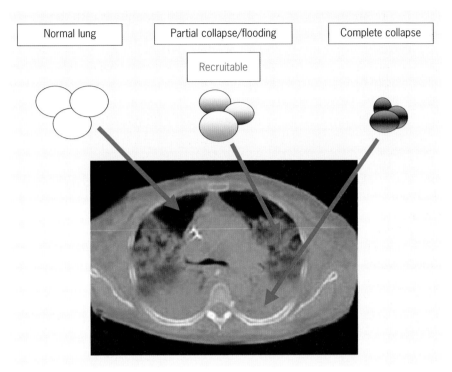

Fig 2 A three compartment model of acute lung injury. In the first (uppermost) compartment alveolar gas exchanging units are normal. In the second intermediate compartment, the units are collapsed or flooded partially but can be recruited back into effective gas exchange by various manoeuvres. In the third (lowest) compartment, the units are injured irreversibly and cannot support gas exchange.

Ventilation induced lung injury

The second fundamental discovery was the fact that mechanical ventilation can cause lung injury.[11] Beginning in the 1970s, many experimental studies showed that even relatively modest tidal volumes, delivered by mechanical ventilators, could cause a picture of lung injury in animals identical to that reported in patients with ARDS. The precise cellular and molecular causes of ventilator induced lung injury (VILI) continue to attract considerable research interest.[2] Clearly, however, the injury is a result of the delivered volume of ventilation. Alveolar damage then may occur because of classic overdistension, repetitive opening and closing of alveoli, or the release of damaging cytokines by a process of mechanotransduction.

By the early 1990s, these research-based ideas were being translated into changes in clinical practice, with a move towards lower tidal volume ventilation. They also produced the necessary clinical climate to conduct important randomised trials. Four major randomised controlled trials were conducted in this decade.[10] All tested the hypothesis that ventilating patients with ARDS at lower tidal volumes – so called 'protective ventilatory strategies' – would improve outcome. More than 1,000 patients in total were recruited into the studies, which produced apparently conflicting findings: two studies reported no difference in outcome, while two (the largest and smallest) found that low tidal volumes improved survival.

Although similar in overall design, the studies differed in a number of details. Of particular note was the fact that the two 'positive' trials used the highest tidal volumes in their control groups, thereby generating the highest airway pressure (Fig 3). This type of analysis has generated subsequent controversy, with claims that the control patients may not have received current standards of ventilatory management. Most agree that the studies show that, at least in established lung injury, high tidal volumes and airway pressures can worsen the injury process. Low(ish) tidal volume strategies generally have been adopted by most critical care units. As a consequence of this deliberate underventilation approach, many patients with ARDS now remain hypercapnic for prolonged periods of time. 'Permissive hypercapnia' seems to be well tolerated as long as oxygenation is maintained.

The ARDS Network trial also challenged the conventional view of acceptable oxygen saturation. Conventionally, oxygen saturations >90% have been the aim in patients with ARDS on the basis of the oxyhaemoglobin dissociation curve. The

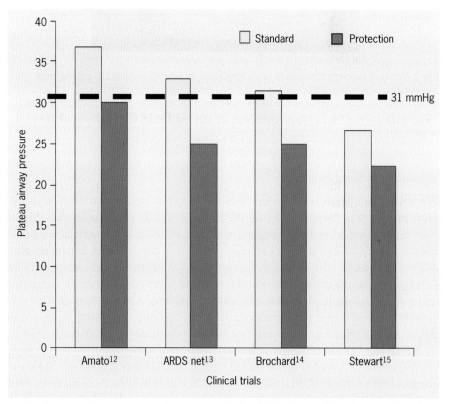

Fig 3 (a) Plateau airway pressures from four randomised clinical trials of low ('protection') and high ('standard') tidal volume ventilation in patients with acute respiratory distress syndrome. The two studies that reported significant differences in outcome used the highest inflation pressures in their control groups.

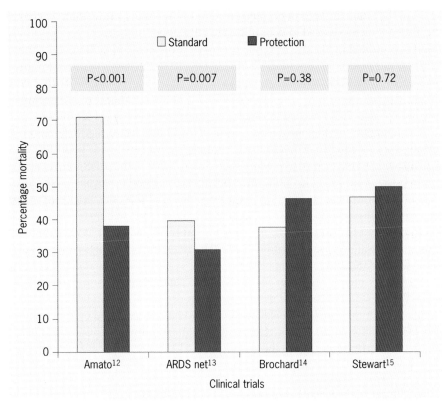

(b) The mortality of patients randomised to either conventional or protective ventilation strategies in four major trials of ARDS. The outcome in two trials (Amato and ARDSnet) was significantly better in patients receiving protective ventilation.

protocol in the ARDS Network trial, however, accepted lower arterial oxygen saturation (SaO_2) (target SaO_2 88–95%); mean SaO_2 was lower in the intervention group in the first few days, but survival was better. As all mountaineers know, cellular oxygen delivery, not SaO_2, is what really matters in maintaining organ function. Current technology, however, does not allow us to monitor this vital variable. The ARDS Network trial and other trials do suggest that when the risk of moderate hypoxaemia is balanced against the risk of overinflation, it is better to tolerate hypoxaemia than to further injure the lung with higher pressures.

Positive end expiratory pressure

Extensive evidence supports a beneficial role of PEEP in patients with lung injury. The addition of PEEP lessens or even prevents the development of VILI in many models. Positive end expiratory pressure also seems to reduce lung injury in a number of other models that involve direct and indirect toxins. An important difference between the four protective ventilation trials was in the use of PEEP.[10] The study that reported the greatest difference in outcome also used the highest levels of

PEEP in the intervention group. Interpretation of the results also is complicated by the different methods used to determine the PEEP used. In the most positive study, PEEP was titrated by the use of ventilator-based measurements of lung mechanics. Whether this method is reproducible or very reliable in the hands of other groups is unclear. In the ARDS Network study, PEEP was titrated pragmatically with a very simple clinical algorithm. The level of PEEP was determined by the fractional inspired oxygen (FiO_2) needed to achieve the target arterial oxygen saturation.

The question of the most effective level of PEEP led the ARDS Network investigators to conduct a randomised control trial of 'low' and 'high' PEEP in patients with established ARDS. More than 500 patients with ARDS were assigned to low (mean 8 cm water) or high (mean 13 cm water) PEEP.[16] Mortality in hospital was similar in the two groups. Unfortunately, this trial does not fully resolve the issues around best PEEP. By chance, the two groups were not well matched (the high PEEP group tended to be more ill), and the protocol had to be revised midway through the trial because separation of PEEP between the two groups was not being achieved at the desired level.

This raises interesting issues in terms of the conduct of trials in patients with ARDS. These studies often take many years from design to final analysis to achieve completion. In this period, clinical practice may change, and good evidence shows that lower tidal volumes and higher positive end expiratory pressures were being adopted by participants during these studies.

Other clinical trials in acute respiratory distress syndrome

A number of other large randomised controlled trials have been conducted in patients with ARDS over the past 15 years. Pharmacological studies include trials of high dose steroids, surfactant, nitric oxide, and a range of anti-inflammatory agents. Other studies include non-conventional ventilation, extracorporeal membrane oxygenation, and prone positioning. Unfortunately, none of these trials produced good evidence in favour of the intervention. Despite the clear inflammatory nature of ARDS, the goal of improving outcome by manipulation of the inflammatory process remains elusive.

□ CONCLUSIONS

The successful management of ARDS remains one of the major challenges in critical care medicine. Our improved understanding of the pathophysiology of acute lung injury has not translated always into better outcomes for patients. Many treatments that seemed promising in the laboratory – including steroids, anti-inflammatory drugs, and nitric oxide – have proved ineffective in large randomised controlled trials.

Good evidence, however, shows that overall outcome in ARDS has improved since the 1970s, with the ARDS Network studies reporting survival >70%. Changes in ventilation have contributed to this, but general improvements in the management of the critically ill also have been considerable. As often is the case, attention to the detail of care is as important as the 'big breakthrough'.

REFERENCES

1 Ware LB, Matthay MA. The acute respiratory distress syndrome. *N Engl J Med* 2000; 342:1334–49.

2 Matthay MA, Zimmerman GA. Acute lung injury and the acute respiratory distress syndrome: four decades of inquiry into pathogenesis and rational management. *Am J Respir Cell Mol Biol* 2005;33:319–27.

3 Donnelly SC, Strieter RM, Kunkel SL *et al.* Interleukin-8 and development of adult respiratory distress syndrome in at-risk patient groups. *Lancet* 1993;341:643–7.

4 Bellingan GJ. The pulmonary physician in critical care * 6: the pathogenesis of ALI/ARDS. *Thorax* 2002;57:540–6.

5 Herridge MS, Cheung AM, Tansey CM *et al.* One-year outcomes in survivors of the acute respiratory distress syndrome. *N Engl J Med* 2003;348:683–93.

6 MacCallum NS, Evans TW. Epidemiology of acute lung injury. *Curr Opin Crit Care* 2005; 11:43–9.

7 Rubenfeld GD, Caldwell E, Peabody E *et al.* Incidence and outcomes of acute lung injury. *N Engl J Med* 2005;353:1685–93.

8 Ware LB. Prognostic determinants of acute respiratory distress syndrome in adults: impact on clinical trial design. *Crit Care Med* 2005;33(3 Suppl):S217–22.

9 Gattinoni L, Caironi P, Carlesso E. How to ventilate patients with acute lung injury and acute respiratory distress syndrome. *Curr Opin Crit Care* 2005;11:69–76.

10 Fan E, Needham DM, Stewart TE. Ventilatory management of acute lung injury and acute respiratory distress syndrome. *JAMA* 2005;294:2889–96.

11 Lionetti V, Recchia FA, Ranieri VM. Overview of ventilator-induced lung injury mechanisms. *Curr Opin Crit Care* 2005;11:82–6.

12 Amato MB, Barbas CS, Medeiros DM *et al.* Effect of a protective-ventilation strategy on mortality in the acute respiratory distress syndrome. *N Engl J Med* 1998;338:347–54.

13 Ventilation with lower tidal volumes as compared with traditional tidal volumes for acute lung injury and the acute respiratory distress syndrome. The Acute Respiratory Distress Syndrome Network. *N Engl J Med* 2000;342:1301–8.

14 Brochard L, Roudot-Thoraval F, Roupie E *et al.* Tidal volume reduction for prevention of ventilator-induced lung injury in acute respiratory distress syndrome. The Multicenter Trail Group on Tidal Volume reduction in ARDS. *Am J Respir Crit Care* 1998;158:1831–8.

15 Stewart TE, Meade MO, Cook DJ *et al.* Evaluation of a ventilation strategy to prevent barotrauma in patients at high risk for acute respiratory distress syndrome. Pressure- and Volume-Limited Ventilation Stategy Group. *N Engl J Med* 1998;338:355–61.

16 Brower RG, Lanken PN, MacIntyre N *et al.* Higher versus lower positive end-expiratory pressures in patients with the acute respiratory distress syndrome. *N Engl J Med* 2004; 351:327–36.

Improving outcomes in lung cancer

Stephen G Spiro

☐ INTRODUCTION

Lung cancer remains the most common cause of death from cancer in men and women in the western world, and the death toll related to tobacco in the developing world is also increasing. In 2003, 38,000 deaths occurred from lung cancer in the United Kingdom and 178,000 deaths in the United States; in China, 15% of deaths in men in 2003 were from tobacco-related causes. Twenty-five years ago, lung cancer killed four times as many adult men as women in Britain, but now about 35% of deaths are in women. Smoking remains the overwhelmingly most important cause of the disease, and the highest prevalence of smokers in Britain is in women aged 15–25 years.

Unlike other common cancers, such as breast cancer and colon cancer, the survival rates at five years for lung cancer have hardly improved over the past 30 years. The United Kingdom has one of the lowest survival rates at five years of all European countries (5–7%); in the United States, the rate is nearer 15%. This may be related to age, as more than 40% of newly diagnosed patients in the United Kingdom are older than 70 years and have a high incidence of coexisting chronic obstructive bronchitis and a considerable incidence of social deprivation, which makes these people a poorer risk for curative treatments. This chapter discusses the possible prognostic value of presenting symptoms, screening of high risk cohorts, and how staging for resection is improving. New treatment strategies that have emerged during the past 2–3 years are discussed.

☐ SYMPTOMS AND SIGNS

The potential list of presenting symptoms and signs for lung cancer encompasses much of general internal medicine, as the symptoms and signs may be caused by the local effects of the primary tumour itself, and by several intrathoracic extra-pulmonary features (usually the mediastinal syndromes, such as superior vena caval obstruction and left recurrent laryngeal nerve palsy) and extrathoracic symptoms and signs, as well as a host of paramalignant syndromes (Table 1).

As with all solid tumours, lung cancer kills after about 40 doublings of volume (when the tumour is 1 kg in size), and most patients die a wasting death. Halfway through the life of a tumour (20 doublings), it is 1 mm in size – far too small for detection. The usual size of presentation on a chest radiograph is 3–4 cm, which represents 36 doublings. This is an exceedingly late presentation, with only 3–4 doublings before

Table 1 Symptoms suggestive of lung cancer.

		Symptom	
Intrapulmonary	**Extrapulmonary intrathoracic**	**Extrathoracic**	**Paramalignant syndromes**
• Haemoptysis	• Superior vena caval obstruction	• Weight loss	• Clubbing or hypertrophic pulmonary osteopathy
• Wheeze	• Hoarseness	• Malaise	• Syndrome of inappropriate antidiuretic hormone secretion
• Cough	• Dysphagia	• Neurological	• Syndrome of adrenocortical hormone sensation
• Dyspnoea	• Arryhthmias	• Bone pain	• Hypercalcaemia
• Pneumonia	• Pericardial effusion	• Skin metastases	• Anaemia
• Chest pain	• Horner's syndrome		• Sensory neuropathy
			• Cerebellar dysfunction
			• Lambert-Eaton syndrome

death. Nevertheless, with the urgency instilled by the *NHS Cancer Plan* in 1997, all patients with cancer need to begin definitive treatment within 62 days of presentation or begin treatment within 31 days of diagnosis. As a result, efforts to identify crucial symptoms that are associated uniquely with the tumour and may have a bearing on a favourable presentation and prognosis have been sought.

Several studies in primary care and of hospital-referred patients have failed to identify good prognostic features at presentation. A general practice study in Exeter, Devon, matched each of 247 new patients with lung cancer to five controls. Although the authors identified haemoptysis, cough, weight loss, loss of appetite and dyspnoea as significantly associated with the presentation of lung cancer, these symptoms had a low positive predictive value, as they were also common in the control population. Many of the symptoms of lung cancer, such as cough, change in cough, and constitutional symptoms, are far too non-specific to predict having the disease or suggest a more favourable outcome.[1] A hospital-based study of 1,200 patients referred over 13 years to a single centre in Italy showed no advantage for any particular presentation, and, indeed, delays in referral for those with key symptoms became longer over the time of the study. The best prognostic feature was a tumour found casually on a chest radiograph.[2] The method of presentation thus is unhelpful, particularly as many of the symptoms are systemic, which indicates metastatic disease.

The late presentation of lung cancer means there has been a re-examination of screening for earlier cases with low dose spiral computed tomography (CT) (annual chest X-ray screening failed through the 1950s, 1960s, and 1970s). Hypothesis-generating studies in various high risk populations – generally those of middle age, with a smoking history of 20 or more packs per year, and the presence of airflow obstruction – have found more cases with CT than routine chest radiography alone (a prevalence of 1.4–2.8%). In most studies, most of these cancers were found at a favourable stage of the TNM classification (usually Stage 1A or B); however, this has not been invariable. Some studies report a very high incidence of benign nodules, which makes investigation and follow up stressful and often difficult. Large randomised controlled studies are in progress in the United States and Europe to determine whether this potentially very expensive protocol will improve mortality sufficiently (if at all) to make these studies cost effective.

☐ IMPROVEMENTS IN STAGING LUNG CANCER

The most common reason for unresectability is spread of the tumour to the mediastinal lymph nodes or direct mediastinal invasion of the primary tumour into the mediastinum. Computed tomography has been the cornerstone of investigating and staging lung cancers, and although it remains the investigation of choice after chest radiography, it is not sufficiently sensitive or specific in reading lymph node enlargement and tumour involvement. Positron emission tomography (PET) has a far higher positive predictive value for mediastinal involvement than CT; however, as up to 15% of cases may be false positive, biopsy of nodes positive on PET is recommended. Nevertheless, PET has had a major effect on patients with tumours deemed resectable by CT and has turned up to 30% into inoperable cases and downstaged just a few others.

Considerable advances have been made in biopsy techniques for the mediastinum that are less interventional than cervical mediastinoscopy or anterior mediastinotomy. Two important developments are transoesophageal ultrasound guided fine needle core biopsy (E-BUS) of the posterior and left lateral mediastinum and transbronchial ultrasound guided fine needle aspiration (TBNA), in which the right paratracheal, subcarinal, and pretracheal nodes can be sampled. These techniques are very dependent on the skill of the operator, but they allow careful ultrasonic examination of the mediastinum and selective nodal biopsy. When mediastinoscopy was used as the arbiter of mediastinal tumour involvement, E-BUS was able to prevent thoracotomy in 70% of patients with lung cancer that needed to be staged by mediastinoscopy. False negatives were seen in only 15 of 242 patients.[3] After CT, TBNA should become a routine examination at diagnostic fibreoptic bronchoscopy to sample the mediastinal nodes where a computed tomogram suggests enlargement. Although dependent on the skill of the operator and having a low sensitivity of around 40%, it will save further invasive tests or thoracotomy.[4] These improved methods of sampling nodes will become very important with the increasing use of PET to stage the mediastinum.

Positron emission tomography is also advancing in its value as a prognostic test. Although CT provides anatomical data on tumour size, invasion, and metastatic spread, PET provides unique data on the metabolic activity of the primary tumour and any metastases. Positron emission tomographic studies of glucose metabolic activity in preoperative patients have been much more discriminating for prognosis than staging by CT, with a high standardised uptake value (SUV) of >5 predicting a poor prognosis as the result of a very active and probably anaplastic tumour. Similar predictive patterns have been seen in studies that assessed responses to neoadjuvant chemotherapy and radical radiotherapy. High glucose metabolic activity according to SUV by PET before treatment heralds a poorer outcome, with shorter disease-free intervals after treatment. Similarly, greater reductions in glucose metabolic activity according to SUV after chemotherapy indicate a shorter period of disease control than with, for example, a 20% reduction in glucose metabolism activity by PET.

☐ ADJUVANT CHEMOTHERAPY IN POSTOPERATIVE NON-SMALL CELL LUNG CARCINOMA

Surgery remains the best chance of cure in patients with non-small cell lung carcinoma (NSCLC), with 65–70% survival at five years for patients with Stage IA disease and 15–20% for patients with Stage IIIA disease. Stages IIIB and IV are advanced and inoperable.

A meta-analysis in 1995 looked at, among other things, the effect of adjuvant and neoadjuvant chemotherapy around surgery in non-small cell lung carcinoma.[5] All included studies were randomised; most evaluated adjuvant chemotherapy and, as long as the regimen contained cisplatin, the addition of chemotherapy produced an almost 5% survival advantage at five years, which just failed to reach significance.

Since this meta-analysis, several studies have assessed the value of adjuvant chemotherapy. Most have been large – for example, 1,200–1,800 patients in two studies and several hundreds in others.[6–10] Six studies have been published in the last four years. All incorporated a 'platin' in the chemotherapy regimen and gave at least three courses. Some of the studies failed to recruit the expected numbers of patients, and others showed a disappointingly poor dose intensity for the administration of chemotherapy; this varied from 49% to 84% of the intended dose. In addition, a few patients developed grade IV toxicity, and occasional deaths related to the treatment occurred. The low dose intensity in mainly fit individuals was disappointing, as were the reported toxicity and, of course, any deaths related to chemotherapy. Furthermore, most studies have concentrated on patients with a better prognosis and a 'good' pathological stage. Some studies included only patients with Stage IB or Stage II disease, while others were open to all postoperative patients. Very few studies included patients with Stage IA disease. The outcome was an overall 4.2% survival advantage at five years for adjuvant chemotherapy (almost identical to that in the meta-analysis from 1995), which is significant statistically (Table 2).

Table 2 Adjuvant trials: summary of survival advantage at five years.

Study	n	Five-year difference (%)	Hazard ratio (95% confidence interval)	Dose intensity (%)	p
Meta-analysis (1995)[5]	1,394	5	0.87 (0.74 to 1.02)	–	0.08
ALPI (2002)[6]	1,209	3	0.96 (0.81 to 1.13)	69	0.6
IALT (2004)[7]	1,867	4	0.86 (0.76 to 0.98)	74	0.03
NCI-C (2005)[8]	482	15	0.70 (0.52 to 0.92)	48	0.01
CALBG (2005)[9]	344	12	0.62 (0.41 to 0.95)	85	0.03
ANITA (2005)[10]	841	8	0.79 (0.66 to 0.95)	76	0.013

The administration of chemotherapy to patients after curative resection thus should become a standard treatment and represents an important advance, although the advantages currently are more clear cut for patients with better stage disease than for those with Stage IIIA disease, which happens to be the most common stage of disease to undergo resection. Potential recipients of adjuvant chemotherapy will have to be prepared and counselled for this before surgery.

☐ ADVANCES IN THE TREATMENT OF ADVANCED NON-SMALL CELL LUNG CARCINOMA

About 60% of all patients with NSCLC present with advanced metastatic disease, and eventually 90–95% of patients reach this stage. It therefore represents a very important area in the treatment of the disease. Chemotherapy has been the only systemic treatment to show some benefit during the last decade, with improvements in median survivals from 4.5 months with best supportive care to about nine months' median survival after chemotherapy and an increase in survival at one year from 28% to 40%. Improvements with chemotherapy have reached a plateau, however, with most patients receiving 4–6 courses of usually platin-containing regimens of two or three agents. Although recent data suggest little difference between platin and non-platin containing regimens, most of those who respond have better performance status and less bulky disease, with those with performance status 3 or 4 being too ill to be given chemotherapy. Patients with performance status 2 tolerate treatment moderately well for relatively short term periods of disease control.

Over the past five years, biological disease modifying drugs have emerged in clinical practice. The best studied are the epidermal growth factor receptor antagonists, which inhibit tyrosine kinase activity in the tumour cell and, in theory, impede tumour growth. The first of these was gefitinib, which has been shown to be well tolerated when given daily as a 250 mg tablet. It has shown no activity in terms of improved survival when given in conjunction with chemotherapy as initial treatment in two large randomised trials. Two Phase II trials using two different doses of gefitinib showed no difference in effect between doses. Both trials showed a 10–20% rate of partial response in terms of reduction of tumour size and an improvement in quality of life. A large randomised trial of gefitinib compared with placebo in patients with advanced disease who had relapsed after chemotherapy or failed to tolerate chemotherapy, however, showed no survival advantage for the addition of the epidermal growth factor receptor antagonist. Secondary endpoints, however, showed significant survival advantages for never smokers, women, and Asian patients.[11]

A second epidermal growth factor receptor antagonist, erlotinib, also has come into practice. As with gefitinib, erlotinib showed no activity when given as first line therapy together with chemotherapy, but in a trial with a similar design to the gefitinib study in previously treated patients, erlotinib had a significant survival advantage and significant improvement in quality of life compared with placebo in patients who had completed chemotherapy for advanced disease. The improvement was most marked in women, never smokers, Asian patients, and those with adenocarcinoma.[12] These drugs still are being evaluated and their mechanisms of action determined. Hopefully, their biological actions can be determined and perhaps patients with an appropriate genetic structure can be identified as potential responders before treatment. Monoclonal antibodies to the epidermal growth factor receptor, such as cetuximab, are also under investigation as another biological modifier, but current data are scanty.

□ CONCLUSIONS

Lung cancer remains the most lethal of malignancies, and little progress in survival at five years has been made during the past 30 years. Early symptoms and signs are hard to distinguish from similar phenomena in other respiratory conditions. The staging of preoperative patients has been much improved with PET, which also can predict outcome by the rate of glucose uptake within the tumour. More sophisticated techniques for sampling mediastinal lymph nodes are emerging. On therapy adjuvant chemotherapy looks as if it will become established, and the role of biological growth modifying agents are being explored urgently. Aside from never starting to smoke, however, quitting smoking before the age of 40 years must be emphasised as the best decision.

REFERENCES

1   Hamilton W, Peters TJ, Round A, Sharp D. What are the clinical features of lung cancer before the diagnosis is made? A population based case-control study. *Thorax* 2005;60:1059–65.

2   Buccheri G, Ferrigno D. Lung cancer: clinical presentation and specialist referral time. *Eur Respir J* 2004;24:898–904.

3   Annema JT, Versteegh MI, Veselic M, Voigt P, Rabe KF. Endoscopic ultrasound-guided fine-needle aspiration in the diagnosis and staging of lung cancer and its impact on surgical staging. *J Clin Oncol* 2005;23:8357–61.

4   Holty J-EC, Keeschner WG, Gould MK. Accuracy of transbronchial needle aspiration for mediastinal staging of non-small cell lung cancer: a meta analysis. *Thorax* 2005;60:949–55.

5   Non-Small Cell Lung Cancer Collaborative Group. Chemotherapy in non-small cell lung cancer: a meta-analysis using updated data on individual patients from 52 randomised clinical trials. *BMJ* 1995;311:899–909.

6   Scagliotti GV. Fossati R, Torri V *et al.* Randomized study of adjuvant chemotherapy for completely resected stage I, II or IIIa non-small cell lung cancer. *J Natl Cancer Inst* 2003;95: 1453–61.

7   The International Adjuvant Lung Cancer Trial Collaborative Group. Cisplatin-based adjuvant chemotherapy in patients with completely resected non-small cell lung cancer. *N Engl J Med* 2004;350:351–60.

8   Winton T, Livingston R, Johnson D *et al.* Vinorelbine plus cisplatin vs. observation in resected non-small-cell lung cancer. *N Engl J Med* 2005;352:2589–97.

9   Strauss GM, Herndon J, Maddaus MA *et al.* Randomised clinical trial of adjuvant chemotherapy with paclitaxel and carboplatin following resection in stage IB non-small cell lung cancer (NSCLC): report of Cancer and Leukemia Group B (CALGB) protocol 9633. *Proc Am Soc Clin Oncol* 2004;23:17 (Abstract 7019).

10 Douillard J-Y, Rosell R, Delena M *et al.* ANITA: phase III adjuvant vinorelbine (N) and cisplatin (P) versus observation (OBS) in completely resected (stage I-III) non-small cell lung cancer (NSCLC) patients (pts): final results after 70-month median follow-up. On behalf of the Adjuvant Navelbine International Trialist Association. *Proc Am Soc Clin Oncol* 2005;23:16s (Abstract 7013).

11 Thatcher N, Chang A, Parekh P *et al.* Gefitinib plus best supportive care in previously treated patients with refractory advanced non-small-cell lung cancer: results from a randomised, placebo-controlled, multicentre study (Iressa Survival Evaluation in Lung Cancer). *Lancet* 2005;366:1527–37.

12 Shepherd FA, Rodrigues Pereira JR, Ciuleanu E *et al.* Erlotinib in previously treated non-small-cell lung cancer. *N Engl J Med* 2005;353:123–32.

☐ RESPIRATORY SELF ASSESSMENT QUESTIONS

Management of acute respiratory distress syndrome

1   Mortality in acute respiratory distress syndrome is:
   (a) Related to patients' age
   (b) Higher in patients with direct lung injury than in those with indirect lung injury
   (c) Independent of case mixture
   (d) Improving over time
   (e) More than 90% in patients with sepsis

2   The following alter outcome in acute respiratory distress syndrome:
   (a) Nitric oxide
   (b) Low tidal volume ventilation
   (c) High dose steroids
   (d) Surfactant
   (e) Positive end expiratory pressure

3   The pathophysiology of acute respiratory distress syndrome includes:
   (a) High pressure pulmonary oedema
   (b) Areas of normal lung
   (c) A predominantly lymphocytic infiltrate
   (d) Late-onset lung fibrosis
   (e) Reduced lung compliance

4   Ventilatory management in acute respiratory distress syndrome includes:
   (a) Maintenance of normocapnia
   (b) Maintenance of arterial oxygen saturation >90%
   (c) Keeping positive end expiratory pressure less than 15 cm water
   (d) High tidal volumes to ensure adequate ventilation
   (e) Titration of positive end expiratory pressure using pressure-volume curves

Improving outcomes in lung cancer

1   Metabolic uptake according to PET:
   (a) Is highest in the most aggressive tumours
   (b) Can be used to predict survival after treatment
   (c) Is less discriminating for prognosis than CT
   (d) Is always truly positive in staging for involvement of the lymph nodes
   (e) Changes preoperative staging by CT in 30% of cases

2   Clinical indicators of lung cancer:
   (a) Help to identify early cases
   (b) Suggest that airways obstruction is a high risk factor
   (c) Suggest haemoptysis merits follow up with a chest X ray

(d) Suggest cough, weight loss, and dyspnoea as indications of early disease

(e) Allow general practitioners to identify most high-risk patients

3   Adjuvant chemotherapy after surgery:
   (a) Is as effective in small cell lung cancer as in non-small cell lung cancer
   (b) Seems to confer a 5% survival advantage at five years compared with surgery alone
   (c) Is easy to give, with a high rate of achieving the prescribed dose intensity
   (d) Will become a treatment of choice after curative resection
   (e) Needs to include a platin as part of the chemotherapy regimen

4   In patients with advanced non-small cell lung cancer:
   (a) About 60% of newly diagnosed patients have advanced disease
   (b) Chemotherapy has improved the median survival
   (c) Chemotherapy improves the quality of life
   (d) Advances with chemotherapy are increasing
   (e) Targeted therapy with EGFR antagonists work particularly in Asians, women, and never smokers with adenocarcinoma

Cardiovascular

Of stents and stem cells – advances in the management of ST elevation myocardial infarction

Michael Fisher

Despite great advances in treatment and prevention, ischaemic heart disease (IHD) continues to be a major cause of premature death and disability in the west and is rapidly increasing in importance in the developing world. Within the spectrum of IHD generally, ST elevation myocardial infarction (STEMI) exerts a particularly malign influence, with about one third of men and one quarter of women dying before reaching hospital and an overall 30-day mortality rate of about 40%.[1] In those who do survive, the resulting ventricular dysfunction and consequent heart failure results in substantial long-term morbidity and mortality. The impact on public health is also substantial: as people with IHD survive longer, the prevalence of ischaemically driven left ventricular (LV) dysfunction rises, swelling the number of those living with heart failure, which is set to become the greatest cardiological cause of morbidity in our community. In light of these considerations, the need for better ways of treating acute MI remains pressing in order to reduce mortality, and we also need new strategies for managing patients who survive their MI but with significantly impaired LV function. A brief consideration of the figures quoted above shows that much of the mortality attributable to STEMI occurs before the patient reaches hospital, which emphasises the crucial roles that primary and secondary prevention have to play in achieving significant reductions in cardiac mortality. Nevertheless, this review will focus on two advancing areas in the hospital management of acute myocardial infarction (AMI) and the resulting ventricular dysfunction.

☐ INTERVENTIONAL TREATMENT OF ACUTE MYOCARDIAL INFARCTION

Since early trials showed that thrombolysis improves mortality in patients with STEMI, several authors have noted the close association between the presence of a patent infarct-related artery (IRA) and a positive prognosis. A review by Gibson *et al* found that patients who achieved grade 2 or 3 flow in the infarct-related artery after thrombolysis had roughly half the mortality of those with no flow (Fig 1).[2]

Despite the use of relatively high-efficiency thrombolytics, one meta-analysis found that short- and long-term death rates overall still averaged around 8% and 12%, respectively, in patients who received lysis,[3] hence it seemed there was significant room for improvement. As the IRA patency rate, as assessed by angiography,

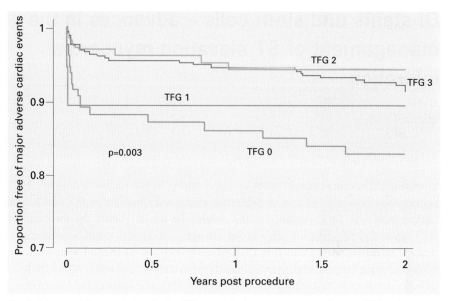

Fig 1 Relation of flow grade (TFG) after PCI to survival over a two-year follow up. TFG 0–3 represents increasing degrees of flow in the IRA from no flow (TFG 0) to normal flow (TFG 3). Reproduced from Gibson *et al* with permission of Lippincott, Williams and Wilkins.[2]

varied between 40% and 70% depending on the thrombolytic used, the question inevitably arose as to whether percutaneous coronary intervention (PCI) might be able to substantially improve on this.

Initial studies of primary PCI seemed encouraging, with IRA patency rates of around 85–90%. These figures need to be treated with some caution, however, as the degree of vessel patency and flow were almost always reported at the end of the angioplasty procedure, whereas equivalent figures in thrombolytic studies were generally taken a minimum of 60 minutes after the drug had been given. It is likely, therefore, that early reocclusion of the vessel would occur in at least some of those who had undergone PCI, so lessening the benefit. This was illustrated by Halkin *et al*, who showed a 10% incidence of late reocclusion of the IRA in patients who had undergone successful PCI for AMI.[4] This paper further showed that the open artery hypothesis applied equally well in those who are treated with PCI – in that the rate of major adverse cardiac events was threefold higher in those in whom the IRA had reoccluded (Fig 2).

Despite the problem with reocclusion, throughout the late 1970s and 1980s, a number of trials of primary PCI showed the strategy to be superior to that of thrombolysis. A meta-analysis of 23 such studies published in 2003 showed the clear superiority of primary PCI in every outcome category other than risk of bleeding (Fig 3).[3]

An obvious practical difficulty with the widespread adoption of primary PCI for the routine treatment of STEMI was the fact that the technique required dedicated and experienced interventional teams and cardiac catheter laboratories to be

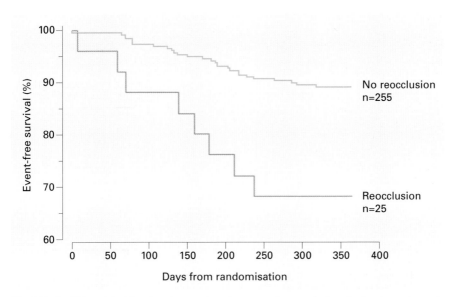

Fig 2 Kaplan-Meier plot of freedom from major adverse cardiac events in patients who underwent primary PCI: comparison of patients with occlusion of the IRA and those with a patent vessel. Reproduced from Halkin *et al* with permission of Excerpta Medica, Inc.[4]

available 24 hours a day. Although this had been possible in the setting of a clinical trial run by highly skilled and motivated individuals, delivering such a service in the 'real world' represented a major logistical and financial task. It was recognition of this fact that led to a strategy of transferring patients from peripheral hospitals to an interventional regional centre capable of offering such a service. This frequently required that patients be transferred by helicopter; however, successful examples of this type of model exist in several European countries, including Denmark and the Czech Republic. Inevitably, transfer of the patient for PCI results in delays in revascularisation compared with a policy of local thrombolysis, and this has led to an examination of the effect of this delay on the relative benefit of primary PCI. One study that looked at death rates concluded that a time delay of greater than one hour in reperfusion achieved by PCI would abolish the benefit of the treatment.[5] These considerations have led to guideline recommendations from bodies such as the European Society of Cardiology and the American Heart Association, which state that primary PCI is overall the preferred strategy for the management of STEMI, but if the expected delay in delivering this is likely to be greater than 90 minutes thrombolysis should be administered immediately.

We performed a similar preliminary analysis looking at the six largest studies that compared angioplasty with lysis and found a similar relation between delay and the most commonly used composite endpoint of death, stroke and revascularisation (Fig 4(a)). Interestingly, in our analysis and that of Nallamothu,[5] although the negative association of delay to PCI with benefit of PCI was significant, the degree of correlation was weak: in our analysis the R^2 value was only 0.27. We also found that if the relation between time to PCI is plotted against absolute outcome, while again

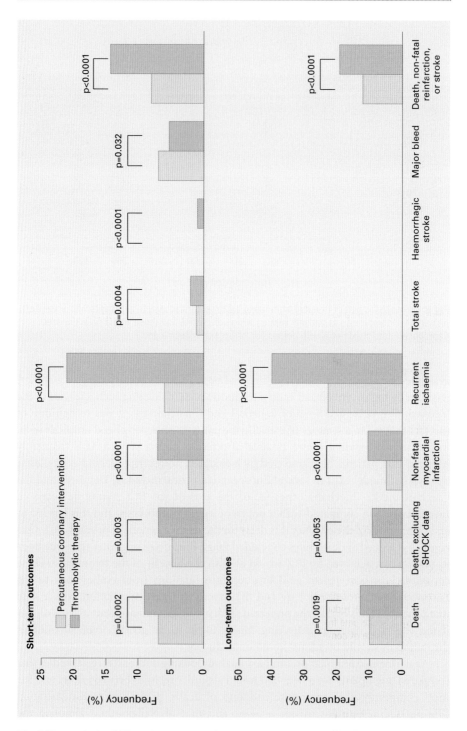

Fig 3 Meta-analysis of 23 studies: analysis of outcome in patients with STEMI who underwent primary percutaneous coronary intervention and those treated with thrombolysis. Reproduced from Keeley *et al* with permission of Elsevier.[3]

(a)

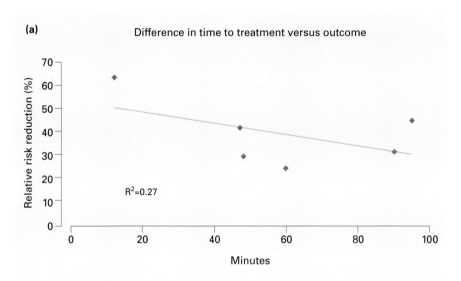

(b)

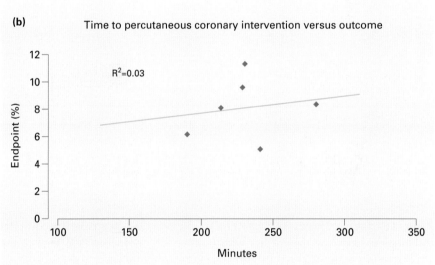

Fig 4 Relation between different time parameters and 30-day outcome after percutaneous coronary intervention (PCI) in the six largest trial published to date of primary PCI versus thrombolysis. **(a)** Delay between time of administration of thrombolysis and first balloon inflation versus the relative risk reduction of composite endpoint of death, stroke and recurrent infarction for PCI. **(b)** Absolute time from onset of symptoms to first balloon inflation versus absolute value for 30-day incidence of composite endpoint.

longer times to treatment equate to a less favourable result, the correlation is very weak and the gradient of the regression line is quite close to 0 (Fig 4(b)). This suggests that, at least over the range of time delays to PCI in these studies (up to 280 minutes), absolute time to treatment has comparatively little effect on the outcome. If it is the case that the 'lateness' of PCI is relatively less important, then perhaps the decline in relative risk reduction for treatment with PCI with increasing time between thrombolysis and mechanical reperfusion may be accounted for by earlier lytic treatment.

Our analysis has also found some support for this notion: a correlation of the absolute time to lysis against the relative risk reduction for the interventional strategy clearly showed that the earlier thrombolysis is administered, the less the benefit for the interventional strategy (Fig 5). This association showed a very high degree of correlation (R^2=0.79), which suggests that the critical factor in determining the potential relative benefit of primary PCI is not so much the delay in time to balloon inflation but the rapidity with which thrombolysis can be administered.

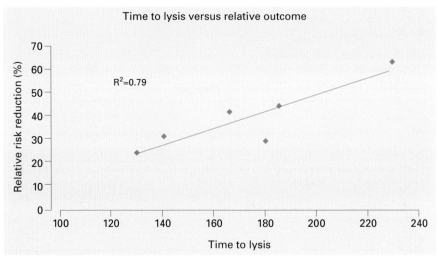

Fig 5 Time from onset of symptoms to administration of throbolysis in minutes compared with relative risk reduction for the interventional strategy. Note the high degree of correlation.

Further evidence for this comes from the recently published Thrombolysis in Acute Myocardial Infarction (CAPTIM) study,[6] which compared prehospital thrombolysis given by paramedics with transfer for immediate PCI. One of the striking results of this trial was that the time from symptom onset to delivery of lysis (130 minutes) was the shortest of any study thus far published. Although the composite endpoint of death, stroke and re-infarction was reduced in those assigned to PCI (6.2% *v* 8.2%), this difference was not significant and, indeed, the mortality rate was actually (non-significantly) higher in the primary PCI group (4.8% *v* 3.8%). It should be pointed out that, in common with many trials that pit primary PCI against a 'conservative' option, the excellent outcome achieved by a strategy of early thrombolysis was accompanied by an extremely low threshold for intervention. This resulted in 85% of the 'conservatively' treated patients having angiography by day 30 and 70% having an angioplasty due to a combination of ongoing or recurrent ischaemia in hospital or evidence of residual ischaemia after discharge. Consequently, CAPTIM does *not* show that early thrombolysis obviates the need for interventional treatment but simply suggests that it may be at least as good as primary PCI when used as the first step in management.

The evidence discussed above suggests that the crucial question is not whether it is better to have thrombolysis or primary PCI as treatment for acute STEMI, rather the important issue is to achieve an open infarct-related artery (and to maintain that patency). Although primary PCI may be the best way of achieving this when the time since onset of symptoms is greater than two hours, lysis with an efficient agent may be just as good in patients with earlier presentations.

☐ STEM-CELL THERAPY FOR VENTRICULAR DYSFUNCTION

Despite the best efforts to achieve a persistently patent IRA at an early stage, inevitably some patients will present too late to have effective reperfusion therapy and will have significant and irreversible myocardial damage. Although a number of treatment options exist for these patients, until recently it has been assumed that regeneration of lost ventricular function was impossible, as the adult heart was considered to be a post-mitotic organ incapable of producing new myocytes.

Over the last few years, this view increasingly has been challenged by papers that have suggested a turnover of cardiomyocytes, with old cells being removed by apoptosis and new cells being produced from progenitor cells believed to be resident in specialised niches within the myocardium.[7] Research has further shown that this process is increased in certain pathological states, such as hypertension, in which an increase in mitotic figures can be observed within the myocardium.[8] This is believed to reflect an upregulation in progenitor cell activity in order to correct the cell loss engendered by pressure overload. The realisation that the heart is, after all, a self-renewing organ was greeted with considerable excitement and indeed scepticism.

Initial enthusiasm was tempered, however, by the realisation that, although this mechanism could repair the damage produced by relatively low-level insults, the massive cell loss produced by myocardial infarction seemed to overwhelm the ability of the stem-cell pool to restore the myocardium.[7] The possibility that myocardial regeneration might be possible resurfaced therapeutically in 2001, when Orlic showed that the myocardial dysfunction associated with experimental infarction in female mice could be reversed by the direct injection of progenitor cells derived from the bone marrow of male donor mice.[9] Using the presence of the Y chromosome and a genetically engineered protein marker (enhanced green fluorescent protein), the authors were able to show that the donor cells repopulated the infarcted territory and seemed to give rise to a functional myocardium.

This work was replicated and extended by several groups;[7] however, several unanswered questions remained in terms of the exact mechanism by which the apparent new myocardium was being produced and the best type of cell and route of administration in order to maximise the therapeutic effect.[10] Indeed, some dissenting voices doubted whether the effect was real at all and suggested that the apparent presence of donor myocardium in these experiments was due to a combination of artefacts of the imaging systems used and cell fusion.[11]

Despite these doubts, the field progressed so rapidly that only one year after the publication of Orlic's paper in *Nature*, the first preliminary study of stem-cell therapy for myocardial regeneration after clinical myocardial infarction was published.[12] This showed that the protocols, which previously had been applied only in experimental animal models, could be emulated in patients after an infarct. Furthermore, the study showed evidence of improved perfusion to the infarct zone and restitution of contraction, which suggests that all the elements necessary for a functional myocardium were being regenerated. Although exciting, these results suffered from the lack of a contemporaneous control group, so a further important development came with the publication of the first randomised human trial.[13] This provided further evidence of the feasibility and efficacy of stem-cell therapy. The primary endpoint in this trial was the increase in global ejection fraction at six months, which increased from a baseline value of 50% to 56.7% in the intervention group compared with 51.3% and 52%, respectively, in controls. This difference, although apparently small, was highly significant.

These results offer great promise for the future treatment of post-infarction myocardial dysfunction, but the current enthusiasm needs to be tempered with caution. Some still have grave misgivings about the whole notion of transdifferentiation of progenitor cells into functional myocardium.[11] The data quoted above seem to show that improvement in myocardial function occurs, but many different possible mechanisms for the effect have been proposed. These include genuine differentiation of stem or progenitor cells into functional myocardium, recruitment of resident stem cells within the myocardium by paracrine effects mediated by the administered cells, or alteration of the physical properties of the scar to beneficially effect remodelling.[7] We need to further understand the basic mechanisms that are operating if we are to be able to fully exploit the potential of this new treatment. Equally, because these mechanisms are poorly understood, we do not even know which types of stem or progenitor cells are likely to be most effective. Finally, very little data is available on long-term follow up to inform us if the apparently beneficial effects of stem-cell treatment are maintained and little is known about potential adverse effects.

☐ CONCLUSIONS

The area of management of acute STEMI is going through an exciting period of change. Clear evidence now shows that primary angioplasty is superior to even the best thrombolytics in most cases. Faced with this evidence, different health economies are struggling with the logistics and costs of delivering the service, and a number of differing models are emerging. Very recently, however, some tantalising evidence has suggested that if lysis is delivered sufficiently early, it can rival and even exceed PCI for outcome. The burgeoning field of myocardial repair by stem-cell therapy is a fascinating example of the speed with which basic research can translate to clinical practice, even though many important issues remain to be solved before this can become an established treatment. In the future, we may see a model in which patients with an MI are treated according to the time from onset of symptoms. Those with very recent onset would receive thrombolysis before transfer to an interventional centre for expectant management, whereas those with later presentation would go straight for primary PCI. Finally, for patients in whom significant myocardial damage occurs despite revascularisation or in those who present too late, stem-cell therapy may allow the opportunity for myocardial repair to prevent the later onset of heart failure, with all of its attendant morbidity and increased mortality.

REFERENCES

1 Birkhead J, Goldacre M, Mason A *et al* (eds). *Health outcome indicators: myocardial infarction. Report of a working group to the Department of Health.* Oxford: National Centre for Health Outcomes Development, 1999.

2 Gibson CM, Cannon CP, Murphy SA *et al.* Relationship of the TIMI myocardial perfusion grades, flow grades, frame count, and percutaneous coronary intervention to long-term outcomes after thrombolytic administration in acute myocardial infarction. *Circulation* 2002;105:1909–13.

3 Keeley EC, Boura JA, Grines CL. Primary angioplasty versus intravenous thrombolytic therapy for acute myocardial infarction: a quantitative review of 23 randomised trials. *Lancet* 2003;361:13–20.

4 Halkin A, Aymong E, Cox DA *et al.* Relation between late patency of the infarct-related artery, left ventricular function, and clinical outcomes after primary percutaneous intervention for acute myocardial infarction (CADILLAC trial). *Am J Cardiol* 2004;93:349–53.

5 Nallamothu BK, Bates ER. Percutaneous coronary intervention versus fibrinolytic therapy in acute myocardial infarction: is timing (almost) everything? *Am J Cardiol* 2003;92:824–6.

6 Bonnefoy E, Lapostolle F, Leizorovicz A *et al.* Primary angioplasty versus prehospital fibrinolysis in acute myocardial infarction: a randomised study. *Lancet* 2002;360:825–9.

7 Leri A, Kajstura J, Anversa P. Cardiac stem cells and mechanisms of myocardial regeneration. *Physiol Rev* 2005;85:1373–416.

8 Anversa P, Kajstura J, Leri A, Bolli R. Life and death of cardiac stem cells: a paradigm shift in cardiac biology. *Circulation* 2006;113:1451–63.

9 Orlic D, Kajstura J, Chimenti S *et al.* Bone marrow cells regenerate infarcted myocardium. *Nature* 2001;410:701–5.

10 Dawn B, Bolli R. Cardiac progenitor cells: the revolution continues. *Circ Res* 2005;97:1080–2.

11 Chien KR. Stem cells: lost in translation. *Nature* 2004;428:607–8.

12 Assmus B, Schachinger V, Teupe C *et al.* Transplantation of progenitor cells and regeneration enhancement in acute myocardial infarction (TOPCARE-AMI). *Circulation* 2002;106: 3009–17.

13 Meyer GP, Wollert KC, Lotz J *et al.* Intracoronary bone marrow cell transfer after myocardial infarction: eighteen months' follow-up data from the randomized, controlled BOOST (bone marrow transfer to enhance ST-elevation infarct regeneration) trial. *Circulation* 2006;113: 1287–94.

Angina pectoris: second wind, warm up and walk through

Rainer Zbinden and Michael S Marber

☐ THE SENSATION OF ANGINA PECTORIS

There is a disorder of the breast marked with strong and peculiar symptoms, considerable for the kind of danger belonging to it and not extremely rare, which deserves to be mentioned more at length. The seat of it, and sense of strangling, and anxiety with which it is attended, may make it not improperly be called angina pectoris.

These are the words of William Heberden (1710–1801) on the syndrome he named without knowledge of the underlying mechanism.

At the turn of the last century, Colbeck proposed that ischaemic cardiac pain might be related to distension of the ventricular wall ('mechanical hypothesis').[1] Three decades later, Lewis hypothesised that ischaemic pain might be elicited by the intramyocardial release of pain-producing substances induced by ischaemia ('chemical hypothesis').[2] About five decades later, Davies *et al* showed that dilation of the ventricle is unlikely to be responsible for angina, because the rate and the magnitude of left ventricular dilation during ergonovine-induced or spontaneous transient ischaemic episodes were found to be similar during painful and painless episodes.[3] The negligible importance of mechanical distortion and distension of ventricular fibres in the genesis of ischaemic cardiac pain is further supported by the observation that ventricular dilation – as it occurs during acute ventricular failure, myocardial biopsy, or valvuloplasty – does not cause any painful sensation. The chemical hypothesis thus prevailed.

In the 1980s, intravenous administration of adenosine was introduced for the detection of coronary artery disease during perfusion scintigraphy or two-dimensional echocardiography and for the treatment of supraventricular tachycardia. During infusion of adenosine, patients without evidence of coronary artery disease often complained of a short-lasting chest pain with features similar to those of ischaemic cardiac pain. Crea *et al* showed subsequently that intracoronary infusion of adenosine in patients with chronic stable angina consistently caused pain with features identical to those experienced during daily life but without detectable signs of myocardial ischaemia.[4] Infusion of a similar dose of adenosine into the right atrium failed to elicit pain, thus proving that the pain elicited by the intracoronary infusion of adenosine originated from the heart. Adenosine-induced cardiac pain is not secondary to myocardial ischaemia, because it typically occurs in the absence of ischaemia-like electrocardiographic changes and can be elicited by adenosine infused into angiographically normal coronary arteries. Substance P (a polypeptide present in perivascular nerves) enhances adenosine-induced pain, which explains the extreme pain during myocardial infarction, when a large amount of substance P is released into the myocardium because of necrosis. The adenosine type 1 (A_1) receptor mainly mediates the pain sensation, while the type 2 (A_2) receptor is primarily responsible for the vasodilatory effects of adenosine.

The localisation of cardiac pain is determined by the convergence of visceral and somatic afferents on the same neurones in the central nervous system. Cardiac pain is typically located in the retrosternal region, but it is also frequently experienced in the left hemithorax, left arm, epigastrium, and neck (Fig 1).[5] It is worth noting that sequential infusions of adenosine into the right or left coronary artery in the same patient result in a similar distribution of pain in 75% of patients, whereas pain distribution is different in the remaining 25%. In contrast, Pasceri *et al* found that 67% of patients who had both anterior and inferior myocardial infarction during their life experienced cardiac ischaemic pain in different body regions, whereas the remaining 33% experienced pain in the same region.[6] Studies of this nature, however, are bound to be biased by distortions introduced by recall of distant events. Anecdotally, the character of chest discomfort during multivessel angioplasty does not seem very dependent on target territory, more in keeping with the findings of Crea *et al*.[4] Chest pain, however, represents only the tip of the iceberg in the ischaemic cascade (Fig 2).

☐ SECOND-WIND ANGINA

Walk-through angina has been recognised for more than 200 years and was also first described by William Heberden (see above) in the 18th century. It is related to warm

Coronary angiogram		Normal (n=65)	Abnormal (n=65)	OR
Site	1	5 (8%)	3 (5%)	1.72
	2	11 (17%)	16 (25%)	0.62
	3	11 (17%)	13 (20%)	0.81
	4	23 (35%)	10 (15%)	3.01*
	5	55 (85%)	41 (63%)	3.22†
	6	38 (58%)	18 (28%)	3.67‡
	7	7 (11%)	3 (5%)	2.49
	8	10 (15%)	7 (11%)	1.51
	9	10 (15%)	3 (5%)	3.76

*p<0.05; †p<0.01; ‡p<0.001. OR = odds ratio.

Fig 1 Location of chest pain in 65 patients with normal coronary arteries and 65 patients with at least one epicardial stenosis >70%: patients with non-cardiac chest pain (normal coronary arteries) more frequently lateralise the pain. Reproduced from Cooke *et al* with permission of the BMJ Publishing Group.[5]

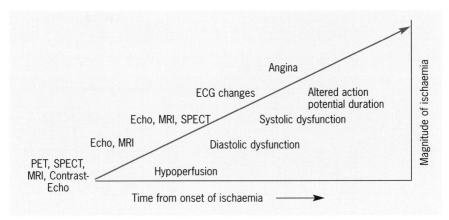

Fig 2 Scheme of the ischaemic cascade and commonly used diagnostic tests. The events are related to the time course of occurrence from left to right over approximately 5 to 10 minutes. The first changes during ischaemia are hypoperfusion, followed by diastolic and systolic contractile dysfunction and then electrocardiographic changes. Many patients experience ischaemia, although there may be no accompanying symptoms (silent ischaemia). If ischaemia is prolonged (greater than about 15 minutes), irreversible injury occurs, with release of intracardiac proteins such as the troponins. Commonly used diagnostic tests appear above the line and relate to the physiological events below the line. ECG = electrocardiogram; ECHO = echocardiography; MRI = magnetic resonance imaging; PET = positron emission tomography; SPECT = single-photon emission computed tomography.

up, or second-wind, angina – a common and intriguing phenomenon in which angina on initial effort is more severe than on subsequent effort. In golfers, this phenomenon is also known as first-hole angina. Second-wind angina can be demonstrated objectively as a significant decrease in electrocardiographic signs of myocardial ischaemia on the second of two exercise tests performed within a short interval (Fig 3). The traditional explanation of warm-up angina has been that myocardial blood flow is enhanced on second effort by the opening of collateral channels (that is, collateral recruitment), vasodilatation of the diseased artery, or subtended vascular bed, or their combination. The observation, however, of increased myocardial resistance to ischaemia after a brief episode of ischaemia – ischaemic preconditioning (IP) – has increased the understanding of warm-up or second-wind angina. In contrast to the traditional view, IP does not depend on an increase in myocardial blood flow but is caused by an increase in the intrinsic resistance of the heart to ischaemia. The exact mechanism of this important attenuation of myocardial ischaemia, however, remains undefined.

☐ ISCHAEMIC PRECONDITIONING AND COLLATERAL RECRUITMENT

In 1986, Murry and coworkers introduced the term ischaemic preconditioning and referred to it as myocardial adaptation to ischaemic stress induced by repetitive brief periods of ischaemia and reperfusion.[7] Ischaemic preconditioning is mediated by receptors, and, in animal models, several ligands are able to precondition the heart in

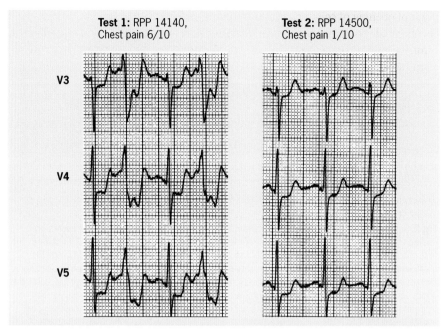

Fig 3 Surface electrocardiograph in a patient with single vessel disease of the left anterior descending coronary artery undergoing repetitive treadmill testing. Test 2 was separated from test 1 by a 15-minute rest period. In test 2, ST-segment depression is almost absent at the same workload, and the patient experiences less chest pain than in test 1 (that is, second-wind or warm-up phenomenon). Note the ventricular bigeminy in test 1, which is absent in test 2. In test 1, the narrow complexes are sinus beats with a QRS morphology similar to that of test 2 but with greater ST depression. RPP = rate–pressure product.

the absence of an initial ischaemic insult (see below). Not all time combinations and durations of ischaemia and reperfusion will trigger the preconditioning phenomenon and afford myocardial protection. Ischaemic preconditioning can be induced by a period of ischaemia as short as 3–5 minutes followed by a minimum of 1 minute of reperfusion, but a brief 1–2-minute period of ischaemia followed by subsequent reperfusion has no protective effect. A single episode of ischaemia is needed to induce preconditioning, but repetitive episodes of brief ischaemia are also effective.

Ischaemic preconditioning is now established as a biphasic phenomenon, with a first window of protection developing within minutes of an ischaemic insult but lasting only 1–2 hours and a second window of protection developing between 12–24 hours but lasting for 3–4 days. This second window of protection has important therapeutic implications because, unlike the first window, it can protect against myocardial stunning and infarction, and, unlike early IP, tolerance does not occur because repeated triggers prolong the effect.[8]

As previously mentioned, the traditional view is that angina is the result of an imbalance between the supply and demand of the myocardium for blood. A component of second-wind angina thus may result from increased resistance to ischaemia in a manner analogous to IP, although another component may be the result of opening of collateral channels (that is, collateral recruitment). This has been documented in humans with the coronary occlusion model during percutanous coronary intervention (PCI) at rest and during exercise, which indicates that collateral recruitment is an additional factor that leads to the second-wind phenomenon.[9]

☐ PHARMACOLOGICAL INDUCTION OF MYOCARDIAL TOLERANCE AND FEATURES COMMON TO ANGINA

Ischaemic preconditioning is mediated by receptors, and a major objective in recent years has been identification of the responsible triggers and end effectors in the myocytes. Several triggers have been described in IP in vitro and in animal models of ischaemia, including adenosine and bradykinin. Like the sensation of angina, it seems likely that A_1 receptors initiate protection. Thus, if the sensation of angina is a surrogate measure of myocardial interstitial adenosine reaching a concentration sufficient to occupy and activate receptors on efferent nerve endings, these same receptors are likely occupied on cardiac myocytes to initiate IP. This suggests that warm-up angina and IP may be linked. Some human studies, however, have failed to show that adenosine receptor activation influences warm-up angina.[10]

A very recent study using sequential treadmill testing to investigate the influence of different drugs on warm-up angina in humans showed that the angiotensin-converting enzyme (ACE) inhibitor enalapril prolonged the protective window after first exertion but had no influence on the magnitude of the warm-up phenomenon.[11] The angiotensin II type 1 receptor (AT_1) blocker losartan did not have any effect on warm up, which suggests that the protective effect of the ACE inhibitor is independent of the AT_1 receptor. Angiotensin-converting enzyme also cleaves bradykinin, and ACE inhibitors therefore result in accumulation of bradykinin. In animal models of IP, inhibition of ACE has been shown to reduce infarct size and decrease reperfusion arrhythmias, while specific bradykinin receptor blockers abolished this effect. This suggests that bradykinin, at least in part, determines the protective duration of the warm-up phenomenon. Nicorandil (a potassium-channel opener) did not have any effect on warm-up angina in the same study, which suggests that opening of adenosine triphosphate (ATP)-sensitive potassium channels is not an essential event in triggering adaptation in humans (Fig 4).

☐ PRECONDITIONING VERSUS POSTCONDITIONING

The prerequisite for salvage of viable myocardium and limitation of infarct size after an acute ischaemic event is timely reperfusion. Restoration of coronary blood flow, however, carries the risk of further myocardial injury (reperfusion injury). Modulation of blood flow on reperfusion (through gradual or intermittent reperfusion) has been shown to reduce experimental infarct size in animals. The protective effect of postconditioning is of similar magnitude to that seen with IP. However, IP is not feasible in clinical practice, because the coronary artery is already occluded at the time of hospital admission in a patient with acute myocardial infarction (AMI). Unlike IP, the experimental design of postconditioning allows

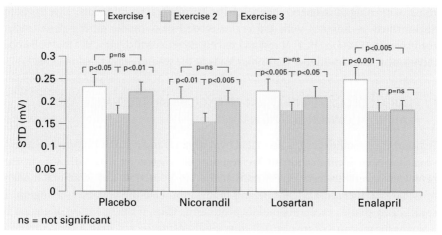

Fig 4 ST-segment depression at equivalent workloads during exercise treadmill testing in patients with coronary artery disease and stable angina. Bar graphs show the mean (standard deviation) values of ST depression at equivalent workloads during three sequential exercise tests. The second exercise test was separated from the first by a 15-minute rest period. The third exercise test was performed after a further 90 minutes of rest. Serial exercise tests were performed while patients were taking the drug indicated. The second test shows a consistent decrease in ST depression compared with the first test, which corresponds to the warm-up (second-wind) phenomenon. This protective effect vanishes in the third test except in the enalapril group, which indicates a prolongation of the protective window of preconditioning with enalapril. Adapted from Edwards *et al* with permission of Oxford University Press.[11]

direct application to the clinical setting, especially during PCI. In this case, inflation and deflation of the angioplasty balloon after reopening of the coronary artery can mimic repetitive coronary artery clamping. Very recent studies showed a 36% reduction in myocardial infarct size in patients with AMI and protection against endothelial ischaemia-reperfusion injury in the forearm of 11 healthy volunteers with a postconditioning protocol.[12,13]

□ SUMMARY

The terms 'angina pectoris' and 'walk-through angina' date back more than 200 years. They were first used by the British physician Heberden. Angina pectoris is the result of release of adenosine (which acts via the A_1 receptor) during (myocardial) ischaemia, whereas substance P potentiates adenosine-induced pain. Chest pain is only the tip of the iceberg in the ischaemic cascade.

Second-wind (or warm-up) angina describes the ability of some patients to exercise to angina, rest, and then continue exercise with reduced symptoms or no symptoms at all. After an episode of exercise-induced angina, significant reductions in severity of angina, exercise limitation, and ST-segment depression are seen. Although the mechanisms that underlie second-wind angina are not yet clearly understood, preconditioning and collateral recruitment in combination are thought to play a role.

Triggers and mediators involved in preconditioning in animal models include adenosine, bradykinin, opioid receptor agonists, ATP-sensitive potassium channels, and protein kinase C. Adenosine and bradykinin seem to have some influence on warm-up angina in humans. Late or delayed preconditioning, which develops 12–24 hours after the first ischaemic stimulus and lasts for 3–4 days, has important clinical relevance, as it can protect against myocardial stunning and infarction.

Post-conditioning refers to the modulation of blood flow on reperfusion through gradual or intermittent reperfusion. The protective effect of post-conditioning is of similar magnitude to that seen with IP and can be applied in a clinical setting of AMI. Postconditioning reduces myocardial infarct size in patients with AMI and protects against endothelial ischaemia-reperfusion injury in humans.

Funding: RZ is supported by a grant from the Swiss National Foundation.

REFERENCES

1   Colbeck E. Angina pectoris: a criticism and a hypothesis. *Lancet* 1903;1:793–5.

2   Lewis T. Pain in muscular ischemia: its relation to anginal pain. *Arch Intern Med* 1932;49: 713–27.

3   Davies GJ, Bencivelli W, Fragasso G *et al.* Sequence and magnitude of ventricular volume changes in painful and painless myocardial ischemia. *Circulation* 1988;78:310–9.

4   Crea F, Pupita G, Galassi AR *et al.* Role of adenosine in pathogenesis of anginal pain. *Circulation* 1990;81:164–72.

5   Cooke RA, Smeeton N, Chambers JB. Comparative study of chest pain characteristics in patients with normal and abnormal coronary angiograms. *Heart* 1997;78:142–6.

6   Pasceri V, Cianflone D, Finocchiaro ML, Crea F, Maseri A. Relation between myocardial infarction site and pain location in Q-wave acute myocardial infarction. *Am J Cardiol* 1995;75: 224–7.

7   Murry CE, Jennings RB, Reimer KA. Preconditioning with ischemia: a delay of lethal cell injury in ischemic myocardium. *Circulation* 1986;74:1124–36.

8   Lambiase PD, Edwards RJ, Cusack MR *et al.* Exercise-induced ischemia initiates the second window of protection in humans independent of collateral recruitment. *J Am Coll Cardiol* 2003;41:1174–82.

9   Zbinden R, Billinger M, Seiler C. Collateral vessel physiology and functional impact – experimental evidence of collateral behaviour. *Coron Artery Dis* 2004;15:389–92.

10   Yellon DM, Baxter GF, Marber MS. Angina reassessed: pain or protector? *Lancet* 1996;347: 1159–62.

11   Edwards RJ, Redwood SR, Lambiase PD, Marber MS. The effect of an angiotensin-converting enzyme inhibitor and a K+(ATP) channel opener on warm up angina. *Eur Heart J* 2005;26: 598–606.

12   Staat P, Rioufol G, Piot C *et al.* Postconditioning the human heart. *Circulation* 2005;112:2143–8.

13   Loukogeorgakis SP, Panagiotidou AT, Yellon DM, Deanfield JE, MacAllister RJ. Postconditioning protects against endothelial ischemia-reperfusion injury in the human forearm. *Circulation* 2006;113:1015–9.

Minimally invasive valve replacement

Louise Coats and Philipp Bonhoeffer

□ INTRODUCTION

Rates of surgery for valvular heart disease are increasing, in part, as a result of the growing population of elderly patients with acquired valve disease and adults with congenital heart disease. Morbidity and mortality related to surgery are significant, and interest in developing a less invasive approach that can avoid cardiopulmonary bypass and reduce hospital stay is emerging. Minimally invasive valve replacement faces many challenges; however, if cardiologists, surgeons, and engineers can find solutions, this approach could transform the management of a rapidly expanding patient group.

□ MINIMALLY INVASIVE PULMONARY VALVE REPLACEMENT

Percutaneous pulmonary valve implantation (PPVI) was first performed in 2000, and, to date, is the largest and most successful clinical programme of minimally invasive valve replacement worldwide.[1,2] It is intended to treat the many patients with repaired congenital heart defects who develop dysfunction of the pulmonary valve as a result of the presence of a transannular patch placed to relieve pulmonary stenosis or degeneration of prosthetic right ventricular to pulmonary artery conduits. In particular, pulmonary regurgitation can cause exercise intolerance, arrhythmia, and an increased risk of sudden death in this patient group. Surgical pulmonary valve replacement can stabilise and, in some cases reverse, these undesirable outcomes; however, a successful transcatheter approach could achieve this while avoiding the morbidity associated with repeat open-heart surgery.

The device used comprises a bovine jugular venous valve sewn inside a balloon-expandable platinum iridium stent (Fig 1(a)). It typically is delivered from a femoral venous approach, under the guidance of biplane angiography, via the right atrium and ventricle. To date, 119 patients – including children as young as seven years and adults in their late fifties – have undergone this procedure. These patients have had a median of three previous sternotomies each for surgical treatment of conditions such as tetralogy of Fallot, pulmonary atresia, transposition of the great arteries, and truncus arteriosus. Percutaneous pulmonary valve implantation is performed under general anaesthesia with a balloon in balloon delivery system that allows two-step deployment of the device in the right ventricular outflow tract (Fig 1(b)). Invasive pressure monitoring and contrast angiography is performed initially to select the most suitable site for device implantation and again at the end of the procedure to

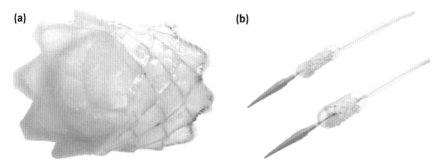

Fig 1 (a) Percutaneous pulmonary valve and **(b)** balloon in balloon delivery system, showing partial (inner balloon) and complete (outer balloon) inflation.

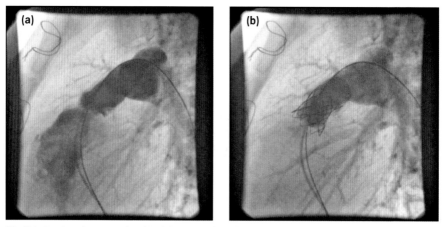

Fig 2 Lateral angiograms showing **(a)** a regurgitant homograft conduit between the right ventricle and pulmonary artery and **(b)** restoration of a competent pulmonary valve as a result of the percutaneous pulmonary valve device.

confirm valve stability and competency (Fig 2). Delivery of the device to the proposed implantation site has been successful in more than 99% of patients in whom it was attempted, and most patients can be discharged home the next day.

Importantly, PPVI reduces pulmonary regurgitation, relieves right ventricular outflow tract obstruction, and improves right ventricular performance. Furthermore, relief of right ventricular volume and pressure overload improves left ventricular filling and function, which may relate to the subjective and objective improvement in exercise capacity that can be seen in these patients within the first few weeks after valve implantation.[2] The success of PPVI is an important clinical step in avoiding multiple operations for this patient population while optimising ventricular haemodynamics. Furthermore, it provides a unique opportunity to study right ventricular behaviour. In a subgroup of patients with right ventricular outflow tract obstruction – a condition traditionally believed to be well tolerated by the myocardium – PPVI showed that the right ventricle in fact is decompensated and unable to generate its expected stroke volume prior to intervention.[3] This new finding supports a growing trend towards earlier intervention in this patient group before right ventricular dysfunction becomes irreversible.

New procedures, however, are not without their difficulties, and PPVI is no exception. Six patients have experienced serious procedural complications. Two patients with borderline outflow tracts experienced device instability soon after implantation, while a third patient's right pulmonary artery was obstructed by the device. All three patients needed removal of the valved stent and surgical conduit replacement. Three-dimensional imaging and careful measurement of the outflow tract is essential to help define suitable morphologies for PPVI and minimise these risks. The current device is appropriate only for outflow tracts <22 mm in diameter because of the size of the biological valve. One patient with complex anatomy experienced coronary artery compression after deployment of the device. Selective coronary angiography with simultaneous balloon inflation in the right ventricular outflow tract has since provided a useful method by which to exclude patients at risk of this complication. Homograft rupture occurred in two patients – one was managed conservatively and one needed surgical haemostasis. This complication remains difficult to predict and avoid, although care should be taken when dilating small conduits.

In terms of morbidity, PPVI compares favourably with surgical pulmonary valve replacement, although the durability of the percutaneous device is unproved as yet.[4] One issue during follow up is the development of stent fractures, which occur in around 15% of patients with these devices. This usually is an incidental finding with no clinical consequence; however, in one case, late dislodgement of the device occurred and required surgical removal. Regular chest X-rays, therefore, form an essential component of the follow up. Early identification of device fracture that affects stent integrity can be treated successfully by implantation of a second valved stent within the first, which reduces the risk of more serious complications and also avoids further surgery.

Patients who are turned down for surgery on account of operative risk can benefit from PPVI. Patients with severe kyphoscoliosis or those with pulmonary valve dysfunction in the setting of pulmonary hypertension have shown marked improvement after restoration of a competent pulmonary valve, although specialist anaesthetic input remains essential. In patients who are 'in extremis', the benefits are less clear; in our population, two patients with end-stage cardiac failure (one with pulmonary regurgitation and one with severe obstruction) underwent PPVI. The first patient – an adult with four previous conduit replacements, chronic atrial fibrillation, ascites, and pleural effusions – underwent a successful procedure but deteriorated six weeks later after a chest infection and died. The second patient – a child with complex left ventricular outflow tract obstruction treated with a Ross operation – presented in a coma with cardiogenic shock related to severe recoarctation and right-ventricular outflow tract obstruction. Despite a technically successful procedure to relieve the coarctation and implant a pulmonary valve, the patient died 24 hours later from irretractable pulmonary oedema. No other mortality – at the time of procedure or during follow up – has occurred in our population.

At present, PPVI cannot be performed in all patients with pulmonary valve dysfunction. The main limitation is the size of the right ventricular outflow tract. Degenerated homograft conduits seem most suited to treatment with this technique, as they tend to calcify circumferentially, which provides a secure environment for stent implantation. Although these patients represent less than a quarter of those who need intervention, PPVI has, nevertheless, become a realistic clinical treatment option for this group. Development of novel devices and new strategies to percutaneously implant valves into dilated (>22 mm) outflow tracts is underway.[5] Mathematical modelling from magnetic resonance datasets can provide new insights into the spectrum of right ventricular outflow tract morphology and allow virtual testing of novel devices before *in vivo* implantation (Fig 3). Hybrid procedures – in which a percutaneous valve is inserted through the right ventricular apex via a mini thoracotomy – avoid cardiopulmonary bypass and may provide an alternative treatment approach for patients with dilated outflow tracts.[6]

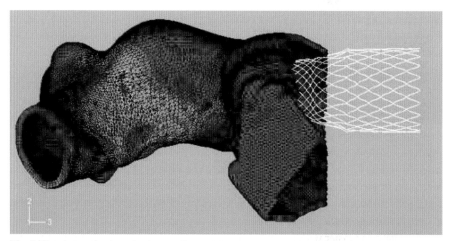

Fig 3 Virtual stent implantation into a dilated right ventricular outflow tract, reconstructed from a real magnetic resonance dataset of a patient with tetralogy of Fallot repaired with a transannular patch. Reproduced courtesy of Miss Silvia Schievano, UCL Institute of Child Health, London.

☐ MINIMALLY INVASIVE AORTIC VALVE REPLACEMENT

The morbidity and mortality associated with calcific aortic valve disease in the growing elderly population have led it to become an important target for minimally invasive catheter technology. High levels of comorbidity in this patient group confer considerable risk for cardiopulmonary bypass and surgery but, equally, add to the complexity of attempting new percutaneous procedures. Furthermore, the aortic valve provides a different and more difficult anatomical challenge to the pulmonary valve for those attempting transcatheter valve implantation. The proximity of the coronary arteries and the fibrous continuity that exists between the aortic and mitral valves requires a different type of device to avoid compromise of these vulnerable adjacent structures. An outer rotational stent that allows orientation with the coronary orifices may offer one solution and has been successful in the experimental setting (Fig 4).[7] Other investigators have used a shorter stent to avoid impinging on surrounding structures; however, paravalvular leak and device stability remain substantial concerns within the high-pressure system of the left heart.[8] Self-expandable valved stents that can be retracted if implantation is suboptimal also have been trialled.[9]

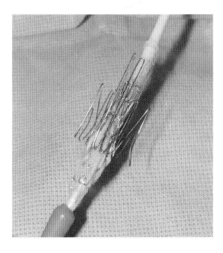

Fig 4 Percutaneous aortic valve composed of outer nitinol stent to orientate with the coronary artery orifices prior to final deployment of inner balloon-expandable valved stent. Reproduced from Boudjemline Y *et al* with permission of Lippincott, Williams and Wilkins.[7]

Most experience in humans has been gathered with a short stainless steel stent with equine pericardial leaflets.[10,11] To date, percutaneous aortic valve implantation (PAVI) has been performed only in the palliative setting, with patients required to have New York Heart Association functional class IV or cardiogenic shock for inclusion. Vascular access presents a challenge, with two options available. The antegrade approach, which requires trans-septal puncture, technically is challenging and risks damage to the mitral valve; however, device implantation into more heavily calcified valves is easier with this approach. The retrograde approach, although faster and simpler, requires cannulation of the femoral artery and negotiation of an often tortuous and atheromatous descending aorta; development of a novel steerable catheter system, however, may make this the preferred approach in the future. Predilatation of the calcified native valve is usually undertaken to facilitate subsequent implantation, while rapid right ventricular pacing is used at the time of device deployment to temporarily lower left ventricular pressure and create a more favourable environment for stable implantation.

The largest clinical experience with PAVI was recently reported.[10] Of 36 patients recruited, 27 underwent successful implantation: 23 with an antegrade approach and four with a retrograde approach. All patients had severe calcific aortic stenosis (valve area <1.0 cm²) and were formally declined for surgery on account of clinical status and comorbidity. After device implantation, improvements in valve area and transvalvular gradient were seen; however, at least moderate paravalvular regurgitation was seen in five patients, with others having a mild or trivial leak. Left ventricular function, measured by echocardiographic parameters, improved within the first week. Despite some of these positive findings, the morbidity at 30 days was significant and included pericardial tamponade, stroke, arrhythmia, septicaemia, and an unexplained death. Only 11 patients survived beyond nine months, with the longest follow up at 26 months. Function of the percutaneous heart valve device remained unchanged during follow up.

A second group of investigators who have favoured the retrograde approach for PAVI and designed a steerable catheter to aid device delivery also recently reported results.[11] Of 18 patients, 14 with surgical risk deemed excessive because of comorbidities underwent successful PAVI. The failed procedures were the result of inability to negotiate the diseased iliac artery in two patients and device embolisation in two cases. All but one patient had evidence of paravalvular regurgitation after device implantation, with three cases being severe. Nevertheless, aortic valve area increased significantly in those whose device implantation was successful. One transient neurological event occurred during the follow up and two patients died: one related to rupture of the iliac artery and the other because of obstruction of the left coronary artery orifice by a native valve leaflet displaced by the implanted device.

Percutaneous aortic valve implantation currently is targeted at a high-risk group of patients who have no conventional surgical option for treatment. Morbidity and mortality have been relatively high compared with the pulmonary experience, as a result of the technical difficulties of placing a percutaneous device in the left side of the heart and the poor health of this patient population. This intervention is in the early stages of development, and much work is needed before it will become a real treatment option for all patients.

☐ MINIMALLY INVASIVE VALVE REPLACEMENT – WHERE DO WE GO FROM HERE?

Percutaneous pulmonary valve implantation is rapidly becoming an accepted clinical strategy for suitable patients with pulmonary valve dysfunction. The challenge will be to extend this procedure to the wide range of outflow tract morphologies that exist after complete repair of congenital heart defects. The encouraging procedural and midterm results seen here, however, have not been mirrored when this technology has been applied to the aortic valve. Despite this, aortic valve disease in the elderly population clearly represents a much greater burden on our health services than pulmonary valve disease, which overall remains relatively rare.

Reliable implantation of devices into a defined anatomical location, with available surgical backup in case of failure, undoubtedly would improve outcomes. One way to achieve this in the aortic position may be to implant devices into failing stented bioprosthetic valves. The crown-like stent structure of the existing surgically placed valve would be visible readily in X-ray, which would allow easy orientation of a new percutaneous valve with the coronary orifices; furthermore, surgical intervention would remain possible. In this situation, minimally invasive valve replacement would be performed as a treatment for biological valve failure rather than primary disease. Nevertheless, if successful, this could have considerable implications for the use of mechanical valves and anticoagulation in surgery.

Minimally invasive valve replacement is one of the most exciting advances in cardiology today. In the experimental setting, attempts have even been made to address percutaneous atrioventricular valve replacement.[12] Application of novel ideas supported by strong cooperation between cardiologists, cardiothoracic surgeons, biomedical engineers, and industry should see this technology progress rapidly over the coming years.

REFERENCES

1   Bonhoeffer P, Boudjemline Y, Saliba Z *et al*. Percutaneous replacement of pulmonary valve in a right-ventricle to pulmonary-artery prosthetic conduit with valve dysfunction. *Lancet* 2000;356:1403–5.

2   Khambadkone S, Coats L, Taylor A *et al*. Percutaneous pulmonary valve implantation in humans: results in 59 consecutive patients. *Circulation* 2005;112:1189–97.

3   Coats L, Khambadkone S, Derrick G *et al*. Physiological and clinical consequences of relief of right ventricular outflow tract obstruction late after repair of congenital heart defects. *Circulation* (in press).

4   Coats L, Tsang V, Khambadkone S *et al*. The potential impact of percutaneous pulmonary valve stent implantation on right ventricular outflow tract re-intervention. *Eur J Cardiothorac Surg* 2005;27:536–43.

5   Boudjemline Y, Agnoletti G, Bonnet D *et al*. Percutaneous pulmonary valve replacement in a large right ventricular outflow tract: an experimental study. *J Am Coll Cardiol* 2004;43:1082–7.

6   Boudjemline Y, Schievano S, Bonnet C *et al*. Off-pump replacement of the pulmonary valve in large right ventricular outflow tracts: a hybrid approach. *J Thorac Cardiovasc Surg* 2005;129: 831–7.

7   Boudjemline Y, Bonhoeffer P. Steps toward percutaneous aortic valve replacement. *Circulation* 2002;105:775–8.

8   Cribier A, Eltchaninoff H, Tron C *et al*. Early experience with percutaneous transcatheter implantation of heart valve prosthesis for the treatment of end-stage inoperable patients with calcific aortic stenosis. *J Am Coll Cardiol* 2004;43:698–703.

9   Laborde JC, Borenstein N, Behr L, Farah B, Fajadet J. Percutaneous implantation of an aortic valve prosthesis. *Catheter Cardiovasc Interv* 2005;65:171–4.

10 Cribier A, Eltchaninoff H, Tron C *et al*. Treatment of calcific aortic stenosis with the percutaneous heart valve: mid-term follow-up from the initial feasibility studies: the French experience. *J Am Coll Cardiol* 2006;47:1214–23.

11 Webb JG, Chandavimol M, Thompson CR *et al*. Percutaneous aortic valve implantation retrograde from the femoral artery. *Circulation* 2006;113:842–50.

12 Boudjemline Y, Agnoletti G, Bonnet D *et al*. Steps toward the percutaneous replacement of atrioventricular valves: an experimental study. *J Am Coll Cardiol* 2005;46:360–5.

Hypertension: lessons from the eponymous syndromes

Isla S Mackenzie and Morris J Brown

☐ INTRODUCTION

Hypertension is a common condition that causes considerable morbidity and mortality. Most cases of hypertension are so-called 'essential hypertension,' or hypertension of unknown cause. A significant minority of cases, however, are the result of underlying secondary causes, and an even smaller minority are the result of rare monogenic syndromes. Little evidence sheds light on the precise molecular basis of essential hypertension. Evidence, however, has strongly supported a simple physiological model, in which two main routes to developing or reversing hypertension are recognised: salt-handling in 'low-renin hypertension' and vasoconstriction in 'high-renin hypertension'.

☐ ESSENTIAL HYPERTENSION

For each of the monogenic syndromes, one single best drug lowers blood pressure much more than the 10 mmHg average achieved with unselected drugs in patients with essential hypertension (Table 1). This led us to ask whether, in reverse, discovery of each patient's best drug in essential hypertension would help elucidate underlying causes. The answer, so far, has been negative for finding molecular causes, but the studies have shown how hypertension itself, and the drugs used to treat it, divide into two opposite categories.

These two types of hypertension are easy to recognise through measurement of levels of renin in plasma. Low-renin hypertension occurs when the kidney recognises an excess of sodium ions reaching the kidney; an arbitrary cut-off level for plasma renin mass of <10 mU/l may be used for diagnosis. As secretion of renin should also be suppressed by high pressure in the glomerular afferent arterioles, high (that is, inappropriately high)-renin hypertension is present in patients whose plasma levels of renin are within or above the upper limit of the normal range (5–80 mU/l). The cut-off level between low- and high-renin types of hypertension is arbitrary, but we have found the levels of renin quoted to be useful in guiding drug treatment in practice. Indeed, recent outcome trials of antihypertensive treatments – such as the Anglo-Scandinavian Cardiac Outcomes Trial (ASCOT), Antihypertensive and Lipid-Lowering Treatment to Prevent Heart Attack Trial (ALLHAT), and Valsartan Antihypertensive Long-Term Use Evaluation (VALUE)[1–3] – have largely supported the fact that two overall forms of essential hypertension exist on the basis of levels of renin by

Table 1 Monogenic syndromes that cause hypertension and other secondary causes of hypertension.

Syndrome	Cause	Treatment
Monogenic syndromes:		
Liddle's syndrome	Epithelial sodium channel (ENaC) (β or γ subunit) mutations	Amiloride
Glucocorticoid-remediable aldosteronism	Aldosterone synthase chimera	Dexamethasone
Apparent mineralocorticoid excess	Liquorice; 11 β HSD mutation	Spironolactone
Gordon's syndrome	WNK1 or WNK4 mutation	Thiazide
Secondary syndromes:		
Conn's syndrome	Adrenal adenoma	Spironolactone or eplerenone
Phaeochromocytoma	Chromaffin tumour	Phenoxybenzamine
Renal artery stenosis	Fibromuscular hyperplasia (or atherosclerotic disease in older patients)	Angiotensin converting enzyme inhibitor or angiotensin receptor antagonist*

*Use with extreme caution in patients with bilateral renal artery stenosis, as renal function may worsen.

showing that a drug acting on the renin system used as the first-line agent in an older population results in a less good outcome than may be achieved with a diuretic or calcium channel blocker as first-line treatment (see below).

☐ ABCD RULE FOR THE TREATMENT OF HYPERTENSION

The concept of classifying hypertension into high-renin and low-renin types, each with different preferred therapies, has been encapsulated for some time within the ABCD rule adopted by the British Hypertension Society in their guidelines for the treatment of hypertension (the abbreviation 'ABCD' derives serendipitously from the initials of the main antihypertensive drug classes).[4] Younger Caucasian patients tend to have high levels of renin and therefore tend to respond better to drugs that suppress the renin system, such as angiotensin-converting enzyme (ACE) inhibitors and angiotensin receptor antagonists (A) and β blockers (B). Older Caucasian patients tend to have low levels of renin and therefore tend to respond better to drugs that cause vasodilatation or natriuresis, such as calcium channel blockers (C) and diuretics (D). Black patients, whatever their age, tend to have low-renin hypertension and therefore respond in a similar way to older Caucasian patients.

If combination treatment is needed, as is often the case, drugs from the A or B classes should be combined with drugs from the C or D classes, as the different groups will counteract any reflex mechanisms induced by the other agent, such as activation of renin caused by thiazide diuretics. Although this approach is very effective overall, it is important to note that exceptions in individual patients do occur – for example, not all young patients will have high levels of renin and will respond well to an A or B drug. In such cases, levels of renin can be measured to guide treatment or the first-choice drug can simply be changed to one from the C or D group, and the clinical response then reassessed.

The ABCD rule has recently been adopted in a modified form by the National Institute for Health and Clinical Excellence (NICE), with the role of drugs from classes B and D downgraded because of increased risk of diabetes. Class B is additionally downgraded because of its reduced ability to prevent stroke (compared to other classes); we believe this stems from its relative failure to lower central as much as peripheral arterial pressure.[5] Because NICE is constrained in its recommendations by the quality of evidence, we would like to broaden the scope of ABCD to incorporate our current practice (Fig 1). As renin (or, more correctly, log-renin) is normally distributed, most patients have plasma levels of renin that are neither high nor low and do not respond as dramatically to single treatment as patients at the extremes. The American and European guidelines already recommend combination treatment for initial management of patients with blood pressure ≥20/10 mmHg above target, and this should particularly be considered in patients with a 'normal' plasma level of renin. Similarly, for patients with resistant (step 4) hypertension, we recommend different additions, as discussed below, for patients at the extremes and those at the middle of the distribution of plasma levels of renin. The British Hypertension Society is planning a study of the 'α,β,Δ' recommendation shown in Fig 1.

☐ RENIN

Renin is produced by the juxtaglomerular apparatus in the kidney, and four main factors regulate its release: the sympathetic supply to the juxtaglomerular apparatus cells via the β_1 adrenoceptor, sodium reabsorption in the macula densa, blood pressure perfusing the arterioles of the kidney, and negative feedback on release of renin by angiotensin II. Renin stimulates the conversion of angiotensinogen to angiotensin I, which is converted to angiotensin II by the enzyme angiotensin converting enzyme (ACE). Angiotensin II is a potent vasoconstrictor and also stimulates the release of aldosterone from the zona glomerulosa of the adrenal gland, which causes sodium and water retention (Fig 2).

☐ MEASUREMENT OF PLASMA LEVELS OF RENIN

Renin can now be measured by a high-throughput immunochemiluminometric assay that allows accurate determination of total renin mass and renin activity for less than the price of a single month's treatment with an antihypertensive agent. It therefore seems sensible to make more use of this measurement in guiding management – at initial diagnosis before treatment is started or in patients in whom hypertension is difficult to control despite multiple drug treatments. At present, the British Hypertension Society guidelines suggest that measurement of renin should be considered in cases of resistant hypertension (that is failure to achieve target blood pressure (usually <140/85 mmHg) despite triple drug treatment) in order to guide further drug treatment. If the level of renin measured when the patient is on

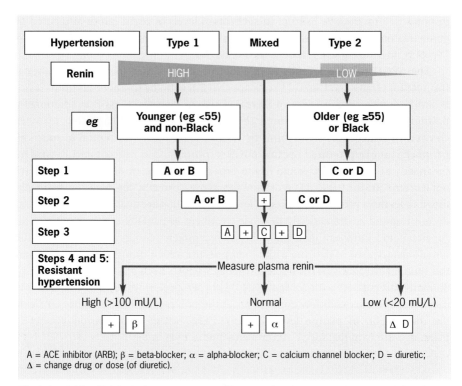

Fig 1 Cambridge AbCd rule for management of hypertension. Younger patients with high-renin hypertension respond better to drugs that act on the renin system (A or B), while older patients with low-renin hypertension (and black patients) respond better to calcium-channel blockers or diuretics (C or D).

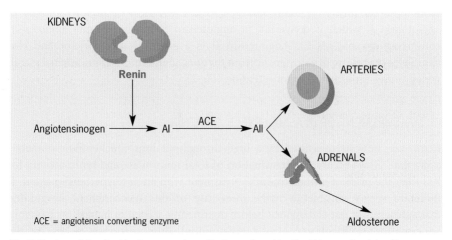

Fig 2 Renin-angiotensin-aldosterone system. Renin produced by the kidneys stimulates the production of angiotensin I (A-I) from angiotensinogen. The A-I is then converted by the action of angiotensin-converting enzyme (ACE) to angiotensin II (A-II), which is a potent vasoconstrictor that also stimulates the production of aldosterone from the adrenal glands, which leads to sodium and water retention.

A, C and D drugs is low (<10 mU/l), options include a trial of spironolactone (or another diuretic) or addition of an α blocker. If the level of renin is high (>100 mU/l), options include the addition of a drug to further block the renin-angiotensin system (for example, double blockade with ACE inhibition and angiotensin receptor antagonism) or addition of a β blocker.

Previously, measurements of renin were often made in a rather prescribed fashion after an overnight hospital admission and bed rest. In practice, as a general screening tool, it is not necessary or indeed practical to implement these conditions. Levels of renin vary widely between individuals and there is only around a 2–3-fold difference between supine and standing or ambulant measurements of levels of renin, which will not affect differentiation between people at the bottom end of the range of levels of renin and those at the top end.

Effects of antihypertensive drugs on measurement of plasma levels of renin

It is important to note that treatment with antihypertensive drugs often affects measurements of levels of renin. β Blockers tend to suppress renin, and ACE inhibitors and angiotensin receptor antagonists significantly increase levels of renin because of reflex stimulation of the renin system. Calcium channel blockers and thiazide diuretics cause smaller increases in levels of renin. Interpretation of levels of renin should therefore be made in the context of current drug treatment, and it may be particularly useful to withdraw β blockers for two weeks before levels of renin are measured, as long as suitable alternative antihypertensive treatment is in place, to allow accurate interpretation of the results.

☐ EPONYMOUS SYNDROMES THAT CAUSE HYPERTENSION

Several eponymous syndromes cause hypertension. Some of these are the result of single gene mutations, while others are less well defined in their origin. Table 1 lists these conditions, along with some other secondary causes of hypertension, their origins, and their preferred drug treatments. Some of these conditions represent extreme examples of low- or high-renin forms of hypertension. In such cases, a single effective drug often significantly reduces the blood pressure and, to some extent, this information can be extrapolated to apply more generally to low- or high-renin forms of essential hypertension.

Liddle's syndrome

Liddle's syndrome is an autosomal dominant condition caused by mutations in the genes that encode the β and γ subunits of the mineralocorticoid-dependent epithelial sodium channel. This results in continuous (constitutive) activation of the channel, even in the absence of mineralocorticoid. Clinically, the condition is characterised by early-onset hypertension, with hypokalaemia and low levels of renin and aldosterone.[6] The condition responds to treatment with the potassium-sparing diuretic amiloride (or triamterene).

Glucocorticoid-remediable aldosteronism

Glucocorticoid-remediable aldosteronism (GRA) is a rare autosomal dominant condition (about 200 known cases) characterised by hypertension associated with low levels of renin but high levels of aldosterone.[7] In this condition, a chromosomal translocation between the genes that encode aldosterone synthase and 11β-hydroxylase – two enzymes involved in steroid biosynthesis – results in a loss of the normal secretory control processes, such that adrenocorticotropic hormone (ACTH), rather than angiotensin II, stimulates secretion of aldosterone. A loss of negative feedback from circulating aldosterone on secretion of ACTH also occurs, which leads to excessive levels of aldosterone, salt and water retention, and hypertension. The hypertension of GRA can be controlled by administration of glucocorticoids such as dexamethasone.

Apparent mineralocorticoid excess

Apparent mineralocorticoid excess (AME)[8] is inherited in an autosomal recessive manner and results from a mutation in the gene that encodes 11β-hydroxysteroid dehydrogenase. This results in a reduction in the normal conversion of cortisol to cortisone, so that levels of cortisol in urine over 24 hours are characteristically elevated. Cortisol (unlike cortisone) is a potent agonist at the mineralocorticoid receptor that leads to hypertension. Apparent mineralocorticoid excess thus results in hypertension associated with high levels of cortisol but low levels of renin and aldosterone. Clinically, AME resembles primary hyperaldosteronism, with the exception that levels of aldosterone are characteristically low. Apparent mineralocorticoid excess can be treated with a combination of high doses of the aldosterone antagonist spironolactone (or the potassium-sparing diuretic amiloride) and dexamethasone, which is used to suppress endogenous secretion of cortisol.

Gordon's syndrome

Gordon's syndrome (or pseudohypoaldosteronism type II) is an autosomal dominant condition caused by mutations in the with-no-lysine (or K) kinase genes *WNK1* or *WNK4*.[9] Clinically, it is characterised by early-onset low-renin hypertension, increased renal reabsorption of sodium, hyperkalaemia, and hyperchloraemia. The metabolic abnormalities and hypertension respond well to treatment with thiazide diuretics.

Other rare monogenic syndromes that cause hypertension

An extremely rare condition that causes hypertension in response to progesterone has been described in up to 10 patients worldwide. It is caused by a mutation in the mineralocorticoid receptor, which makes it exquisitely sensitive to stimulation by progesterone and results in cyclical hypertension in women who have menstrual cycles and severe exacerbations of hypertension during pregnancy as a result of the increased levels of progesterone. Another extremely rare autosomal dominant condition caused by a mutation of a gene on chromosome 12 results in a syndrome of hypertension and brachydactyly.

☐ OTHER SYNDROMES THAT CAUSE HYPERTENSION AND RESPOND TO SPECIFIC ANTIHYPERTENSIVE DRUG TREATMENTS

In several other syndromes that cause hypertension, a specific drug treatment is preferred, but the exact genetic basis of the condition is not fully understood.

Conn's syndrome

The classic clues are hypertension with a level of sodium ions in the plasma >140 mmol/l and levels of potassium ions <3.5 mmol/l or bicarbonate >30 mmol/l. The low levels of potassium may be apparent only during diuretic treatment, which increases delivery of sodium ions to the site of sodium and potassium ion exchange. The diagnosis is confirmed by an increased level of aldosterone (>400 pmol/l) in plasma in the presence of a suppressed (often undetectable) level of renin in plasma – hence the correct name for the syndrome is primary hyperaldosteronism. Unfortunately, low levels of potassium are often ignored or attributed to diuretic treatment and not investigated further. A high level of aldosterone may be absent in patients with uncorrected low levels of potassium; hypokalaemia and high levels of aldosterone may be masked by calcium channel blockers, which can suppress the calcium ion entry-dependent secretion of aldosterone.[10]

Conn's syndrome classically is the result of a benign aldosterone-secreting adenoma in one of the adrenal glands. The diagnosis is confirmed by computed tomography (CT) (Fig 3) or magnetic resonance imaging (MRI) (Fig 4) of the adrenal glands, followed by selective adrenal venous sampling to confirm excessive aldosterone secretion from the suspected abnormal adrenal gland. The latter is essential in most patients, as 4% of healthy people have non-functioning incidentalomas of the adrenal that cannot easily be distinguished radiologically from aldosteronomas. Some enthusiasts have even advocated adrenal vein sampling in all patients with biochemical evidence of Conn's syndrome, on the basis that small adenomas (typically 1–2 cm, but sometimes <0.5 cm) can be missed. Adrenal vein sampling, however, is not trivial – especially because of the required cannulation of the right adrenal vein – and should probably be undertaken only in a few tertiary centres with considerable experience. In the future, positron emission tomography (PET) with ^{11}C-metomidate may become a useful investigation that obviates the need for the more invasive procedure of selective adrenal venous sampling. Whether an invasive or non-invasive method is used for lateralisation, it may be necessary to reduce temporarily the dose of spironolactone in order to avoid desuppression of the contralateral normal adrenal and a consequently false-negative finding. Our practice is to check, before sampling, that plasma levels of renin are no higher than one third of the upper limit of normal for the assay used.

The definitive treatment for Conn's syndrome is surgical removal of the adenoma (Fig 5), usually laparoscopically. Before surgery, or if medical management is

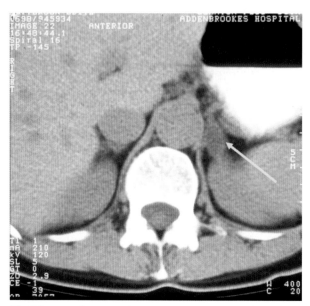

Fig 3 Computed tomograph showing left adrenal Conn's adenoma. An abnormality of the left adrenal gland (arrow) is suggestive of an adrenal adenoma. Computed tomography should be performed with and without contrast enhancement, with an adenoma appearing slightly less vascular than the rest of the gland. As 4% of healthy people have a non-functioning adrenal adenoma, the diagnosis of aldosteronoma must be proved by further investigations such as selective venous sampling. In patients with surgically curable primary hyperaldosteronism, the sampling should show an increased ratio of aldosterone:cortisol secretion by the adrenal gland on the side of the lesion compared with the contralateral adrenal gland.

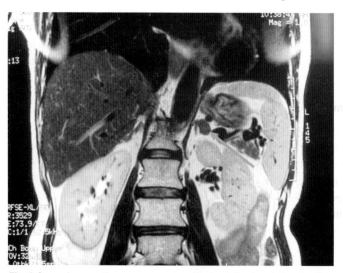

Fig 4 Coronal magnetic resonance scan showing left adrenal Conn's adenoma. Magnetic resonance imaging is often useful in localising Conn's adenomas as a primary investigation or where adrenal computed tomography is equivocal. This scan shows an abnormality of the left adrenal gland (arrow) consistent with a Conn's adenoma. Occasionally, an adenoma is convincingly seen only in the coronal view. Thin patients who lack much peri-adrenal fat seem to have an increased chance of false-negative scans.

preferred, hypertension and metabolic abnormalities may be treated with the aldosterone antagonist spironolactone; if this is not tolerated, high-dose amiloride can be substituted. The newer aldosterone antagonist, eplerenone, is less effective at licensed doses than spironolactone. Spironolactone or amiloride are also useful in the management of the related condition, bilateral adrenal hyperplasia, in which both adrenal glands contain nodules that produce too much aldosterone. This condition is managed medically, as both adrenals are affected.

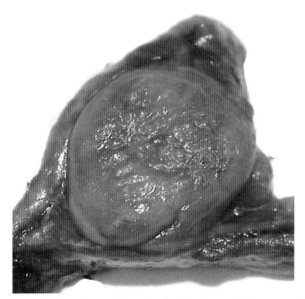

Fig 5 Pathological specimen showing the characteristic canary-yellow appearance of the cut surface of a Conn's adenoma. The adenoma is surrounded by the remnants of the normal adrenal gland.

Phaeochromocytoma

Phaeochromocytoma is a tumour of chromaffin tissue that produces excessive levels of catecholamines (usually norepinephrine or epinephrine, or both) (Fig 6). Although many phaeochromocytomas are apparently sporadic, a significant proportion are the result of recognised genetic syndromes, including multiple endocrine neoplasia type 2 (MEN-2), von Hippel Lindau syndrome, and neurofibromatosis type 1. Diagnosis is confirmed by finding high levels of catecholamine and then localising the lesion through scanning, which may include CT, MRI, I-123 metaiodobenzylguanidine (^{123}I-MIBG) scanning, or ^{18}F-dopamine PET. Treatment starts with an α blocker, such as phenoxybenzamine (an irreversible α blocker), for at least six weeks before surgery to allow the intravascular volume to expand adequately before surgical removal of the source of catecholamines. Combined treatment with β blockade may also be needed in the preparation for surgery depending on the resulting tachycardia secondary to phenoxybenzamine treatment, which is largely determined by the level of epinephrine secretion from the tumour.

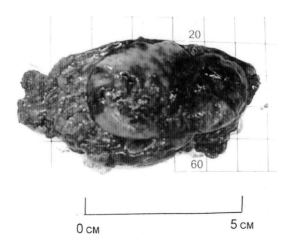

Fig 6 Pathological specimen showing an adrenal phaeochromocytoma with characteristic areas of haemorrhage and necrosis within the tumour. Phaeochromocytomas are usually benign; however, 10–20% prove to be malignant, even when the initial histology shows no particularly malignant features. Malignancy is more likely in extra-adrenal phaeochromocytoma in patients with mutations of the SDHB gene.

Renal artery stenosis

Two distinct forms of renal artery stenosis exist. Fibromuscular dysplasia tends to affect young people and results in a corkscrew appearance of the renal arteries on MRI or conventional angiography. Atherosclerotic disease is the more common form in older patients and is characterised by tight stenoses, often near the origin of the renal arteries (Fig 7). Both forms are associated with the clinical presence of renal bruits and high levels of renin in plasma, although these indicators are not present in all cases. Both forms respond best to treatment with drugs that block the renin system, particularly angiotensin II receptor antagonists; however, these should be used only under specialist supervision, as they have the potential to worsen the situation, particularly in patients with bilateral renal artery stenosis, in whom renal function may deteriorate in the presence of ACE inhibitors or angiotensin II receptor antagonists. Angioplasty may be particularly successful in the treatment of fibromuscular dysplasia and can also be used in patients with atherosclerotic disease but with much higher associated risks of renal artery dissection or restenosis. Medical management of hypertension with a combination of antihypertensive drugs is often preferred in patients with atherosclerotic disease, unless renal function is deteriorating or the level of blood pressure is very difficult to control.

Excessive ingestion of liquorice

It is important to remember that excessive ingestion of liquorice may result in hypertension with associated metabolic abnormalities. Liquorice contains glycyrrhizinic acid, a substance that, in addition to binding weakly to mineralocorticoid receptors, also inhibits 11β-hydroxysteroid dehydrogenase type 2 in the kidney, which leads to changes in the metabolism of cortisol and increased effects of cortisol on the mineralocorticoid receptor. Typically, patients present with hypertension, hypokalaemia, hypernatraemia, and high levels of bicarbonate with metabolic alkalosis, which may initially resemble Conn's syndrome. When levels of

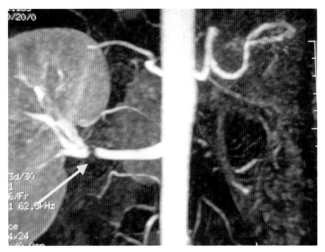

Fig 7 Magnetic resonance renal angiogram showing renal artery stenosis. A tight stenosis is seen in the right renal artery of this 22-year-old man with hypertension. The level of renin in plasma was 23 mU/l (normal range 9–56 mU/l) when measured while the patient was on atenolol but 578 mU/l when repeated when the patient was on candesartan, showing the importance of knowing about drug treatment when interpreting levels of renin. β Blockers suppress levels of renin, while angiotensin receptor antagonists increase levels of renin.

renin and aldosterone are measured, however, both are found to be suppressed. The hypertension and metabolic abnormalities usually improve after withdrawal of liquorice.

☐ CONCLUSIONS

In terms of the response to drug treatment, hypertension is of two main types, high- and low-renin hypertension, with the type largely determined by the age and race of the patient but also occasionally by the underlying cause of the hypertension. With modern assays, levels of renin in plasma can now be measured relatively easily at a reasonable cost. The level of renin may be helpful in guiding appropriate drug treatment, particularly in cases of resistant hypertension. A high level of renin in patients with hypertension suggests that drugs that act on the renin system may be the most effective, while a suppressed level of renin often means that drugs that act to increase sodium excretion or vasodilators will be most effective. Unusual metabolic findings in a patient with hypertension should always prompt the consideration of a secondary cause of hypertension, and further investigations may be warranted.

REFERENCES

1   Dahlof B, Sever PS, Poulter NR *et al.* Prevention of cardiovascular events with an antihypertensive regimen of amlodipine adding perindopril as required versus atenolol adding bendroflumethiazide as required, in the Anglo-Scandinavian Cardiac Outcomes Trial-Blood Pressure Lowering Arm (ASCOT-BPLA): a multicentre randomised controlled trial. *Lancet* 2005;366:895–906.

2   ALLHAT Officers and Coordinators for the ALLHAT Collaborative Research Group. Major outcomes in high-risk hypertensive patients randomized to angiotensin-converting enzyme inhibitor or calcium channel blocker vs diuretic: the Antihypertensive and Lipid-Lowering Treatment to Prevent Heart Attack Trial (ALLHAT). *JAMA* 2002;288:2981–97.

3   Julius S, Kjeldsen SE, Weber M *et al.* Outcomes in hypertensive patients at high cardiovascular risk treated with regimens based on valsartan or amlodipine: the VALUE randomised trial. *Lancet* 2004;363:2022–31.

4   Williams B, Poulter NR, Brown MJ *et al.* Guidelines for management of hypertension: report of the fourth working party of the British Hypertension Society, 2004-BHS IV. *J Hum Hypertens* 2004;18:139–85.

5   Deary AJ, Schumann AL, Murfet H *et al.* Influence of drugs and gender on the arterial pulse wave and natriuretic peptide secretion in untreated patients with essential hypertension. *Clin Sci (Lond)* 2002;103:493–9.

6   Liddle GW, Bledsoe T, Coppage WS. A familial renal disorder simulating primary aldosteronism but with negligible aldosterone secretion. *Trans Assoc Physicians* 1966;76: 199–213.

7   Sutherland DJ, Ruse JL, Laidlaw JC. Hypertension, increased aldosterone secretion and low plasma renin activity relieved by dexamethasone. *Can Med Assoc J* 1966;95:1109–19.

8   Stewart PM, Corrie JE, Shackleton CH, Edwards CR. Syndrome of apparent mineralocorticoid excess. A defect in the cortisol-cortisone shuttle. *J Clin Invest* 1988;82:340–9.

9   Wilson FH, Disse-Nicodeme S, Choate KA *et al.* Human hypertension caused by mutations in WNK kinases. *Science* 2001;293:1107–12.

10   Brown MJ, Hopper RV. Calcium-channel blockade can mask the diagnosis of Conn's syndrome. *Postgrad Med J* 1999;75:235–6.

☐ CARDIOVASCULAR SELF ASSESSMENT QUESTIONS

Of stents and stem cells – advances in the management of ST elevation myocardial infarction

1   Randomised trials of PCI in MI have shown PCI confers benefit in:
(a) Total mortality
(b) Recurrent MI
(c) Stroke
(d) Bleeding
(e) Recurrent ischaemia

2   Regarding primary PCI, the following are true:
(a) Initial IRA patency rates are about the same as with thrombolysis
(b) IRA reocclusion occurs in less than 5% of cases
(c) IRA reocclusion is associated with a poorer prognosis
(d) Time from symptom onset to treatment is a strong predictor of outcome
(e) Guidelines recommend that thrombolysis is preferable if transfer for PCI is liable to result in a treatment delay of greater than three hours

3   Stem cells for treating infarcted myocardium in humans:
(a) May be derived from the bone marrow
(b) May be derived from the spleen
(c) May be derived from a circulating cell population
(d) May promote the division of mature cardiomyocytes
(e) May release local factors that recruit local progenitor cells

4   Stem cell therapy for MI in humans has been shown to:
(a) Prolong life
(b) Reduce reinfarction
(c) Improve ejection fraction
(d) Increase perfusion to the infarcted zone
(e) Result in the formation of new cardiomyocytes

Angina pectoris: second wind, warm up and walk through

1   What elicits the sensation of discomfort during angina pectoris?
(a) Distension of the left ventricular wall
(b) Release of adenosine
(c) Release of substance P
(d) Distension of the coronary vessels
(e) Epinephrine

2   Which of the following contribute to the second wind phenomenon?
(a) Opening of collateral channels (that is, collateral recruitment)
(b) Post-conditioning

(c) Pre-conditioning
(d) Norepinephrine
(e) Bradykinin

3   Which of the following factors or substances are thought to be involved in the preconditioning process?
(a) Adenosine
(b) Bradykinin
(c) Opioid receptor agonists
(d) Mitochondrial ATP-sensitive potassium channel
(e) Protein kinase C

Minimally invasive valve replacement

1   A percutaneous approach to valve replacement:
(a) Avoids the need for cardiopulmonary bypass
(b) Requires longer hospital inpatient stays
(c) Is the preferred method for primary repair of tetralogy of Fallot
(d) May be used in patients too ill for aortic valve surgery
(e) Is altering surgical approaches to valvular heart disease

2   Transcatheter placement of a valved stent in the right ventricular outflow tract:
(a) Could avoid repeat operations in patients with congenital heart disease
(b) Can be complicated by coronary artery compression
(c) Can be performed only once before surgery is needed
(d) Is indicated only for the treatment of pulmonary regurgitation
(e) Has been performed in more than 100 patients

3   Minimally invasive replacement of the aortic valve is challenging because:
(a) Of the potential risk of coronary artery obstruction
(b) The target population often is elderly and has other comorbidities
(c) Only one type of percutaneous device has been developed
(d) Of the proximity of the mitral valve
(e) It has not been shown to improve ventricular function

4   Percutaneous aortic valve implantation in humans:
(a) Improves valve area in patients with calcific aortic stenosis
(b) Requires trans-septal puncture for delivery of the device
(c) Is an acceptable alternative to surgical valve replacement
(d) Often is complicated by paravalvular leak
(e) Could be used to treat failed bioprosthetic valves

Hypertension: lessons from the eponymous syndromes

1   Characteristic biochemical abnormalities in Conn's syndrome include:
(a) Hypokalaemia

(b) Hyponatraemia
(c) Metabolic acidosis
(d) High levels of aldosterone
(e) Suppressed levels of renin

2   Plasma aldosterone level is typically low in the following conditions:
(a) Liddle's syndrome
(b) Glucocorticoid-remediable aldosteronism
(c) Apparent mineralocorticoid excess
(d) Conn's syndrome
(e) Bilateral adrenal hyperplasia

3   Excessive liquorice ingestion may lead to:
(a) Hypertension
(b) Hypokalaemia
(c) Hypernatraemia
(d) Metabolic alkalosis
(e) High levels of aldosterone in plasma

Gastroenterology

Recent progress in inflammatory bowel disease: from bench to bedside

Daniel R Gaya, Charles W Lees and Jack Satsangi

☐ FROM THE BENCH: PATHOGENIC MECHANISMS IN INFLAMMATORY BOWEL DISEASE

The precise aetiology of the chronic inflammatory bowel diseases – Crohn's disease (CD) and ulcerative colitis (UC) – remains unknown. Recent advances in basic molecular science, animal models, and clinical studies, however, have highlighted the importance of genetic and environmental contributions to the pathogenesis of inflammatory bowel disease (IBD) (Fig 1).[1] The currently accepted hypothesis is that specific defects in barrier function, dysregulated immune responses, or ineffective bacterial clearance in genetically susceptible hosts, or their combination, may lead to the establishment of T cell-mediated chronic mucosal inflammation. Gene–environment interactions seem critical to initiation of the exaggerated and inappropriate inflammatory response that characterises these relapsing and remitting inflammatory disorders.

The mucosal interface in which commensal and pathogenic bacterial antigens interact directly and indirectly with the epithelium is the front line to a healthy, well-regulated mucosal immune system. Defects in barrier genes and those that interact directly with bacterial antigen may predispose to the development of IBD. Dysregulation of innate immune signals is increasingly recognised to be important in pathogenesis. Epithelial–mesenchymal interactions via a raft of cytokines and chemokines initiate further downstream immune responses, which, in the healthy state, bring about resolution of the inflammatory episode. In patients with CD and UC, however, a loss of immune tolerance leads to a breakdown in this homeostasis and paves the way for chronic inflammation and its sequelae.

Importance of gene-environment interactions

Perhaps the most compelling recent evidence in support of gene–environment interactions comes from Sartor's work in animal models of colitis.[2] Mice with targeted deletions of the interleukin (IL) 10 gene (*IL-10–/–*) and human leucocyte antigen (HLA)-B27 transgenic rats develop colitis in specific pathogen-free conditions but not when kept completely germ-free. It is now clear, however, that selective colonisation with different bacterial species critically affects aspects of disease phenotype – notably severity and anatomical location. In *IL-10–/–* mice monoassociated with *Enterococcus faecalis* or *Escherichia coli*, a progressive chronic

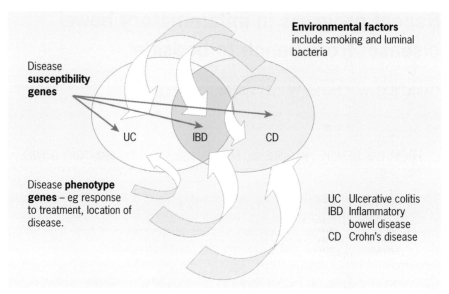

Fig 1 Model of pathogenesis of inflammatory bowel disease. Ulcerative colitis and Crohn's disease can be thought of as overlapping syndromes that share some phenotypes and also share some genetic and environmental susceptibility and modifying stimuli. Some phenotypic features and environmental/genetic factors, however, are specific to one or other disorder. CD = Crohn's disease; IBD = inflammatory bowel disease; UC = ulcerative colitis. Reproduced from Gaya *et al* with permission of Elsevier.[1]

colitis develops, although the regional distribution and kinetics of this colitis vary with the bacteria. That secretion of interferon gamma (IFN-γ) from mesenteric lymph-node CD4+ T cells precedes the onset of microscopic inflammation is noteworthy. Mice monoassociated with *Pseudomonas fluorescens* or *Bacteroides vulgatus* do not develop colitis. In stark contrast, HLA-B27 transgenic rats monoassociated with *B. vulgatus* develop an aggressive colitis but no inflammation with *E. coli*. Clearly, the interaction of genetic factors (*IL-10–/–* or HLA-B27) and environmental factors (*E. coli* or *B. vulgatus*) is fundamentally important for the establishment of colitis in these animal models.

Genetics

Susceptibility loci for IBD have been identified by genomewide scanning on chromosomes 1, 2, 5 (IBD5), 6 (IBD3), 12 (IBD2), 14 (IBD4), 16 (IBD1), and 19 (IBD6) (Fig 2[3]) (for a detailed current review see Gaya *et al*[1]). The susceptibility gene within the consistently replicated IBD1 locus was identified as *NOD2/CARD15* in 2001. Structural changes are induced in the muramyl dipeptide-sensing NOD2 protein by two single nucleotide polymorphisms (Gly908Arg and Arg702Trp) and one frameshift mutation (Leu1007fsincC). Carriage of a *NOD2* mutation is associated with susceptibility to CD. This has been replicated widely, but of great interest is that significant heterogeneity is seen between different populations. Carriage rates vary greatly (0–50%), with the highest rates seen in central Europe.

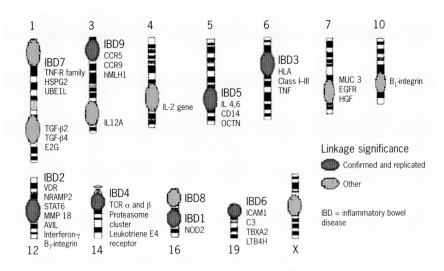

Fig 2 Susceptibility loci for inflammatory bowel disease as identified on genomewide scanning. Reproduced from Ahmad et al with permission of Blackwell Publishing.[3]

The contribution of *NOD2* to disease susceptibility is relatively lower in Northern European (Scottish and Scandinavian) populations, where the population-attributable risk ranges from 7.9% (Scottish patients with early-onset CD) to 11.4% (Swedish patients with CD). In Japanese, Chinese, and South Korean populations, mutations in *NOD2* (Gly908Arg, Arg702Trp, and Leu1007fsincC) are absent.

Much debate has arisen from experimental data that apparently are conflicting about whether *NOD2* mutations represent a 'loss-of-function' or 'gain-of-function' phenotype. Two different animal models (*NOD2–/–* and 3020insC transgenic) published simultaneously in *Science* last year,[4,5] added extra insight but failed to resolve this unsettling paradox. Neither mutant developed chronic intestinal inflammation spontaneously. *NOD2–/–* mice responded less well to challenge with oral *Listeria monocytogenes* than wildtype mice – an observation that may be related to decreased antimicrobial activity of Paneth cells.[4] Peripheral blood monocytes from patients with mutations related to CD have defective cytokine production and NF-kappaB activity in response to muramyl dipeptide, which lends support to the loss of function hypothesis. Further discussion of this complex subject is beyond the scope of this chapter (see Gaya *et al*[1] and Watanabe *et al*[6]).

New IBD genes

Many genes currently are under active investigation as IBD susceptibility genes. Some of the most promising genes include *DLG5, OCTN, MDR1 (ABCB1), NOD1*, and *CCL20/MIP-3α*. In 2004, consecutive *Nature Genetics* papers generated much interest in two new candidate susceptibility genes – *DLG5* (Drosophila discs large homologue 5) and the organic cation transporter (OCTN) cluster in IBD5.[7,8] The confirmation of a candidate gene as a true disease susceptibility gene requires a combination of data that replicate the findings and confirmation of relevance to biomolecular function – as illustrated for *NOD2/CARD15* above.

These two new candidates have generated substantial controversy and debate over the past two years, but for different reasons. Fine mapping of a susceptibility locus on chromosome 10 led Stoll and colleagues to *DLG5*.[7] A risk haplotype ('D') for IBD and a protective haplotype ('A') in the *DLG5* gene originally were described in this German population, but replication has proved frustrating. Although two of three European derived populations replicated an association with risk haplotype D (but not haplotype A), a Scottish population with patients with adult-onset IBD and a Flemish population of patients with IBD have shown no association with *DLG5*. These differences may reflect one or a combination of statistical power, population heterogeneity, lack of consistency of phenotyping across studies, and sampling inconsistencies. In order to replicate Stoll's original findings with a statistical power of >90% to detect p<0.01, it has been calculated that several thousand IBD cases and controls will be needed. This has important implications for current and future studies, as no individual centres have genotyped populations of this size. Where populations of patients with IBD are combined to increase the power of individual studies or in meta-analyses of genetics datasets (which are being seen with increasing frequency), consistency of phenotyping will be vital. The newly described Montreal classification of IBD, which was produced by a working party at the World Congress of Gastroenterology in 2005, will go a long way towards achieving this, if it is adopted widely.[9]

The *OCTN* cluster is located in the IBD5 region on chromosome 5q31. Association of this locus with IBD susceptibility (mostly CD but also UC) has been replicated widely since the original finding in a Canadian population. Peltekova and colleagues reported that two causal single nucleotide polymorphisms in the *OCTN* cluster were associated with CD, forming a two-allele risk haplotype (TC haplotype).[8] Many other genes within this area are involved in IBD pathogenesis and therefore make attractive candidate genes for inherited susceptibility to IBD. Singling out any one particular gene as being related to IBD susceptibility is very difficult, however, as very large chromosomal areas are inherited together. This tight linkage-disequilibrium has been central to the debate about *OCTN*. Although many groups have replicated the original dataset's association with the *OCTN*-TC risk haplotype, none has been able to show a stronger association with IBD or independence with other alleles on the extended haplotype. In the absence of any convincing data on expression or function to implicate the *OCTN* genes in the pathogenesis of IBD, the only conclusion is that a strong signal comes from the IBD5 locus, but no current evidence supports the cation transporters as IBD susceptibility genes. Studies to dissect the IBD5 signal will need several thousand patients with IBD and controls to overcome the tight linkage-disequilibrium.

Defective acute inflammation in Crohn's disease

Catalysed by the discovery of *NOD2*, innate immunity has risen to the forefront of research into the pathogenesis of CD. The NOD2 protein principally is expressed in one of two key cell types: monocytes and Paneth cells. Much interest in recent years has centred on the role of the Paneth cell in pathogenesis. Paneth cells – secretory epithelial cells located in small intestinal crypts – synthesise a range of antimicrobial proteins, including the human α-defensins 5 and 6 (HD5 and HD6). Human α-defensin 5 transgenic mice are protected against usually lethal infection with *Salmonella*. Mice unable to produce mature α-defensins are susceptible to a range of pathogens when challenged orally with bacteria. It now is apparent that patients with ileal CD may have decreased α-defensin function that largely corresponds to decreased expression.[10] This is not simply a consequence of ongoing inflammation and is not seen in patients with purely colonic CD or UC.

Most recently, Marks and colleagues published an extensive report that provides compelling evidence for a constitutive defect in acute inflammation in CD.[11] Mechanical trauma induced in the rectum and skin was characterised by reduced accumulation of neutrophils and production of IL-8 in patients with CD compared with those with UC and healthy controls. In addition, macrophages cultured from peripheral blood of patients with CD secreted significantly less IL-8 than healthy controls after exposure to wound fluid (from acute surgical incision in healthy controls undergoing hernia repair), C5a or tumour necrosis factor alpha (TNFα). No difference in IL-8 secretion was seen between patients with CD who had mutations of *NOD2/CARD15* and patients with wild-type *NOD2/CARD15*. The same investigators also injected heat-killed *E. coli* subcutaneously in healthy controls, patients with CD, and patients with UC. As well as discomfort, erythema, and swelling, healthy controls had a ninefold increase in blood flow at the injection site at 24 hours. The increase in blood flow was substantially smaller in patients with CD, particularly those with purely colonic disease. These phenotypes were not influenced by the *NOD2/CARD15* genotype.

These data suggest that patients with CD may not have a sufficiently responsive acute inflammatory response to deal with bacterial insults from commensal bacteria or pathogens and that these manifest as intestinal lesions. The authors point out that this hypothesis is consistent with the hygiene hypothesis, in that a relatively unstimulated bowel coupled with a subprimed immune system will respond less effectively to bacterial insult. The constitutive nature of this acute inflammatory defect may reflect simply the lower extreme of a normally distributed population immune response. Indeed, the wisdom of the widespread use of immunosuppressive drugs in the treatment of CD may need re-examination, with the realisation that treatment of the secondary inflammation exacerbates the underlying immunodeficiency.

☐ TO THE BEDSIDE: NOVEL APPROACHES IN TREATMENT

The aim of therapy in IBD is the induction and maintenance of remission with minimal side effects. The hope in achieving this is to alter disease course and reduce long-term morbidity – this objective is not easy to prove, as the diseases are characterised by spontaneous remissions and relapses.

The 'traditional' treatment options for the management of IBD consist of 5-aminosalicylates, corticosteroids, immunosuppressant drugs, and surgery (Fig 3).

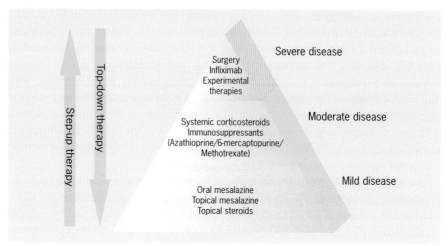

Fig 3 Treatment pyramid in Crohn's disease – 'step up' or 'top down'? Recent developments in treatments for Crohn's disease have resulted in reassessment of the management strategies currently used for treatment of the disease. Can the natural history of Crohn's disease be altered by the introduction, earlier in the disease course, of treatments currently reserved for the top of the treatment pyramid. Is it possible to prevent the occurrence of chronic complications, such as fibrosis, stricture, and possibly fistulae, by early use of agents that promote mucosal healing (such as infliximab)? As discussed in the text, however, biological treatments have potentially serious side effects, invariably are more expensive than conventional treatments, and long term safety data is not available. In addition, it is important to note that the course of Crohn's disease is relatively mild in a significant proportion of patients. An aggressive approach of using more toxic treatments early on during treatment thus may not be necessary for all patients with Crohn's disease, who instead could be effectively treated with milder and less toxic agents such as oral mesalazine. The development of an improved classification system that would allow identification of particular subgroups with differing disease phenotypes and prognoses could play a factor in deciding between a 'step-up' or 'top-down' approach.

Although steroids are well recognised to have rapid and beneficial effects in a proportion of patients with CD and UC, side effects are an important consideration in management. Furthermore, not all patients respond (steroid resistance), and some who respond are unable to taper the dose or relapse shortly after steroid discontinuation (steroid dependence). In unpublished work, we have shown that rates of steroid dependence in patients with IBD are 31–35% at 30 days after diagnosis and 17–23% after one year.

The thiopurine analogues (azathioprine and 6-mercaptopurine) are the most commonly prescribed immunosuppressives for IBD and are of great benefit to many patients (numbers needed to treat in patients with CD: 3–5). Serious side effects (including sepsis, hepatotoxicity, pancreatitis, and myelosuppression) often limit these drugs, however (number needed to harm: 16–20). The first widespread clinical use of pharmacogenetics in the day-to-day practice of gastroenterology has been assessment of the activity of thiopurine methyltransferase – a key enzyme in the catabolism of azathioprine and 6-mercaptopurine – to predict patients at higher risk of myelotoxicity. Unfortunately, most cases of bone marrow suppression associated with these drugs occur in the setting of normal activity of thiopurine methyltransferase, so routine monitoring of blood counts still is recommended. Although surgery can be lifesaving for patients with toxic megacolon and the septic complications of CD, it is not curative in this condition. Indeed, even in patients with UC, quality of life often does not return to normal after colectomy with an ileoanal pouch or end ileostomy. As a result, massive investment in the search for novel medical treatments for patients with medically refractory disease is underway. It is critically important that all new treatment options are evaluated carefully before traditional treatments are replaced, especially as these novel options invariably are more expensive and long-term safety data initially will not be available.

Despite the large number of new biological agents being investigated for the treatment of IBD (Table 1), infliximab received renewed attention in the gastrointestinal literature in the past 12 months. Infliximab is a chimeric (75% human, 25% murine) monoclonal antibody that binds to and neutralises membrane-bound and soluble TNFα – the proinflammatory cytokine that evidently is central to the pathogenesis of IBD. Although now established as an effective treatment for severe and fistulising CD, its effectiveness in UC previously has been disputed. Two key publications in 2005 supported the notion that infliximab indeed was effective in a proportion of patients with UC.[12,13] Data from Rutgeerts and colleagues, which analysed the results of two clinical trials involving 728 patients (active ulcerative colitis trial (ACT) 1 and ACT 2), showed that moderately active UC was more likely to respond to infliximab than placebo with respect to clinical response (ACT 1: 69% v 37%, p<0.001; ACT 2: 64% vs 29%, p<0.001), mucosal healing (ACT 1: 62% v 34%, p<0.001; ACT 2: 60% vs 31%, p<0.001), and rates of steroid discontinuation.[12] No significant differences were seen between the two doses of infliximab used (5 and 10 mg/kg). Unfortunately, rates of colectomy, which is a critical endpoint for treatment for many patients, are not reported in the follow-up period.[14] Although rates of steroid discontinuation were higher in the infliximab group, only around 25% of patients on infliximab maintenance treatment were free of steroids at one year's follow up. A further concern is that although the paper discusses patients with 'moderate–severe' UC, patients treated only with oral mesalazine were deemed eligible for ACT 2 – such patients would not be classified as 'severe' with validated colitis scoring systems.

Another study addressed the use of infliximab in the setting of severe colitis unresponsive to intravenous steroids.[13] Forty-five patients were randomised to receive a single infusion of 5 mg/kg infliximab or placebo at day 3. The rate of colectomy with inflixmab was 50% of the rate for patients who received placebo (7 v 14, p=0.017). Infliximab may challenge ciclosporin as the medical salvage treatment of choice in patients with severe colitis who are heading towards colectomy.

The prevailing view of the pathogenesis of Crohn's disease involves an overactive T cell-driven immune response to an unknown stimulus – most putative biological agents aim to suppress this aberrant immune response. An alternative hypothesis suggests that CD is an immunodeficiency disorder that primarily affects the innate immune system (see Marks et al[11]). This theory is consistent with much of the NOD2 functional data discussed and also with other data – the increased adherence

Table 1 Monoclonal antibody treatments for IBD. In the past decade, multiple potent biological treatments have been developed to selectively target components of the inflammatory cascade thought critical to the pathogenesis of IBD. These have varied from cytokine inhibitors (such as adalimumab) to inhibitors of lymphocyte tracking (such as natalizumab). Thus far, only infliximab has been licensed for the treatment of IBD.

Drug	Structure	Clinical data/future development
Infliximab	Chimeric (75% human, 25% murine) IgG1 antibody to TNFα	• Confirmed efficacy and licensed for patients with refractory and fistulating CD • Recently licensed by Food and Drug Administration for UC on the back of data from ACT 1 and ACT 2 studies
Adalimumab	Fully human IgG1 antibody to TNFα	• Licensed for rheumatoid arthritis • Phase III trials in patients with CD (CLASSIC I and II): induction data (CLASSIC I) similar to that of infliximab • Preliminary studies also support efficacy in patients who become intolerant to or lose response to infliximab • Licence in CD likely to be forthcoming
Certolizumab pegol (CDP-870)	Humanised anti-TNFα Fab antibody fragment linked to a polyethylene glycol molecule	• Phase III data in patients with CD (PRECiSE I and II) suggested benefit • Licensing application in progress
CDP 571	Humanised IgG4 antibody to TNFα	• Data suggest relative lack of efficacy in patients with CD
Etanercept	p75 fusion protein to TNFα	• Licensed for rheumatoid arthritis • Lack of efficacy in patients with CD
Onercept	p55 receptor monomer to TNFα	• Lack of efficacy in patients with CD
Anti-IL-12 (ABT 874)	Fully human IgG1 antibody to the common p40 subunit of interleukins 12 and 23	• Phase II trial data shows efficacy for patients with CD • Phase III trials underway
Visilizumab	Humanised IgG2 antibody to CD3 (component of T-cell receptor)	• Phase II data suggest benefit in patients with steroid-refractory UC • Phase III studies recruiting
Fontolizumab	Humanised IgG1 antibody to interferon γ	• Post-hoc analysis showed significant benefit in subgroup of patients with CD with elevated C-reactive protein in phase II study
Basiliximab	Chimeric IgG1 anti-CD25 (IL-2 receptor) antibody	• Open label study suggested efficacy in patients with UC
Daclizumab	Humanised IgG1 anti-CD25 (IL-2 receptor) antibody	• Open label study suggested efficacy in patients with UC • Placebo-controlled data failed to show benefit
Natalizumab	Humanised IgG4 antibody to α4 integrin	• Large phase III trials (ENACT 1 and 2) showed efficacy in induction and maintenance of remission in patients with CD • Had been licensed for multiple sclerosis before being withdrawn by manufacturers after the drug was linked to three cases of progressive multifocal leucoencephalopathy • Currently undergoing further safety evaluation
MLN-02	Humanised IgG1 antibody to α4β7 integrin	• Phase II study in patients with CD failed to meet primary endpoints • Small, placebo-controlled, short-term study in patients with UC showed benefits in clinical and endoscopic endpoints

ACT = active ulcerative colitis trial; CD = Crohn's disease; CLASSIC = clinical assessment of adalimumab safety and efficacy studied as an induction therapy in Crohn's; ENACT = evaluation of natalizumab as continuous therapy; Ig = immunoglobulin; PRECiSE = pegylated antibody fragment evaluation in Crohn's disease; TNFα = tumour necrosis factor alpha.

of strains of *E. coli* on mucosa affected by Crohn's disease. On this background, Korzenik and colleagues have investigated the effect of granulocyte-macrophage colony stimulating factor (GM-CSF) in the treatment of CD.[15] After small preliminary open-label studies suggested that such treatment was safe and effective, a placebo-controlled, randomised, controlled study was performed. Although the primary endpoint of a 70-point reduction in the Crohn's disease activity index (CDAI) from baseline was not reached and bone pain was a significant side effect in the GM-CSF arm, this potential treatment cannot be discounted at this stage. Rates of secondary endpoints (100-point reduction in CDAI, clinical remission (CDAI <150), and mucosal healing) were all significantly greater in the GM-CSF arm. Further data are awaited eagerly.

Another treatment option to have emerged in recent years for the treatment of IBD is apheresis.[16] The term refers to the removal of cells or protein from the circulatory system via an extracorporeal method. Venous blood is pumped from one antecubital vein, passed through a filter, and returned to the circulation via another vein, with concomitant systemic anticoagulation. Relapse and clinical activity of IBD correlates with the appearance of excess neutrophils and macrophages in the intestinal mucosa; furthermore, the degree of influx correlates with the risk of relapse in IBD. Selective removal of such cells from the circulation of patients with IBD thus may be of therapeutic potential. Two such relatively selective apheresis units, Cellsorba and Adacolumn, are now available; they differ in the type and proportion of cells removed. Adacolumn removes mainly granulocytes and monocytes, whereas Cellsorba removes granulocytes, lymphocytes, and platelets. Although apheresis is used widely to treat IBD in Japan, no sham-controlled trials have been published, so definitive evidence of benefit remains to be proved. Numerous small, uncontrolled case series (most available only in abstract form) with varying durations and intensities of apheresis have reported almost universally positive results, with little in the way of side effects. The clinical benefit observed cannot be explained fully on the basis of granulocyte and monocyte reduction alone, especially as the decrease is transient. Leucocyte trafficking as a result of the activated cells being replaced by immature inactivated cells may be the key mechanism of putative efficacy. The results of North American sham-controlled studies hopefully will give more concrete information about the intensity and effectiveness of apheresis as a treatment for IBD.

A novel and potentially high-risk strategy to treat refractory CD is to consider autologous stem-cell transplant in order to 'reset' the patient's immune system with antigenically naïve stem cells harvested from the patient before conditioning chemotherapy. After a series of case reports highlighted the course of patients whose CD went into remission after stem cell transplantation for haematological malignancies, investigators in Chicago went on to perform a phase I study of autologous stem-cell transplant in 12 patients with medically refractory CD.[17] Eleven patients achieved a sustained remission and were able to stop immunosuppressants, no patient died in relation to the transplant, and the authors concluded that a randomised controlled trial now should be considered. Although these preliminary results are impressive, they must be taken in context: Crohn's disease has a very low mortality; the mortality with autologous stem-cell transplantation is nearly 10% overall (largely because of neutropenia-related sepsis and comorbid illness).

Inflammatory bowel disease is well documented to be primarily an urban and Western disease. As countries become more 'westernised', the incidence of IBD rises. A lack of exposure to intestinal helminths during childhood has been postulated to adversely affect the development of the mucosal immune system and predispose to immunological disease, including IBD. This has led investigators to explore helminthic treatment in the context of IBD. It was shown recently that helminths protect mice against experimental colitis, and an open-label study in patients with CD subsequently suggested this treatment to be safe and effective. The same group then published the first double-blind, placebo-controlled study of helminth treatment for patients with UC.[18] Patients with active UC (n=54) were allocated randomly to placebo or ova of the pig whipworm (*Trichuris suis*) at two-weekly intervals for 12 weeks. Clinical response (defined by a four-point reduction in the UC disease activity index) was seen in 43% of patients in the ova group and 16% in the placebo group (p=0.04). Furthermore, no adverse events were reported despite concomitant immunosuppression. Although real concerns exist about the validity of the activity indices used in the study and whether the benefit shown is relevant clinically, the data are clearly provocative and further trials are merited.

The diversity of novel treatments emerging in the field of IBD is testament to the complexity of and difficulty involved in managing these diseases and the need for more effective treatments. At present, most patients can be managed with traditional oral aminosalicylates, steroids, immunosuppressants, and, if necessary, surgery. An important minority, however, have medically resistant and refractory disease and require a disproportionate amount of medical and nursing support. For such patients, the novel therapies are most welcome.

REFERENCES

1   Gaya DR, Russell RK, Nimmo ER, Satsangi J. New genes in inflammatory bowel disease: lessons for complex diseases. *Lancet* 2006;367:1271–84.

2   Kim SC, Tonkonogy SL, Albright CA *et al*. Variable phenotypes of enterocolitis in interleukin 10-deficient mice monoassociated with two different commensal bacteria. *Gastroenterology* 2005;128:891–906.

3   Ahmad T, Satsangi J, McGovern D *et al*. The genetics of inflammatory bowel disease. *Aliment Pharmacol Ther* 2001;15:731–48.

4   Kobayashi KS, Chamaillard M, Ogura Y *et al*. Nod2-dependent regulation of innate and adaptive immunity in the intestinal tract. *Science* 2005;307:731–4.

5   Maeda S, Hsu L-C, Brankston LA *et al*. Nod2 mutation in Crohn's disease potentiates NF-kB activity and IL-1 processing. *Science* 2005;307:734–8.

6   Watanabe T, Kitani A, Strober W. NOD2 regulation of toll-like receptor responses and the pathogenesis of Crohn's disease. *Gut* 2005;54:1515–8.

7   Stoll M, Corneliussen B, Costello CM *et al*. Genetic variation in DLG5 is associated with inflammatory bowel disease. *Nat Genet* 2004;36:476-80.

8   Peltekova VD, Wintle RF, Rubin LA *et al*. Functional variants of OCTN cation transporter genes are associated with Crohn disease. *Nat Genet* 2004;36:471–5.

9   Silverberg MS, Satsangi J, Ahmad T *et al*. Toward an integrated clinical, molecular and serological classification of inflammatory bowel disease: report of a working party of the 2005 Montreal World Congress of Gastroenterology. *Can J Gastroenterol* 2005;19 (Suppl A):5–36.

10 Wehkamp J, Salzman NH, Porter E *et al*. Reduced Paneth cell alpha-defensins in ileal Crohn's disease. *Proc Natl Acad Sci USA* 2005;102:18129–34.

11 Marks DJ, Harbord MW, MacAllister R *et al*. Defective acute inflammation in Crohn's disease: a clinical investigation. *Lancet* 2006;367:668–78.

12 Rutgeerts P, Sandborn WJ, Feagan BG *et al*. Infliximab for induction and maintenance therapy for ulcerative colitis. *N Engl J Med* 2005;353:2462–76.

13 Jarnerot G, Hertervig E, Friis-Liby I *et al*. Infliximab as rescue therapy in severe to moderately severe ulcerative colitis: a randomized, placebo-controlled study. *Gastroenterology* 2005;128: 1805–11.

14 Lees C, Shand A, Penman I, Satsangi J, Arnott I. Role of infliximab in ulcerative colitis: further questions. *Inflamm Bowel Dis* 2006;12(4).

15 Korzenik JR, Dieckgraefe BK, Valentine JF, Hausman DF, Gilbert MJ. Sargramostim for active Crohn's disease. *N Engl J Med* 2005;352:2193–201.

16 Sandborn WJ. Preliminary data on the use of apheresis in inflammatory bowel disease. *Inflamm Bowel Dis* 2006;12 (Suppl 1):S15–21.

17 Oyama Y, Craig RM, Traynor AE *et al*. Autologous hematopoietic stem cell transplantation in patients with refractory Crohn's disease. *Gastroenterology* 2005;128:552–63.

18 Summers RW, Elliott DE, Urban JF Jr, Thompson RA, Weinstock JV. Trichuris suis therapy for active ulcerative colitis: a randomized controlled trial. *Gastroenterology* 2005;128:825–32.

Progress in understanding and managing functional gastrointestinal disorders

Abhishek Sharma and Qasim Aziz

☐ BACKGROUND

Despite remarkable advances in our understanding and management of 'organic' gastroenterological complaints such as peptic ulcer disease, inflammatory bowel disease, and even cancer over the past 30 years, our knowledge of what is going on in the hordes of patients that fill up our clinics with unexplained symptoms of presumed gastroenterological origin remains poor. People in this medical no-man's land are labelled as having one of almost 30 functional gastrointestinal disorders, depending on the nature and pattern of symptom involvement.[1] Chronic episodic pain is the most common presenting complaint in functional gastrointestinal disorders such as functional dyspepsia, irritable bowel syndrome (IBS) and non-cardiac chest pain (NCCP), which are characterised by recurrent, unexplained symptoms for which extensive investigations often fail to identify a cause. Over the last few decades, however, research has provided novel insights into the mechanisms that may be involved in the pathophysiology of these disorders, which has resulted in new treatment options becoming available for these patients.

☐ PROGRESS IN UNDERSTANDING FUNCTIONAL GASTROINTESTINAL DISORDERS

Role of visceral hypersensitivity

Although patients with functional gastrointestinal disorders are a very heterogeneous group, research has shown that they often share certain pathophysiological features. Trimble *et al* showed heightened sensitivity to rectal distension in patients with IBS and functional dyspepsia, with both groups of patients being hypersensitive to oesophageal distension.[2] This heightened pain sensitivity to experimental gut stimulation – a phenomenon known as visceral hypersensitivity – has been shown repeatedly in patients with functional gastrointestinal disorders and is not specific to the gut organ that is involved symptomatically. What causes and maintains this visceral pain hypersensitivity has been the subject of intense research and, according to current wisdom, involves peripheral and central mechanisms as described below (Fig 1).

During tissue inflammation or injury, peripheral nociceptor terminals are known to be exposed to a number of immune and inflammatory mediators, such as prostaglandins, serotonin, cytokines, and neurotrophic factors.[3] These inflammatory

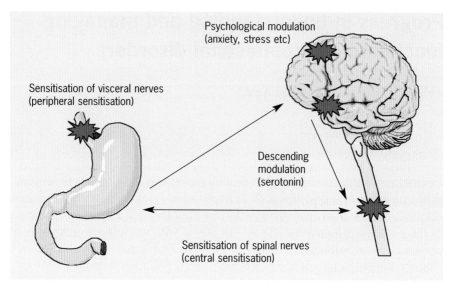

Fig 1 Potential factors involved in the development and maintenance of visceral pain hypersensitivity. During injury, inflammatory and immune mediators can sensitise peripheral sensory nerves, reducing their transduction thresholds (peripheral sensitisation). The increase in nociceptive transmission to the spinal cord can upregulate dorsal horn neuronal activity, with a widening of their receptive fields and the recruitment of previously silent nociceptors (central sensitisation). Nociceptive transmission is further subject to modulation by spinal, supraspinal, and cortical facilitatory and inhibitory influences.

mediators can facilitate the transduction properties of peripheral nociceptor terminals – a phenomenon termed 'peripheral sensitisation'. This modifiable synaptic activity ('synaptic plasticity') is an essential feature of the nervous system that allows it to adapt to adverse stimuli. Peripheral sensitisation is believed to cause pain hypersensitivity at the site of injury or inflammation, which results in a heightened awareness of painful stimuli (primary hyperalgesia) and the perception of innocuous stimuli as being painful (primary allodynia).

Hypersensitivity to painful and non-painful stimuli can also be shown in areas surrounding the inflamed or injured tissue in somatic pain models – so-called 'secondary hyperalgesia' and 'secondary allodynia,' respectively. These phenomena are believed to result from the increase in nociceptive information arriving at the spinal cord due to peripheral sensitisation, which results in an increased excitability and widening of receptive fields of dorsal horn neurones and the recruitment of previously silent nociceptors. This process is called 'central sensitisation.'[3] Co-localisation of peripheral sensory afferent nerve terminals from the gut and skin on the same spinal dorsal horn neurones means that heightened somatic referral of visceral sensation occurs in the presence of central sensitisation.

Whereas the peripheral changes associated with peripheral sensitisation are detectable very soon after tissue injury and persist for the duration of the inflammation, the associated central changes may persist for considerably longer as a result of transcriptional changes in genes involved in determining afferent excitability and translational changes in membrane receptors and ion channels. This results in ongoing pain hypersensitivity despite the subsidence of the peripheral event.[3] Under certain conditions, susceptible individuals can develop prolonged pain hypersensitivity after tissue injury.

Role of inflammation

Visceral inflammation and injury in animal models have been associated with chronic visceral hypersensitivity and gut dysfunction. A similar process may be involved in a subset of patients with functional gastrointestinal disorders, as around one third of patients with IBS give a history of gut injury in the form of gastroenteritis. Chronic pain can also develop after surgery and may result from the peripheral sensitisation of primary afferents as a result of direct injury, which in turn can lead to upregulation of spinal pain processing.[3] Potentially injurious agents may be relevant in other functional gastrointestinal disorders, because, for example, acid reflux is the most common cause of NCCP.[4]

Most work in patients to assess the role of infection on the subsequent development of symptoms has focussed on IBS. Increased gut permeability and altered mucosal characteristics, such as increased rectal mucosal enteroendocrine cells and T lymphocytes, have been documented and discussed in patients with post-infectious IBS.[5] The presence of increased numbers of inflammatory cells in these patients after resolution of the infection is likely to translate to an altered nociceptor terminal milieu. Ongoing peripheral nociceptive input may result in prolonged spinal hyperexcitability, which, in turn, may be related to the persisting visceral pain hypersensitivity seen in these patients.

Role of motility

Motility disturbances originally were thought to be the cause of symptoms in many functional gastrointestinal disorders, including globus sensation, functional heartburn, functional dyspepsia, NCCP, and IBS (to name but a few), and the evidence for dysmotility in these disorders has been reviewed extensively by the Rome II committee.[1] Oesophageal manometry is now performed routinely in the work-up of patients with functional oesophageal disorders who fail to respond to antacid treatment or in whom pH studies fail to identify excessive acid reflux or a positive temporal relation between symptoms and episodes of reflux.[4]

Role of psychological state and stress

The previous adherence to a purely biomedical model of disease understanding and the lack of readily identifiable biological markers indicative of underlying pathology in functional gastrointestinal disorders initially led them to be thought of as a manifestation of psychoneurosis, such as a reflection of anxiety or depression. Research, particularly epidemiological, has shown that psychopathology does play an important role in a subset of patients with functional gastrointestinal disorders.

This is not surprising, as perception of visceral sensation is mediated at a cortical level and therefore is influenced by cognitive mechanisms, such as stress, attention, and anxiety. The development of an integrated biopsychosocial model of illness has increased understanding of the pathophysiological disturbances in functional gastrointestinal disorders, as it couples changes in biological factors (for example, changes in physiology) with psychological state (for example, alterations in brain processing), and has ushered in the concept of the 'brain–gut axis'.

Stress – both pathophysiological (infection and inflammation) and psychological (anxiety) – can activate a number of physiological response systems, such as the autonomic nervous system and hypothalamic-pituitary-adrenal axis, which leads to an altered internal environment and a psychological state more adept at dealing with the threat ('fight or flight') and re-establishing homeostasis. After this, these effector systems rapidly are turned off, as prolonged exposure to their effects (such as high levels of cortisol, catecholamines, and blood glucose; hypertension; and tachycardia) can be harmful. These systems have been implicated in the activation of endogenous pain modulation circuits (as described below) and the reactivity of immune cells and, therefore, inflammatory mediators.[5] Evidence for dysregulation of these effector systems in functional gastrointestinal disorders has been shown, and it is suggested that altered autonomic and neuroendocrine reactivity may be relevant in mediating visceral sensitivity, particularly after gut injury.[5]

Role of spinal descending inhibition in pain modulation

The brain has long been known to be able to modulate spinal pain processing via descending tracts that terminate in the spinal cord. These tracts originate from sites in the midbrain and brainstem and can inhibit or excite spinal ascending nociceptive transmission by their proximity to the central terminals of primary afferent nociceptors and dorsal horn neurons that respond to noxious stimulation. This modulation is effected via a number of neurotransmitters, such as endogenous opioids, catecholamines, and serotonin. The spinal and supraspinal modulation of pain transmission has been reviewed extensively and may be relevant to the prolonged hyperalgesia in clinical pain states, including functional gastrointestinal disorders.[6] Patients with IBS have been shown to have less activation of brain regions concerned with antinociception (such as the periaqueductal grey) after sigmoid colon distension than controls. This imbalance in the endogenous pain modulatory system has been postulated to relate to the observed hyperalgesia via increased spinal cord excitability.[6]

Role of serotonin

Serotonin (5-HT) plays an important role in gut function and sensory signalling in the brain–gut axis. As 95% of 5-HT in the body is found in the gastrointestinal tract and, so far, seven subtypes of 5-HT receptors have been identified differentiated on the basis of structure and function, it is easy to see why it is such an important neurotransmitter and signalling molecule. Recent work has highlighted the important role of 5-HT in descending pain modulatory pathways, and further work has shown how 5-HT_3 receptor antagonists can modulate hyperalgesia and allodynia (the characteristics of central neuronal sensitisation) in animal models.[7] High levels of 5-HT in the postprandial period have been documented in a subset of patients with diarrhoea-predominant IBS (D-IBS), while levels may be lower in the same period in patients with constipation-predominant IBS (C-IBS).[8]

Role of genotype

Considerable variability exists between individuals in their sensitivity to experimental pain. Whether or not these interindividual differences can predict the magnitude and temporal extent of pain hypersensitivity after visceral inflammation or injury remains to be seen. This is an interesting prospect, as the variation is explained incompletely by environmental and cultural factors and, therefore, hints at an underlying genetic component.

Anecdotally, functional gastrointestinal disorders seem to cluster in families, and research has confirmed these impressions. A recent, large, questionnaire-based study found a greater concordance for IBS in monozygotic twins than dizygotic twins (17.2% *v* 8.4%, p=0.03), which supports a genetic contribution to IBS.[9] Further analysis, however, suggested that having a parent with IBS was an independent predictor of IBS status (p<0.001) and a stronger predictor than having a twin with IBS. Although heredity thus certainly contributes to the development of IBS, social learning has an equal or greater influence.

Recent work has suggested that certain functionally distinct polymorphisms of the serotonin transporter protein and α2 adrenoceptor are associated with constipation and high somatic symptom scores in certain functional gastrointestinal disorders.[10] In addition, certain allelic variants of the catechol-O-methyl-transferase polymorphism (*val*[158]*met*) have been shown to predict human somatic pain sensitivity in association with more negative affective ratings and distinct psychophysiological response traits during pain.[11] Catechol-O-methyl-transferase is one of the enzymes involved in the metabolism of catecholamines and, therefore, can modulate noradrenergic and dopaminergic neurotransmission. Although not investigated in any great detail, these and other polymorphisms may be responsible to some extent for the differences in pain responsiveness and adaptation to stressful stimuli.

☐ PROGRESS IN MANAGING FUNCTIONAL GASTROINTESTINAL DISORDERS

The lack of one common pathogenic mechanism generally has hindered the development of causal treatments in patients with functional gastrointestinal disorders. This is changing slowly now, however, as appreciation of the above pathophysiological mechanisms has resulted in the identification of a number of potential therapeutic targets. A number of excellent review articles has highlighted current treatment options in functional gastrointestinal disorders, as described below.[4,12,13]

Smooth muscle relaxants

Antispasmodics such as mebeverine long have been used in the management of functional gastrointestinal disorders, particularly IBS, as motility disturbances have been proposed as a cause of symptoms such as abdominal pain, bloating, and change in bowel habit in a proportion of patients. A number of studies have found such smooth muscle relaxants to be efficacious in patients with IBS, particularly when pain is reported as a significant feature.[13] Smooth muscle relaxants such as calcium channel blockers have been shown to decrease oesophageal pressures in healthy volunteers and in patients with NCCP with diffuse oesophageal spasm and nutcracker oesophagus.[1] Despite this, the overall experience with these agents has been poor, as they do not provide significant or prolonged symptomatic relief. Furthermore, these studies have been criticised for limitations of their methods.

Antidepressants

Antidepressants are among the most widely used drugs in functional gastrointestinal disorders, with well-established evidence of their efficacy.[4,12,13] The doses used are often much lower than would be used for their antidepressant effect, they thus are believed to have visceral analgesic properties. Tricyclic antidepressants have actions on the noradrenaline and serotonin reuptake transporters and have had better results than newer agents, such as the selective serotonin receptor inhibitors, perhaps suggesting that pathways other than serotonin (such as those involving noradrenaline) are important in the maintenance of chronic visceral pain.

Serotonin receptor

A number of trials have evaluated the role of the 5-HT_4 receptor agonist tegaserod in patients with IBS. The fact that this drug increases bowel transit, reduces visceral sensitivity, and stimulates the peristaltic reflex has gained it favour in the management of C-IBS.[13] The 5-HT_3 antagonist alosetron, on the other hand, although also modulating visceral sensitivity, has the opposite effect of slowing colonic transit and therefore has been evaluated in a number of studies for D-IBS.[13] Concerns were raised about its safety because of the possibility of ischaemic colitis, so it has restricted approval in the United States for the management of women with severe D-IBS that has failed to respond to conventional treatment.

Psychological therapy

As has been mentioned, psychological comorbidity is common in patients with functional gastrointestinal disorders, particularly when patients are seen in secondary and tertiary care settings. A number of studies therefore have evaluated the efficacy of behavioural therapy in ameliorating the symptoms of these disorders.[13] Relaxation therapy, hypnotherapy, biofeedback, cognitive behavioural therapy, and psychotherapy all have been reported to offer some benefit in patients with symptoms of IBS, although a number of these trials have been criticised for poor research methods. Further studies of these interventions are needed before conclusive guidance can be issued.

Other agents

A number of other agents have been proposed for the treatment of IBS, including somatostatin, the α_2 adrenoceptor agonist clonidine, peripherally acting opioids, tachykinin antagonists, oxytocin, and cholecystokinin. More detailed work with these compounds, however, is ongoing and results are awaited.

☐ SUMMARY

This very brief summary of the advances in our understanding of the pathophysiology of functional gastrointestinal disorders highlights exactly why progress has not been as rapid as desired – their complexity. The highly complex interactions of a number of integrated biological systems over a long period of time, weighted variably by genetic and psychosocial biases, is likely to be responsible for the huge spectrum of clinical disease in patients with functional gastrointestinal disorders (Fig 2). This is among the most rapidly evolving fields of gastroenterology, and as our knowledge of these disorders increases and the web of functional gastrointestinal disorders slowly is disentangled, new treatment options are likely to be developed to reduce the considerable morbidity associated with these conditions.

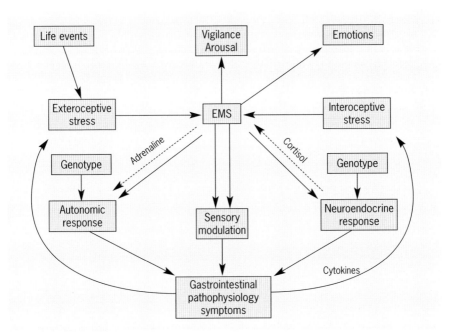

Fig 2 Potential factors that may interact with the emotional motor system (EMS) to govern an individual's visceral pain sensitivity. Stress – exteroceptive (psychological) or interoceptive (such as infection or inflammation) – can activate the emotional motor system, and the resulting autonomic and neuroendocrine responses may modulate pain sensitivity. Dysfunction of these systems may be relevant in the pathophysiology of the visceral pain hypersensitivity seen in functional gastrointestinal disorders. Adapted and reproduced from Mayer with permission of BMJ Publishing Group.[5]

REFERENCES

1 Drossman DA, Corazziari E, Talley NJ *et al.* Rome II. *The functional gastrointestinal disorders. Diagnosis, pathophysiology and treatment: A multinational consensus.* McLean, VA: Degnon Associates, 2000.

2 Trimble KC, Farouk R, Pryde A, Douglas S, Heading RC. Heightened visceral sensation in functional gastrointestinal disease is not site-specific. Evidence for a generalized disorder of gut sensitivity. *Dig Dis Sci* 1995;40:1607–13.

3 Mayer EA, Gebhart GF. Basic and clinical aspects of visceral hyperalgesia. *Gastroenterology* 1994;107:271–93.

4 Dekel R, Fass R. Current perspectives on the diagnosis and treatment of functional esophageal disorders. *Curr Gastroenterol Rep* 2003;5:314–22. .

5 Mayer EA. The neurobiology of stress and gastrointestinal disease. *Gut* 2000;47:861–9.

6 Mayer EA. Spinal and supraspinal modulation of visceral sensation. *Gut* 2000;47(Suppl 4): iv69–72; discussion iv76.

7 Suzuki R, Rygh LJ, Dickenson AH. Bad news from the brain: descending 5-HT pathways that control spinal pain processing. *Trends Pharmacol Sci* 2004;25:613–7.

8 Tack J, Broekaert D, Corsetti M, Fischler B, Janssens J. Influence of acute serotonin reuptake inhibition on colonic sensorimotor function in man. *Aliment Pharmacol Ther* 2006;23:265–74.

9 Levy RL, Jones KR, Whitehead WE *et al.* Irritable bowel syndrome in twins: heredity and social learning both contribute to etiology. *Gastroenterology* 2001;121:799–804.

10 Kim HJ, Camilleri M, Carlson PJ *et al.* Association of distinct alpha(2) adrenoceptor and serotonin transporter polymorphisms with constipation and somatic symptoms in functional gastrointestinal disorders. *Gut* 2004;53:829–37.

11 Zubieta JK, Heitzeg MM, Smith YR *et al.* COMT val158met genotype affects mu-opioid neurotransmitter responses to a pain stressor. *Science* 2003;299:1240–3.

12 Spiller R. Pharmacotherapy: non-serotonergic mechanisms. *Gut* 2002;51(Suppl 1):i87–90.

13 Brandt LJ, Bjorkman D, Fennerty MB *et al.* Systematic review on the management of irritable bowel syndrome in North America. *Am J Gastroenterol* 2002;97(11 Suppl):S7–26.

Neuroendocrine tumours of the gastrointestinal tract and pancreas

D Mark Pritchard

☐ INTRODUCTION

Neuroendocrine tumours are relatively rare, but in many cases they are slow growing and therefore represent a significant burden of disease. The first neuroendocrine tumours of the intestine were described by Siegfried Oberndorfer in 1907 and termed 'karzinoide', because they were believed to behave in a more benign fashion than carcinomas.[1] This chapter gives an overview of clinical aspects of the neuroendocrine tumours that arise in the gastrointestinal tract and pancreas. Interested readers should refer to a number of excellent recently published review articles and guidelines for a more comprehensive discussion and for primary source references.[1–4]

☐ NOMENCLATURE AND CLASSIFICATION SYSTEMS

Neuroendocrine tumours can occur at many sites in the body and include neoplasms as diverse as medullary carcinoma of the thyroid, phaeochromocytoma, and small cell lung cancer. They are sometimes classified as a single tumour type because they express pathological markers such as chromogranin A, synaptophysin, and neuron-specific enolase and because they have clinical similarities, such as being relatively slow growing and having a good prognosis. This has led to several attempts to classify these tumours as a single entity, including the now obsolete APUDoma (amine precursor uptake and decarboxylation) concept. Neuro-endocrine tumours are heterogeneous, however, and current practice therefore classifies these neoplasms on the basis of their anatomical location and the nature of their hormone production.

Neuroendocrine tumours that arise within the gastrointestinal system (gastroenteropancreatic neuroendocrine tumours) can be subdivided according to whether they occur in the gastrointestinal tract or pancreas (Fig 1). Most tumours within the gastrointestinal tract do not produce hormones; however, hormone secreting tumours (such as gastrinomas in the duodenum) can occur in the intestine. In addition, carcinoids can occur at sites (especially the lung) outside the gastrointestinal tract. Tumours that arise within the pancreas sometimes are referred to as 'endocrine' or 'islet cell' tumours; they should no longer be called carcinoids. About 50% of pancreatic tumours are non-functioning, while the other 50% produce a variety of hormones (Table 1).

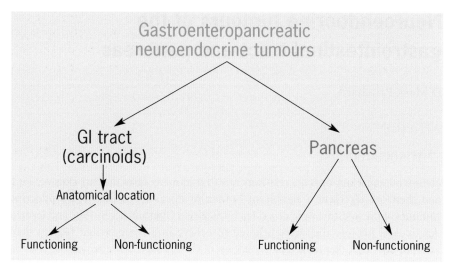

Fig 1 Classification of gastroenteropancreatic neuroendocrine tumours.

Table 1 Clinical features of pancreatic endocrine tumours.

Tumour type	Pancreatic endocrine tumours (%)	Associated with MEN-1 (%)	Clinical features
Non-functioning	50	20	• Pancreatic mass or liver metastases
Insulinoma	25–30	5	• Recurrent hypoglycaemia
Gastrinoma	10–15	25–35	• Zollinger-Ellison syndrome (peptic ulceration and diarrhoea)
VIPoma	2–3	5	• Secretory diarrhoea • Hypokalaemia
Glucagonoma	1–2	1–20	• Necrolytic migratory erythema • Diabetes mellitus • Weight loss
Somatostatinoma	<1	45	• Diabetes mellitus • Steatorrhoea • Gallstones • Weight loss

☐ EPIDEMIOLOGY OF GASTROENTEROPANCREATIC NEUROENDOCRINE TUMOURS

The incidence of gastroenteropancreatic neuroendocrine tumours is low (3–4 cases per 100,000 per annum). The prevalence is much higher, however, because of the relatively good prognosis of many of these tumours. Gastrointestinal carcinoids mostly are sporadic and can occur throughout the gastrointestinal tract, with the most common sites being the small intestine, colon, and appendix.[5] Pancreatic endocrine tumours also are rare and represent 1–2% of all pancreatic tumours.[3] The most common subtype is the non-functioning tumour (50%); of the secretory tumours, insulinomas comprise 25–30%, gastrinoma 10–15%, VIPoma 2–3%, glucagonoma 1–2%, and somatostatinoma <1% (see Table 1). Most pancreatic endocrine tumours also occur sporadically, but some are associated with genetically inherited conditions.

Inherited predisposition

Pancreatic endocrine tumours occur frequently in multiple endocrine neoplasia (MEN) type 1, which also predisposes to primary hyperparathyroidism and pituitary adenomas. This condition is inherited autosomally dominantly and recently has been shown to result from mutations in the *MEN-1* (menin) gene.[6] About 25–35% of gastrinomas occur in patients with MEN-1, and, in this condition, the tumours often are multiple and may be located in the duodenal wall rather than the pancreas. Pancreatic endocrine tumours are not usually a feature of MEN-2, but they do occur more frequently in patients with tuberous sclerosis, von Hippel Lindau syndrome, and neurofibromatosis type 1.[7]

☐ CLINICAL PRESENTATION

Gastrointestinal carcinoids

Gastrointestinal carcinoids may present with local symptoms according to their anatomical location (for example, bowel obstruction from a small intestinal tumour or rectal bleeding from a rectal tumour).[1] Many patients, however, are asymptomatic until they present with evidence of metastases and associated non-specific symptoms, such as anorexia and weight loss. The actual carcinoid syndrome, which is characterised by flushing, diarrhoea, bronchoconstriction, and right sided valvular heart disease, occurs in only <10% of patients. It results usually from secretion of serotonin, tachykinins, and other vasoactive compounds into the bloodstream from hepatic metastases. The carcinoid syndrome more commonly results from metastatic small bowel carcinoid than from tumours originating at other sites in the gastrointestinal tract, although it has been described for tumours arising at all locations. Patients who have carcinoid syndrome themselves are prone to carcinoid crises, which are characterised by bronchoconstriction, tachycardia, and rapidly fluctuating blood pressure. This can occur as a result of anaesthesia, intraoperative handling of the tumour, or interventional radiological procedures, such as embolisation or radiofrequency ablation. Susceptible patients should undergo prophylaxis with an intravenous infusion of octreotide (50 µg/hour) for 12 hours before until 48 hours after a possible precipitating event.[4]

Three types of gastric carcinoids exist.[8] Type 1 gastric carcinoids (70%) arise as a result of hypergastrinaemia caused by achlorhydria and autoimmune atrophic gastritis (Fig 2). They therefore are associated with pernicious anaemia. Type 2 gastric carcinoids (10%) also are associated with hypergastrinaemia in the setting of Zollinger-Ellison syndrome and MEN-1, while type 3 tumours (20%) are sporadic and are not associated with hypergastrinaemia. Type 1 and 2 tumours often are

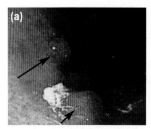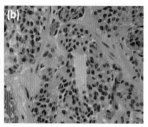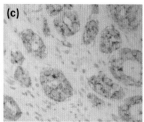

Fig 2 Type 1 gastric carcinoid: **(a)** endoscopic features, **(b)** haematoxylin and eosin histology, and **(c)** chromogranin A immunohistochemistry.

multiple and indolent, sometimes do not require treatment, and have a good prognosis, whereas type 3 tumours often are more aggressive.

Small intestinal carcinoids may present with local symptoms, such as bleeding (resulting in anaemia) or small bowel obstruction. The latter frequently is a result of an intense fibrotic (desmoplastic) reaction in the mesentery rather than the result of the tumour itself. Appendiceal carcinoids often present incidentally and most are benign. The risk of malignancy is higher for large tumours (>2 cm) and for those located near the base of the appendix. Such tumours should be removed by right hemicolectomy rather than conventional appendicectomy.[4] Colonic carcinoids usually appear as sessile polyps and present with the same local symptoms as those caused by colonic adenomas. If small, they may be amenable to colonoscopic polypectomy.

Pancreatic endocrine tumours

Non-functioning pancreatic endocrine tumours often present late with symptoms of a pancreatic mass or metastases. The functioning tumours of the pancreas present with well known endocrinological syndromes, such as recurrent hypoglycaemia (insulinoma) or Zollinger-Ellison syndrome (gastrinoma) (see Table 1).

□ INVESTIGATIONS

On diagnosis of a tumour that is suspected to be a gastroenteropancreatic neuroendocrine tumour, several investigations are indicated for further characterisation before a decision on the most appropriate form of treatment is made (Fig 3). Any hormones produced by the tumour should be characterised carefully, the tumour should be staged with a range of complementary imaging techniques, and consideration should be given to whether an underlying cause (such as MEN-1) exists. Such investigations often are conducted best by a multi-disciplinary team with expertise in endocrinology, endoscopy, radiology, and nuclear medicine.

Biochemical

Biochemical tests should include an assessment of serum levels of chromogranin A, which are increased in >90% of tumours (with the exception of insulinomas, in

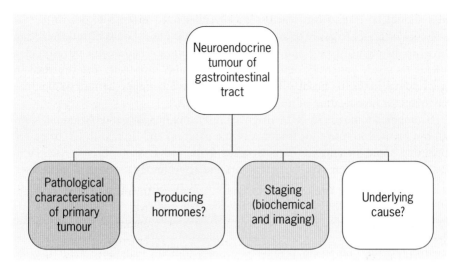

Fig 3 Investigation of gastroenteropancreatic neuroendocrine tumours.

which increased serum levels are less common). Levels of serum chromogranin A show some correlation with tumour burden, and sequential measurements are useful for monitoring disease progression in some patients. Elevated levels also can be found in patients with renal and hepatic impairment, hypergastrinaemia associated with achlorhydria, and inflammatory bowel disease.[4] Assessment of levels of 5-hydroxyindoleacetic acid (5-HIAA) in a urine sample collected over 24 hours also should be performed. During the collection, the patient should avoid eating foods rich in serotonin, such as bananas and avocado.

For assessment of pancreatic tumours, a fasting gut hormone profile also should be performed. This will provide measurements of serum levels of insulin, gastrin, glucagon, somatostatin, and vasoactive intestinal peptide (VIP). In some cases, provocative tests (such as 72 hour fasts for insulinoma or a secretin test for gastrinoma) also may be needed. If MEN-1 is suspected, additional endocrinological investigations (such as pituitary and parathyroid function) also are indicated. Genetic assessment for germline mutations in the menin gene is now possible and can be used to screen family members within a MEN-1 kindred. Measurement of fasting levels of serum gastrin also should be performed in all cases of gastric carcinoid in order to determine the type of tumour. Ideally, this blood test should be performed after discontinuing acid suppressing drugs (such as proton pump inhibitors and H2 antagonists), but in some patients with severe Zollinger-Ellison syndrome, this may not be safe or possible.

Imaging

Several imaging methods may be helpful in the diagnosis and staging of gastroenteropancreatic neuroendocrine tumours. Upper gastrointestinal endoscopy and colonoscopy are useful for assessment of tumours at appropriate locations, and they also allow biopsy to be performed. For assessment of gastric carcinoids, biopsies also should be taken from macroscopically unaffected mucosa to determine the presence of atrophic gastritis, and the pH of gastric juice should be ascertained in order to distinguish type 1 and type 2 gastric carcinoids. Endoscopic ultrasound is useful to assess pancreatic endocrine tumours and investigate the presence of gastrinomas in the duodenal wall. Small bowel enteroscopy and barium studies may be useful for investigation of small bowel carcinoids.

Computed tomography (CT), magnetic resonance imaging, and ultrasound scans all can be used to assess for tumours in the pancreas and liver, with CT being the preferred initial investigation in most cases. Radionuclide scans also are essential to determine the location of primary tumours and assess for the presence of metastases. The ^{111}In octreotide scan detects about 80% of tumours (with the exception of insulinomas) and is positive if the tumour has type 2 (and to a lesser extent type 5) somatostatin receptors (Fig 4). ^{123}I-meta-iodobenzylguandidine (MIBG) scans also sometimes are useful. Although they detect only about 50% of gastroenteropancreatic neuroendocrine tumours, a positive scan does indicate that the tumour may be amenable to targeted radionuclide therapy with ^{131}I-MIBG (see below).

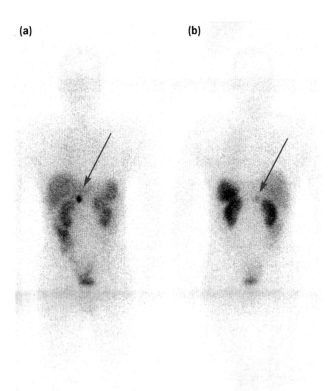

(a)   **(b)**

Fig 4 ^{111}In octreotide scan from a patient with a gastrinoma in the duodenal wall (arrow): **(a)** anterior view, **(b)** posterior view.

Pathological assessment of tumours

Biopsy and resection specimens should be assessed by an expert pathologist. Specimens should undergo immunohistochemistry for markers including chromogranin A, PGP4.5, and synaptophysin; peptide hormones; and Ki67.[4] The World Health Organization recently devised a classification system for these tumours,[4,9] but it is not currently in widespread everyday use.

☐ TREATMENT

Gastroenteropancreatic tumours are unusual and interesting, in that multiple methods of treatment are possible and effective (Fig 5). Many patients, particularly those with metastatic disease, receive multiple treatments sequentially during the course of their illness. The somatostatin analogues have revolutionised the symptomatic management of these patients, particularly those with carcinoid syndrome.

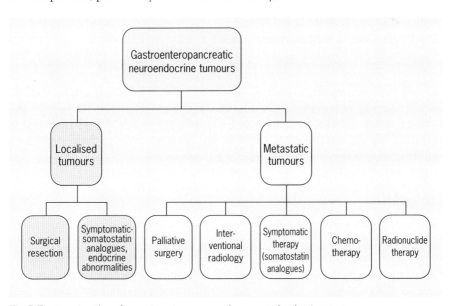

Fig 5 Treatment options for gastroenteropancreatic neuroendocrine tumours.

Symptomatic treatments

Somatostatin analogues lead to symptomatic improvement in 40–80% of patients and biochemical response in 40–70% of patients. An antiproliferative effect upon the tumour, however, is seen in only about 10% of patients. Long-acting injectable formulations of somatostatin analogues, such as octreotide acetate and lanreotide, now allow for intermittent (monthly) dosing rather than the more frequent dosing required by short-acting octreotide. This has resulted in increased compliance and improved symptom control. Somatostatin analogues generally are well tolerated, but some patients do experience side effects such as abdominal discomfort and steatorrhoea, and a proportion will develop gallstones after long-term use.

Symptomatic treatments also are important for several of the hormone producing pancreatic endocrine tumours. In particular, high doses of proton pump inhibitors have improved dramatically the care of patients with Zollinger-Ellison syndrome. Measures such as rehydration and potassium replacement are important in patients with VIPoma, and management of diabetes mellitus is often an important component of the management of patients with glucagonoma and somatostatinoma.

Surgery

Resection of the primary tumour with the intent of cure may be appropriate for some tumours if staging investigations show no evidence of tumour spread. For type 1 gastric carcinoid tumours, antrectomy to remove the source of hypergastrinaemia may be preferred to removal of the gastric carcinoid tumour itself.[10] Palliative surgery (such as enteroenterostomy for obstructing small bowel carcinoid and debulking liver surgery for metastases) also may be appropriate. Liver transplantation has been used for metastatic carcinoid tumours, but the results are relatively disappointing, and this is no longer a widely used treatment option.[4]

Interventional radiology

Interventional radiological techniques, such as chemoembolisation and radiofrequency ablation, have been used successfully for the palliative treatment of carcinoid hepatic metastases. Susceptible patients who undergo these procedures should receive prophylaxis with intravenous octreotide.

Chemotherapy

Systemic chemotherapy generally gives disappointing results in most gastrointestinal tract carcinoids and therefore generally is not used. Chemotherapy (especially streptozocin-based chemotherapy) is useful in some pancreatic endocrine tumours, however, especially those with a high proliferative index. Interferon-α also has been used in some centres, but it does not seem to convey additional benefits over somatostatin analogues and has a generally less well tolerated side effect profile.[4]

Targeted radionuclide treatments

Targeted radionuclide treatments represent a recent significant advance in the management of metastatic gastroenteropancreatic neuroendocrine tumours. The basis of these treatments is that the gamma emitting radionuclides used for imaging are replaced by beta emitting radionuclides that will have a therapeutic effect. The only currently licensed treatment is ^{131}I-MIBG. This is suitable only for a few patients with gastroenteropancreatic neuroendocrine tumours, but 20–45% of suitable patients show a tumour response and 45–65% show symptomatic improvement. This treatment requires admission to a dedicated isolation facility and needs treatment to prevent uptake of radioiodine by the thyroid. ^{90}Y-DOTATOC

(^{90}Y-[DOTA]^0-Tyr^3-octreotide) is a novel treatment in which the radionuclide is conjugated to a somatostatin analogue.[11] Clinical trials are in progress in several centres, and preliminary results suggest a complete or partial tumour response rate of 20–35%.

☐ PROGNOSIS

Gastroenteropancreatic neuroendocrine tumours have a relatively good prognosis, certainly compared with adenocarcinomas located at the same anatomical site. As with other tumours, increased tumour size, the presence of metastases, increased patient age, and an increased tumour proliferative index all are associated with a worse prognosis. For gastrointestinal carcinoids, the prognosis is best for appendiceal and type 1 gastric tumours (>90% survival at five years), but the outlook is good for all types if the tumour has not metastasised at presentation. For pancreatic endocrine tumours, the prognosis is worst for non-functioning tumours, because they usually present at a more advanced stage. The prognosis for certain tumours, such as insulinoma and gastrinoma, is excellent (>90% survival at five years) and in many cases, because of recent advances in symptomatic treatments, patients with metastatic disease often can survive for many years.

☐ CONCLUSIONS

Although gastroenteropancreatic neuroendocrine tumours are rare, they should not be considered as a single tumour type, and each tumour should be managed individually on the basis of its anatomical location, degree of metastatic spread, and nature of hormone production. Several methods of investigation are useful to characterise these tumours fully, and multiple methods of sequential treatment may be appropriate for individual patients. Recent major advances have included the development of radionuclide scans and targeted treatments and the widespread availability of long acting somatostatin analogues. These tumours therefore are managed optimally as part of a multidisciplinary team. The rarity of these tumours means that they are relatively underresearched, and much work is still needed to understand the molecular pathogenesis of these tumours, with a view to developing novel treatments.

ACKNOWLEDGMENTS

Mark Pritchard is funded by a Wellcome Trust Advanced Fellowship for clinicians. I thank members of the neuroendocrine tumour multidisciplinary team at Royal Liverpool and Broadgreen University Hospitals NHS Trust for useful discussions.

REFERENCES

1   Modlin IM, Kidd M, Latich I, Zikusoka MN, Shapiro MD. Current status of gastrointestinal carcinoids. *Gastroenterology* 2005;128:1717–51.

2   Barakat MT, Meeran K, Bloom SR. Neuroendocrine tumours. *Endocr Relat Cancer* 2004;11:1–18.

3   Warner RR. Enteroendocrine tumors other than carcinoid: a review of clinically significant advances. *Gastroenterology* 2005;128:1668–4.

4   Ramage JK, Davies AH, Ardill J *et al.* Guidelines for the management of gastro-enteropancreatic neuroendocrine (including carcinoid) tumours. *Gut* 2005;54(Suppl 4): iv1–16.

5   Modlin IM, Lye KD, Kidd M. A 5-decade analysis of 13,715 carcinoid tumors. *Cancer* 2003;97: 934–59.

6   Brandi ML, Gagel RF, Angeli A *et al.* Guidelines for diagnosis and therapy of MEN type 1 and type 2. *J Clin Endocrinol Metab* 2001;86:5658–71.

7   Alexakis N, Connor S, Ghaneh P *et al.* Hereditary pancreatic endocrine tumours. *Pancreatology* 2004;4:417–33.

8   Modlin IM, Lye KD, Kidd M. Carcinoid tumors of the stomach. *Surg Oncol* 2003;12:153–72.

9   Arnold R. Endocrine tumours of the gastrointestinal tract. Introduction: definition, historical aspects, classification, staging, prognosis and therapeutic options. *Best Pract Res Clin Gastroenterol* 2005;19:491–505.

10 Higham AD, Dimaline R, Varro A *et al.* Octreotide suppression test predicts beneficial outcome from antrectomy in a patient with gastric carcinoid tumor. *Gastroenterology* 1998;114:817–22.

11 Bodei L, Cremonesi M, Grana C *et al.* Receptor radionuclide therapy with 90Y-[DOTA]0-Tyr3-octreotide (90Y-DOTATOC) in neuroendocrine tumours. *Eur J Nucl Med Mol Imaging* 2004;31:1038–46.

Biomedical review – inflammation and cancer

Mairi Macarthur and Emad M El-Omar

☐ INTRODUCTION

Rudolph Virchow was the first to suggest a link between inflammation and cancer when he demonstrated leucocytes in neoplastic tissue in 1863. Since then, an impressive body of evidence has accumulated to corroborate inflammation-mediated oncogenesis. The gastrointestinal system is the site of a significant proportion of such tumours. The aetiology of the inflammation varies and can be infective, such as a virus, bacteria or parasite, or a non-infective irritant, either physical or chemical. For example, Epstein-Barr virus is the aetiological agent responsible for the progression of early dysplastic change into severe dysplasia in nasopharyngeal carcinoma. Hepatitis B virus (HBV) and hepatitis C virus (HCV) account for more than 80% of cases of hepatocellular carcinoma worldwide, and human papilloma virus (HPV) infection is the leading cause of anogenital cancer. The Gram-negative bacterium *Helicobacter pylori* has been identified as the major aetiological factor in gastric adenocarcinoma, and it is also known to significantly increase the risk of gastric mucosa-associated lymphoid tissue (MALT) lymphoma. Parasites such as *Clonorchis sinensis* cause a chronic inflammatory infiltrate of the biliary tract and are linked to subsequent cholangiocarcinoma.[1]

Numerous examples show that non-infective irritants are associated with the development of malignant disease. Within the gastrointestinal tract, chronic oesophagitis (including Barrett's metaplasia), chronic pancreatitis, and chronic cholecystitis are all inflammatory conditions that increase the risk of cancer. It thus is apparent that chronic inflammation is a common underlying theme in the development of many gastrointestinal malignancies. But what are the mechanisms through which these inflammatory stimuli may act to induce cancer? To examine this, we must first give a brief outline of chronic inflammation.

☐ CHRONIC INFLAMMATION

Chronic inflammation may progress from acute inflammation if the injurious agent persists, but, more often than not, the response is chronic from the outset. In contrast to the largely vascular changes of acute inflammation, chronic inflammation is characterised by infiltration of damaged tissue by mononuclear cells such as macrophages, lymphocytes and plasma cells, together with tissue destruction and attempts at repair. The macrophage is the key player of the chronic inflammatory response. This is because of the great number of bioactive products it releases, including proteases, elastase, collagenases, plasminogen activator, hydrolases, phosphatases, lipases, complement components, coagulation factors (for example, factors V, VIII, and tissue factor), reactive metabolites of oxygen, eicosanoids, cytokines (interleukin (IL) 1α, IL-β, and tumour necrosis factor (TNF) α), chemokines (IL-8), growth factors, and nitric oxide.

These mediators form part of the body's powerful defence against invasion and injury. The downside, however, is that persistent or pathological macrophage activation can result in continued tissue damage. This underlies a variety of disease processes from rheumatoid arthritis to atherosclerosis. Three of the most important players in inflammation that have relevance to tissue damage and cancer risk are reactive oxygen species, nitric oxide, and cyclooxygenase (COX) 2.

☐ REACTIVE OXYGEN SPECIES, NITRIC OXIDE, AND CYCLOOXYGENASE 2

A cardinal feature of inflamed tissues, including those of the gastrointestinal tract, is the generation of nitric oxide (NO) through inducible nitric oxide synthase (iNOS). Nitric oxide reacts with superoxide to form peroxynitrite ($ONOO^-$) and nitrosating species, such as NO_3^- (nitrates), NO_2^- (nitrites), and N_2O_3. Nitric oxide and its products may exert oncogenic effects via several mechanisms, including direct damage to DNA and proteins, inhibition of apoptosis, mutation of DNA, cellular repair functions (such as p53), and promotion of angiogenesis.[2]

Another inducible enzyme with carcinogenic properties that is active within inflamed and malignant tissues is COX 2. Several mechanisms of COX 2-mediated intestinal carcinogenesis have been elucidated. These include inhibition of apoptosis, modulation of cellular adhesion and motility, promotion of angiogenesis, and immunosuppression. Strong epidemiological evidence also implicates COX 2 in the pathogenesis of a number of epithelial malignancies, including gastric and colorectal cancer.[3,4] Inhibitors of the enzyme are associated with a reduction of up to 50% in the morbidity and mortality of colorectal cancer.[5] Among the most potent inducers of COX 2 are the key proinflammatory cytokines IL-1α, IL-1β, and TNF-α.

☐ IMMUNE RESPONSE AND CYTOKINES IN GASTROINTESTINAL MALIGNANCY

Immune response undoubtedly has a significant impact on the potential for malignancy, and this is highlighted by the findings that severe combined immunodeficiency (SCID) and T cell-deficient mice infected with *Helicobacter* do not develop the same degree of tissue injury despite high levels of gastric bacterial colonisation. The importance of CD4 lymphocytes, in particular, is also demonstrated by experiments that show that B cell-deficient *Helicobacter*-infected mice are not protected from severe atrophy and metaplasia.[6]

A focus on individual cytokines has generated further evidence to support the role of inflammation in gastrointestinal carcinogenesis. For example, interferon (IFN) γ knockout mice are protected from gastric atrophy, while IL-10-deficient mice develop severe atrophic gastritis and a chronic enterocolitis. Interestingly, many of the IL-10-

deficient mice with chronic enterocolitis go on to develop colorectal cancer similar to human inflammatory bowel disease-associated neoplasia.

The molecular mechanisms involved in the pathogenesis of hepatitis C-associated hepatocellular carcinoma also depend on cytokines. Hepatitis C virus core protein interacts with the signal transducer and activator of transcription 3 protein (STAT3), which mediates cytokine signalling and the local cytokine profile. Nuclear factor kappa B (NF-κB), another transcription factor that is known to activate inflammatory pathways and proinflammatory cytokines, is also stimulated in patients infected with HCV. Both of these factors have additional tumour-promoting potential, in that STAT-3 has growth stimulatory effects and NF-κB can inhibit apoptosis.

☐ NUCLEAR FACTOR-κB

Reactive oxygen species, COX 2, and cytokines interact in a complex manner in the development and progression of an inflammatory environment. They share several intracellular pathways and mediators through which their physiological and pathological effects are exerted. One such mediator is NF-κB, a ubiquitous transcription factor involved in the regulation of various inflammatory, apoptotic, and oncogenic genes. It often has been described as a central mediator of the immune response, particularly as a large variety of bacteria and viruses can lead to its activation. The activation of NF-κB leads to the expression of inflammatory cytokines, chemokines, immune receptors, and cell-surface adhesion molecules.

Further evidence to support inflammation's role in the initiation and promotion of gastrointestinal malignancy comes from the fact that constitutive expression of NF-κB has been identified in a number of gastrointestinal malignancies, including hepatocellular carcinoma and colorectal cancer. For an excellent review of this topic, please refer to Karin and Greten.[7]

☐ CYTOKINE POLYMORPHISMS AND GASTROINTESTINAL MALIGNANCY

Genetic polymorphisms have emerged in recent years as important determinants of disease susceptibility and severity. Perhaps the most compelling evidence for the role of inflammation in gastrointestinal malignancy comes from studies that show that proinflammatory cytokine gene polymorphisms increase the risk of cancer and its precursors. An excellent example of this is the role of these polymorphisms in the pathogenesis of *H. pylori*-induced gastric cancer. *Helicobacter pylori* causes damage by initiating chronic inflammation in the gastric mucosa. This inflammation is mediated by an array of proinflammatory and anti-inflammatory cytokines. Genetic poly-morphisms directly influence interindividual variation in the magnitude of cytokine response, and this clearly contributes to an individual's ultimate clinical outcome. In the case of infection with *H. pylori*, we speculated that the most relevant candidate genes would be those whose products were involved in handling the *H. pylori* attack (innate and adaptive immune responses) and those that mediated the resulting inflammation. Because such a list of candidate genes would be prohibitively extensive, we further narrowed the search by selecting genes that were most relevant to gastric physiology and, in particular, gastric acid secretion.

Helicobacter pylori-induced gastritis is associated with three phenotypes that correlate closely with clinical outcome. The first is an antrum-predominant/corpus-sparing pattern associated with high acid secretion and increased risk of duodenal ulcer disease. The second is mild mixed antrum/corpus gastritis with no major effect on acid secretion and, generally, no serious clinical outcome. Last is a corpus-predominant or severe pangastritis pattern that is associated with gastric atrophy, hypochlorhydria, and an increased risk of gastric cancer. Pharmacological inhibition of gastric acid can lead to a shift from an antrum-predominant pattern to a corpus-predominant pattern with onset of gastric atrophy. It thus was clear that an endogenous agent that was upregulated in the presence of *H. pylori* has a profound proinflammatory effect and was also an acid inhibitor would be the most relevant host genetic factor to be studied. Interleukin 1β (IL-1β) fitted this profile perfectly – for not only is it one of the earliest and most important proinflammatory cytokines in the context of *H. pylori* infection, but it is also the most powerful acid inhibitor known.[8] We have shown that proinflammatory *IL-1* gene cluster polymorphisms (*IL-1B* encoding IL-1β and *IL-1RN* encoding its naturally occurring receptor antagonist) increase the risk of gastric cancer and its precursors in the presence of *H. pylori*.[9] People with the *IL-1B-31*C* or *−511*T* and *IL-1RN*2/*2* genotypes (all of which correlate with high levels of IL-1β) are at increased risk of developing hypochlorhydria and gastric atrophy in response to *H. pylori* infection. This risk extends to gastric cancer itself, with a 2–3-fold increased risk of malignancy compared with people who have the less proinflammatory genotypes. The association of *IL-1* gene cluster polymorphisms and gastric cancer has been confirmed in other reports.[10]

In addition to IL-1 gene cluster polymorphisms, proinflammatory genotypes of *TNF-A* and *IL-10* have also been identified as risk factors for gastric cancer, and, as is the case with *IL-1* gene cluster polymorphisms, this is restricted to non-cardia adenocarcinomas.[11] We have shown that having an increasing number of proinflammatory genotypes (*IL-1B-511*T*, *IL-1RN*2*2*, *TNF-A-308*A*, and *IL-10* ATA/ATA) progressively increases the risk of gastric cancer. Indeed, by the time three or four of these polymorphisms are present, the risk of gastric cancer is increased to 27-fold.[11] The fact that *H. pylori* is a prerequisite for the association of these polymorphisms with malignancy shows that, in this situation, inflammation is indeed driving carcinogenesis. It is likely that other proinflammatory cytokine gene polymorphisms will be relevant to the initiation and progression of gastric cancer. This exciting field has expanded greatly over the past few years and the search is now fully on for the full complement of risk genotypes that dictate an individual's likelihood of developing cancer.

☐ MECHANISMS OF INFLAMMATION-ASSOCIATED TUMOUR DEVELOPMENT IN THE GASTROINTESTINAL TRACT

The mechanisms that mediate inflammation-induced malignancy include direct damage to DNA, inhibition of apoptosis, subversion of immunity, and stimulation of angiogenesis. In addition, chronic inflammation in the gastrointestinal tract is also known to affect proliferation, adhesion, and cellular transformation. For an excellent review of the topic, please refer to Balkwill *et al.*[12] Figure 1 provides an overview of mechanisms of inflammation-associated gastrointestinal carcinogenesis.

The deregulation of cellular proliferation is one of the hallmarks of cancer cells and is the outcome of interaction between a variety of endogenous and exogenous factors active during the inflammatory process. These include luminal contents, bacteria, inflammatory cytokines, and mediators such as the matrix metalloproteinases. Direct mechanical irritation can also lead to epithelial proliferation, and when this is combined with the effects of an additional

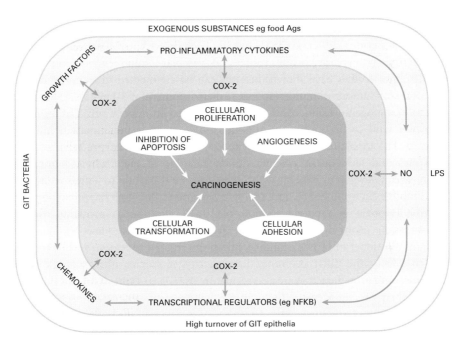

Fig 1 Overview of mechanisms of inflammation-associated gastrointestinal carcinogenesis. This diagram illustrates the complex interactions between inflammatory mediators and the common cellular processes that could lead to cancer. Considering the factors in layers, the environment within the gastrointestinal tract forms the outermost layer. The presence of a rapidly proliferating mucosa exposed to exogenous substances and a vast quantity of lipopolysaccharide (LPS)-rich bacteria, provides an ideal environment for chronic inflammation to get established. Moving inwards, the next layer involves the release of mediators sich as pro-inflammatory cytokines, chemokines, growth factors and nitric oxide, many of which share transcriptional factors such as HIF-1α and NFκB. These may act independently or in combination, leading to the activation of COX-2. At the centres are 5 cellular mechanisms that could form a pathway to malignant transformation, either independently or more likely in concert. COX-2 is known to impact on each of them and is placed in an inner layer because of the growing evidence supporting its central role in gastrointestinal carcinogenesis. However, the relationships between NO, cytokines, activation of COX-2 and their impact on cellular mechanisms are not purely linear. All of tbes factors are capable of exerting effects independent of COX-2 and thus, this layer may not always be a necessary component in revealing the final core of pathways to cancer. Reproduced from Macarthur et al with permission of American Physiological Society.[1]

inflammatory stimulus, such as a bacterium for example, the resulting hyperproliferation can push the tissue further along the pathway towards cancer. Infection with *H. pylori*, while initially enhancing apoptosis, ultimately leads to a compensatory proliferation. Pathways through which *H. pylori* may influence apoptosis include those involving COX 2 and peroxisome proliferator-activated receptor γ (PPARγ). Proinflammatory cytokines, in particular TNF-α, are also able to modulate apoptosis by altering the levels of the pro- and anti-apoptotic proteins Bcl-2 and Bax.

As well as affecting proliferation and apoptosis, the same mediators impact on cellular adhesion and angiogenesis. Cancer cells that respond to proinflammatory cytokines released from macrophages may exploit the same mechanism used by leucocytes to migrate through the vasculature. Upregulation of cell adhesion molecule (CAM) expression is seen on exposure of colon cancer cells to lipopolysaccharide (LPS), and COX 2 has also been shown to promote cell adhesion.

Macrophages are important sources of vascular endothelial growth factor (VEGF), and studies have shown that this can be augmented in tumours by the humoral anti-tumour immune response. An environment of T-helper 2 (Th2) cells promotes angiogenesis, and, conversely, cell-mediated immune (CMI)/Th1 immune responses tend to be inhibitory. Although, infection and inflammation initially generate Th1 cytokines, a cycle involving COX 2 mediated upregulation of Th2 cytokines and subsequent chronic downregulation of the Th1/CMI immune response can develop in patients with neoplasia. The transition to a predominantly Th2 immune environment favours angiogenesis, and COX 2 itself has proangiogenic activity. Hypoxia is a potent inducer of VEGF, and this is mediated by the transcription factor hypoxia-inducible factor-1α (HIF-1α). The VEGF gene contains a number of HIF-1α-binding sites in its regulatory region, and HIF-1α is able to activate the VEGF promoter. Reactive oxygen species, nitric oxide, certain cytokines, and growth factors are also regulators of HIF-1α expression, and this may explain their proangiogenic activity. In the low oxygen concentration of injured, inflamed, or neoplastic tissue, HIF-1α is needed to generate adenosine triphosphate (ATP) in leucocytes and thus enable them to function. It also increases the production of nitric oxide, which acts back to further increase HIF-1α activity. Thus, acting through HIF-1α in a hypoxic environment, various inflammatory mediators – including growth factors, NO, cytokines, chemokines, and COX 2 and its products – may 'switch' on angiogenesis. They may do this via the generation of VEGF – directly or indirectly – and may also aid the process by activating other factors such as proteases, which degrade the extracellular matrix. Therefore, it is not difficult to see that in chronic gastrointestinal inflammation, the development of hypoxic areas may increase the generation of proangiogenic stimuli that tip the balance in favour of angiogenesis and further drive tissues towards carcinogenesis.

Finally, in addition to impacting on cellular proliferation, apoptosis, adhesion, and angiogenesis, the stimuli and mediators of chronic inflammation can cause cellular transformation. A number of viruses such as hepatitis B virus (HBV), Epstein-Barr virus (EBV), and human papillomavirus (HPV) are known to directly bind to certain genes and affect protein activity, including transcriptional factors and oncogenes. Animal models have also shown that bacteria can lead to ultrastructural changes within the colonic epithelia and subsequent hyperplasia. This may precede the development of colonic adenomas.

☐ SUMMARY

This review has discussed the links between chronic inflammation and carcinogenesis of the gastrointestinal tract. Ample epidemiological evidence supports this link, but, increasingly, the basic molecular pathways of this association are being uncovered. Inflammatory cells produce a wide range of mediators, including proinflammatory cytokines, chemokines, reactive oxygen species, growth factors, and eicosanoids. Cyclooxygenase 2 may be a linchpin in orchestrating many of the mutagenic effects of these products, and this is supported by the studies that show the chemopreventative benefits of COX inhibitors. Cytokine gene polymorphisms undoubtedly contribute to an individual's risk of malignancy, but their importance lies in their contribution to the understanding of inflammation-mediated carcinogenesis. The fact that chronic inflammation impacts on crucial cellular processes such as proliferation, adhesion, apoptosis, angiogenesis, and transformation highlights its pivotal role in the pathogenesis of gastrointestinal malignancy.

REFERENCES

1   Macarthur M, Hold GL, El-Omar EM. Inflammation and cancer II. Role of chronic inflammation and cytokine gene polymorphisms in the pathogenesis of gastrointestinal malignancy. *Am J Physiol Gastrointest Liver Physiol* 2004;286:G515–20.

2   Jaiswal M, LaRusso NF, Gores GJ. Nitric oxide in gastrointestinal epithelial cell carcinogenesis: linking inflammation to oncogenesis. *Am J Physiol Gastrointest Liver Physiol* 2001;281: G626–34.

3   Marnett LJ, DuBois RN. COX-2: a target for colon cancer prevention. *Annu Rev Pharmacol Toxicol* 2002;42:55–80.

4   Wang D, Mann JR, DuBois RN. The role of prostaglandins and other eicosanoids in the gastrointestinal tract. *Gastroenterology* 2005;128:1445–61.

5   Gupta RA, DuBois RN. Colorectal cancer prevention and treatment by inhibition of cyclooxygenase-2. *Nat Rev Cancer* 2001;1:11–21.

6   Roth KA, Kapadia SB, Martin SM, Lorenz RG. Cellular immune responses are essential for the development of *Helicobacter felis*-associated gastric pathology. *J Immunol* 1999;163:1490–7.

7   Karin M, Greten FR. NF-kappaB: linking inflammation and immunity to cancer development and progression. *Nat Rev Immunol* 2005;5:749–59.

8   El-Omar EM. The importance of interleukin 1beta in *Helicobacter pylori* associated disease. *Gut* 2001;48:743–7.

9   El-Omar EM, Carrington M, Chow WH *et al*. Interleukin-1 polymorphisms associated with increased risk of gastric cancer. *Nature* 2000;404:398–402.

10 Figueiredo C, Machado JC, Pharoah P *et al*. *Helicobacter pylori* and interleukin 1 genotyping: an opportunity to identify high-risk individuals for gastric carcinoma. *J Natl Cancer Inst* 2002;94:1680–7.

11 El-Omar EM, Rabkin CS, Gammon MD *et al*. Increased risk of noncardia gastric cancer associated with proinflammatory cytokine gene polymorphisms. *Gastroenterology* 2003; 124:1193–201.

12 Balkwill F, Charles KA, Mantovani A. Smoldering and polarized inflammation in the initiation and promotion of malignant disease. *Cancer Cell* 2005;7:211–7.

☐ GASTROENTEROLOGY SELF ASSESSMENT QUESTIONS

Recent progress in inflammatory bowel disease: from bench to bedside

1   The following have been proved to be of benefit in the treatment of IBD in randomised controlled trials:
(a) Infliximab in Crohn's disease
(b) Infliximab in ulcerative colitis
(c) GM-CSF in ulcerative colitis
(d) Apheresis in IBD
(e) Helminths in Crohn's disease

2   Regarding IBD:
(a) Infliximab is 25% human
(b) Infliximab is one of several biological agents currently licensed for the treatment of IBD
(c) GM-CSF may be therapeutic as an immunostimulant
(d) Treatment with invasive helminths has been shown to be of benefit
(e) Autologous stem cell transplant is now widely used as a treatment

Progress in understanding and managing functional gastrointestinal disorders

1   Regarding functional gastrointestinal disorders:
(a) The absence of visceral pain hypersensitivity makes a diagnosis of functional gastrointestinal disorders unlikely.
(b) The sensitisation of dorsal horn neurones after peripheral visceral nerve injury is responsible for heightened referral of pain to somatic areas
(c) Patients with non-cardiac chest pain can be hypersensitive to rectal balloon distension
(d) Proton pump inhibitors are efficacious in subsets of patients with non-cardiac chest pain
(e) Dysregulation of spinal pain modulatory circuits may be relevant for prolonged hyperalgesia in functional gastrointestinal disorders

2   The following are true about the treatment of irritable bowel syndrome:
(a) Mebeverine should be first line if constipation is the main feature
(b) Amitriptyline should be reserved for when psychological comorbidity can be elicited
(c) $5\text{-}HT_3$ agonists have proved efficacy for patients with diarrhoea-predominant irritable bowel syndrome
(d) Tegaserod is efficacious for patients with constipation-predominant irritable bowel syndrome
(e) Most patients with irritable bowel syndrome become asymptomatic within 10 years of diagnosis

3   Which of the following are true about irritable bowel syndrome?
(a) Polymorphisms of the serotonin transporter protein that reduce synaptic sensory signalling have been implicated

(b) A parent with irritable bowel syndrome is a risk factor for irritable bowel syndrome in the offspring

(c) Gastroenteritis is a risk factor for subsequent irritable bowel syndrome

(d) Strong evidence supports relaxation therapy in patients with irritable bowel syndrome with significant anxiety

(e) Dysfunction of the autonomic nervous system has been documented

Neuroendocrine tumours of the gastrointestinal tract and pancreas

1   Which of the following inherited conditions is associated with an increased incidence of pancreatic endocrine tumours?
(a) Multiple endocrine neoplasia type 1
(b) Von Hippel Lindau disease
(c) Type 1 neurofibromatosis
(d) Multiple endocrine neoplasia type 2
(e) Familial adenomatous polyposis

2   Which of the following investigations is likely to be useful for assessment of a gastric carcinoid tumour?
(a) Ultrasound scan
(b) Endoscopy with biopsy
(c) Assessment of gastric pH
(d) Measurement of fasting serum gastrin
(e) ^{123}I-MIBG scan

3   Which of the following treatments should be considered in a patient with a small bowel carcinoid tumour and liver metastases?
(a) Long acting somatostatin analogues
(b) Radiofrequency ablation of liver metastases
(c) Systemic chemotherapy
(d) Resection of small bowel tumour
(e) ^{90}Y-DOTATOC treatment

Biomedical review – inflammation and cancer

1   Inflammatory mediators may increase the risk of neoplasia by:
(a) Downregulating COX-2 expression
(b) Upregulating HIF-α expression in hypoxic tissues
(c) Increasing apoptosis and cellular proliferation
(d) Direct damage to the DNA of resident stem cells
(e) Setting up cytokine networks that promote transformed cells

2   *Helicobacter pylori*-induced gastric cancer is:
(a) Increasing at an alarming rate in the developed world
(b) Associated with gastric atrophy and hypochlorhydria

(c) More common in people with a history of duodenal ulcers

(d) Increased in people with proinflammatory cytokine gene polymorphisms

(e) Potentially preventable if *H. pylori* is eradicated at an early stage

3   Inflammation-induced cancers of the gastrointestinal tract

(a) May be prevented with COX-2 inhibitors

(b) Are invariably associated with an infective aetiology

(c) Respond better to chemotherapy

(d) Commonly share pathways with a prominent role for NF-ÎB

(e) Are a major burden on health resources in the world

Neurology

Stroke: advances in acute treatment and secondary prevention

Peter Sandercock

Recently, it has become clear that patients with transient ischaemic attacks (TIA) and suspected acute stroke should be treated much more rapidly that at present – that is, with assessment, diagnosis, and intervention completed within hours rather than days or weeks. This review covers the evidence that has emerged over the past two years or so to support this major change in clinical practice. Increased investment will be needed not only in acute stroke care services but also in stroke research – two areas that are underfunded compared with heart disease.[1,2]

☐ BURDEN OF ACUTE DISEASE

The Oxford Vascular Study (OXVASC) recently showed that the age-specific rates of non-fatal stroke are higher than those for acute myocardial infarction and acute events related to peripheral vascular disease.[1] The OXVASC study also confirmed that the incidences of stroke and TIA rise steeply with age.

☐ EARLY RISK AFTER MINOR STROKE AND TRANSIENT ISCHAEMIC ATTACK

The OXVASC study applied very careful epidemiological methods to the assessment of prognosis after TIA and minor ischaemic stroke. This study clearly showed that:[3]

- ☐ the early risk of stroke is much higher than was previously thought

- ☐ the risk of stroke is higher for patients with a minor stroke than those with a transient ischaemic attack (about 12% risk of stroke within seven days of a minor stroke and 8% within seven days of a TIA).

If services for acute cerebrovascular disease are to be effective, and disabling stroke to be prevented, patients clearly will need to be assessed and treated on the day of the event. This will need considerable efforts to educate the public, primary care teams, and staff in emergency departments.[2] To meet this need, the Stroke Association has launched a campaign 'Stroke is a medical emergency'. Much more needs to be done, however – general practitioners will need their local hospitals to provide better systems for rapid referral and emergency departments will need to be given altered priorities. If patients are discharged home only after a brief triage assessment, they are at considerable risk of having a disabling stroke while waiting for an appointment at the TIA clinic.[4] The need to achieve 'four hour wait targets' in emergency departments and the pressure to assess and discharge patients as quickly as possible thus must be balanced against the need for an appropriately complete 'on the spot' cerebrovascular assessment (including 'same-day' computed tomography and Doppler examination) to maximise the chance of preventing major stroke.

☐ PATIENTS MOST LIKELY TO BENEFIT FROM CAROTID ENDARTERECTOMY

Patients with a TIA or minor ischaemic stroke related to a severe stenosis of the relevant carotid artery are likely to benefit from carotid endarterectomy. A pooled analysis of the carotid endarterectomy trials, however, showed quite clearly that the net benefit from carotid endarterectomy declines very steeply with time from the index event.[5] Patients with the most severe degree of stenosis (70–99% stenosis measured by the method of the North American Symptomatic Carotid Endarter-ectomy Trial) benefit if surgery is done 2–4 weeks after the index event. For patients with a lesser degree of stenosis (50–69%), however, surgery must be done within two weeks for them to gain a net benefit. A recent audit of time to assessment, imaging, and endarterectomy in Oxfordshire showed that the median time to assessment was nine days, to imaging of the carotid 33 days, and to surgery 100 days. These figures are likely to be moderately representative of the situation in many other parts of the country. If this is the case, many patients are having entirely preventable strokes merely because the system is operating so slowly.[4] Furthermore, many carotid endarterectomies are being done at a time when there is little or no scope for benefit from the operation.

☐ PATIENTS MOST LIKELY TO BENEFIT FROM SURGERY

Detailed modelling studies have helped to identify patients at highest risk of stroke without surgery, and colour-coded risk charts have been drawn up.[6] These take into account the patient's age and sex, the nature of their attack (TIA, stroke, or episode of ocular ischaemia), the type of carotid stenosis (smooth or ulcerated), the degree of stenosis, and time since their most recent event (measured in weeks). These charts enable doctors to identify patients at highest risk of stroke while on medical treatment. Patients at highest risk derive the greatest absolute benefit from surgery, as the risk of operative stroke is relatively constant across all the above risk categories.[6]

☐ CAROTID STENTING, ANGIOPLASTY, AND CAROTID ENDARTERECTOMY

Five completed trials have compared endovascular treatment with carotid endarter-ectomy.[7] The Cochrane systematic review of these trials, which included 1,157 patients, showed that endovascular treatment and carotid endarterectomy have similar early risks of death and stroke and similar long-term benefits and that carotid angioplasty and stenting avoid cranial neuropathy.[7] Uncertainties exist about the safety of carotid stenting, however, and at least one trial has been stopped early because of concerns over this issue. Concern also exists that endovascular treatment has the potential for restenosis, with an associated risk of recurrent stroke. The authors concluded that current evidence does not support a widespread change in clinical practice away from recommending carotid endarterectomy as the treatment of choice for suitable carotid artery stenosis. They also recommended that current randomised trials that are comparing carotid stenting with endarterectomy should continue to recruit patients (Box 1).

Box 1 Current randomised trials comparing carotid stenting with endarterectomy.

- Carotid Revascularization Endarterectomy versus Stenting Trial (CREST)
- Endarterectomy versus Angioplasty in Patients with Symptomatic Severe Carotid Stenosis (EVA 3S)
- International Carotid Stenting Study (ICSS)
- Stentgeschützte Perkutane Angioplastie der Carotis versus Endarterektomie (SPACE)

☐ ORGANISING IMMEDIATE ASSESSMENT

Suspected transient ischaemic attacks

Good evidence shows that patients who present to hospital with suspected TIA or stroke should be assessed and investigated promptly. If possible, this should be on the day that the patient first makes contact with the hospital system. Referral to a 'fast track neurovascular clinic' will – even in the best of circumstances – merely introduce a delay of a week or so, during which a disabling stroke may occur. For patients whose symptoms have completely recovered or are recovering very rapidly at the time of presentation, any patient considered at high early risk of stroke should be admitted immediately. If validated in an independent cohort, the ABCD score has the promise of identifying such patients (Box 2).[8]

Box 2 ABCD score.

- **A**ge of patients
- **B**lood pressure
- **C**linical features with which patients present
- **D**uration of symptoms of transient ischaemic attack

Suspected stroke

For patients whose symptoms are not resolving rapidly by the time they reach hospital, immediate triage in the emergency department is needed to select patients with ischaemic stroke who may be candidates for thrombolytic therapy. In centres with well organised services for stroke thrombolysis, paramedics already will have performed an initial screening of the patient with a simple clinical screening tool during the ambulance journey to hospital and will have prealerted the thrombolysis team to meet the ambulance when it arrives. The face, arm and speech test (FAST) is simple and easy to use and has been validated for use by paramedics and triage nurses.[9]

If the patient has an acute focal neurological deficit, the time of onset is known with certainty, and the patient has no obvious contraindications for thrombolysis (for example, very high or very low blood levels of glucose), the patient should be fast tracked for computed tomography. A member of the thrombolysis team should assess the patient briefly as they are going into the scanner. Acute stroke doctors must be able to detect mimics of stroke on clinical examination and should be sufficiently competent with interpretation of computed tomograms to reliably exclude intracranial haemorrhage (an absolute contraindication to thrombolytic treatment) and detect the presence of subtle early ischaemic changes. Such changes are not necessarily a contraindication to thrombolytic treatment, but they are helpful and provide some reassurance that the patient's focal neurological deficit is indeed the result of an ischaemic stroke and not the result of some other mechanism that would not necessarily be helped by thrombolysis (such as migraine). For training in interpretation of computed tomograms, see the British Association of Stroke Physicians' website (www.neuroimage.co.uk/basp/).

☐ THROMBOLYTIC TREATMENT

Thrombolytic treatment within European licence

If the patient is younger than 80 years and meets all the criteria set out in the licence (Box 3), they can be considered for treatment. The patient should accept that, although they have a strong likelihood of net benefit, the risk of fatal intracranial haemorrhage associated with treatment is 3%. The usual regimen is intravenous recombinant plasminogen activator (rt-PA), given at a dose of 0.9 mg/kg (10% as bolus over one minute and the remainder as an infusion over one hour). Treatment should be administered in an environment with adequate levels of nursing staff and facilities to monitor the patient's clinical and physiological state during and shortly after the infusion. Medical and nursing staff must be familiar with the relevant neurological assessments and the management of complications of thrombolytic treatment (bleeding, life threatening angioneurotic oedema, etc).

Substantial variation exists in the use of rt-PA for the treatment of acute ischaemic stroke 'within licence' across Europe, with a more than 50-fold variation in the number of patients treated per million population. The register of the Safe Implementation of Thrombolysis in Stroke Monitoring Study (SITS-MOST) indicates that about 85 patients per million are treated in Finland, but about only one or two per million apparently are treated in France (www.acutestroke.org/). This variation in implementation does not necessarily represent variation in the quality of medical care between these two countries. A plausible explanation is that the use of thrombolytic treatment in France is underreported, but anecdotal reports suggest that the figures for the United Kingdom, Greece, and Portugal probably are accurate.

Remaining research questions

At least some of the variation in use must represent uncertainties about the place of thrombolytic treatment in routine clinical practice. Uncertainty exists about

Box 3 Brief summary of criteria in licence for thrombolysis for patients younger than 80 years.

- No recognised contraindications to thrombolysis
- Clinical and radiological features consistent with an acute ischaemic stroke
- Reliably known time of stroke onset
- Treatment can be started within three hours of onset

whether to treat patients presenting within three hours who do not exactly meet the current terms of the licence. Substantial controversy exists over whether and how the extent and severity of 'early ischaemic change' on computed tomograms should guide selection for treatment. Considerable debate surrounds whether more advanced imaging methods (for example, magnetic resonance diffusion and perfusion weighted imaging, computed tomographic perfusion imaging, magnetic resonance angiography) may provide more effective selection criteria than plain computed tomography. These technologies are not available widely in many countries, however, and even if they are available, they certainly often are not available to most patients with acute stroke. Computed tomography therefore must remain the 'workhorse' imaging method for acute stroke in most centres.

Current trials

Four main trials of intravenous thrombolytic therapy are underway (Box 4). Of these, the Medical Research Council (MRC)'s Third International Stroke Trial (IST-3) is the only 'cardiological scale' trial that is comparable with the large-scale trials of thrombolytic therapy in acute myocardial infarction undertaken in the 1980s. The preliminary phase of the trial began in 2000, and the phase funded by the MRC began in 2005. It is an international, multicentre, prospective, randomised, open blinded, endpoint study of intravenous rt-PA compared with control in 6,000 patients with acute ischaemic stroke within six hours of onset. Full details of the protocol are available at www.ist3.com. Final results are expected in 2009–10.

Box 4 Main trials of intravenous thrombolytic therapy.

- Third International Stroke Trial (IST-3)
- Echoplanar Imaging Thrombolysis Evaluation Trial (EPITHET)
- Desmoteplase in Acute Ischemic Stroke-2 (DIAS-2)
- European Cooperative Acute Stroke Study-3 (ECASS-3)

☐ OTHER ASPECTS OF ACUTE STROKE CARE

Other aspects of acute stroke care are being researched actively. A recent Phase III trial has shown promising benefit for the neuroprotectant NXY-059 in acute ischaemic stroke. Recombinant factor VII seems promising for the treatment of primary intracerebral haemorrhage, although some uncertainties about the risk of thromboembolic complications remain, and confirmatory trials are underway. The recent Surgical Trial in Intracerebral Haemorrhage (STICH) of surgery to remove acute intracerebral haematomas did not provide evidence to support a policy of routine evacuation of acute spontaneous intracerebral haematomas. For patients who experience massive swelling of the cerebral hemisphere after major middle cerebral artery occlusion, hemicraniectomy may be a lifesaving procedure, but the balance of risk and benefit is being assessed in a number of trials (Box 5).

Box 5 Trials of hemicraniectomy.

- Hemicraniectomy and Durotomy Upon Deterioration From Infarction Related Swelling (HEADFIRST)
- Hemicraniectomy After MCA infarction with Life-threatening Edema Trial (HAMLET)
- Hemicraniectomy For Malignant Middle Cerebral Artery Infarcts (HeMMI)
- Decompressive Surgery for the Treatment of Malignant Infarction of the Middle Cerebral Artery (DESTINY)

The use of intravenous fluids and the optimal feeding strategy (none, nasogastric feeding, or percutaneous gastrostomy) were recently evaluated in the Feed Or Ordinary Diet (FOOD) trials. Management of blood pressure in the acute phase of stroke is under evaluation (Box 6). Evidence suggests that glucose insulin therapy is helpful in the acute phase of myocardial infarction, and the Glucose Insulin Stroke Trial (GIST) is evaluating this in acute stroke. Graded compression stockings often are recommended for patients at risk of deep vein thrombosis and pulmonary embolism after stroke, but the evidence base is very limited. The MRC's Clots in Legs Or TEDs after Stroke (CLOTS) trials are evaluating graded compression stockings: stockings compared with no stockings and below knee stockings compared with above knee stockings (www.dcn.ed.ac.uk/clots/).

Box 6 Trials of management of blood pressure in the acute phase of stroke.

- Efficacy of Nitric Oxide in Stroke (ENOS)
- Continue Or Stop post-Stroke Antihypertensives Collaborative Study (COSSACS)
- Controlling Hypertension and Hypotension Immediately Post-Stroke Trial (CHHIPS)
- Scandinavian Candesartan Acute Stroke Trial (SCAST)

☐ DEVELOPMENT IN SERVICES

The management of patients with acute cerebrovascular syndromes is changing very rapidly. Transient ischaemic attacks and stroke now clearly should be treated as an emergency, and indeed are being treated as such in some places. If all patients in the United Kingdom are to receive care to the standards suggested by the evidence, however, an enormous increase in capacity will be needed in the acute stroke care systems in almost all acute hospitals in the United Kingdom. The capacity to deliver thrombolytic therapy is thin and patchy at present, and major changes in the delivery of acute stroke care will be needed if we are to implement thrombolytic therapy in an evidence-based and equitable manner. Further investment in acute stroke services may be needed if IST-3 shows that a wider range of patients can benefit from thrombolysis. All doctors with an interest in stroke management hope that the government will continue to invest in building capacity in cerebrovascular services and cerebrovascular research to ensure that services for patients with acute cerebrovascular syndromes are as well resourced as services (and research efforts) for acute forms of heart disease.[10]

REFERENCES

1 Rothwell PM, Coull AJ, Silver LE *et al.* Population-based study of event-rate, incidence, case fatality, and mortality for all acute vascular events in all arterial territories (Oxford Vascular Study). *Lancet* 2005;366:1773–83.

2 National Audit Office. *Reducing brain damage: faster access to better stroke care.* London: Stationery Office, 2005.

3 Coull AJ, Lovett JK, Rothwell PM. Population based study of early risk of stroke after transient ischaemic attack or minor stroke: implications for public education and organisation of services. *BMJ* 2004;328:326.

4 Fairhead JF, Mehta Z, Rothwell PM. Population-based study of delays in carotid imaging and surgery and the risk of recurrent stroke. *Neurology* 2005;65:371–5.

5 Rothwell PM, Eliasziw M, Gutnikov SA, Warlow CP, Barnett HJ. Endarterectomy for symptomatic carotid stenosis in relation to clinical subgroups and timing of surgery. *Lancet* 2004;363:915–24.

6 Rothwell PM, Mehta Z, Howard SC, Gutnikov SA, Warlow CP. Treating individuals 3: from subgroups to individuals: general principles and the example of carotid endarterectomy. *Lancet* 2005;365:256–65.

7 Coward LJ, Featherstone RL, Brown MM. Safety and efficacy of endovascular treatment of carotid artery stenosis compared with carotid endarterectomy: a Cochrane systematic review of the randomized evidence. *Stroke* 2005;36:905–11.

8 Rothwell PM, Giles MF, Flossmann E *et al.* A simple score (ABCD) to identify individuals at high early risk of stroke after transient ischaemic attack. *Lancet* 2005;366:29–36.

9 Nor AM, McAllister C, Louw SJ *et al.* Agreement between ambulance paramedic- and physician-recorded neurological signs with Face Arm Speech Test (FAST) in acute stroke patients. *Stroke* 2004;35:1355–9.

10 Jenkinson D, Ford GA. Research and development in stroke services. *BMJ* 2006;332:318.

Mitochondrial disorders – more common than you thought?

Patrick F Chinnery

☐ INTRODUCTION

Until relatively recently, mitochondrial disorders were considered to be obscure, exceptionally rare diseases that affected perhaps one or two per million of the population. Only a limited number of centres throughout the world had clinical and laboratory expertise in mitochondrial medicine, and a general lack of awareness of mitochondrial disease by non-specialist doctors left many patients undiagnosed. The complete sequencing of the human mitochondrial genome (mtDNA) in 1981, followed by the identification of pathogenic mtDNA mutations in 1989, however, led to a surge of interest in human mitochondrial disease in the early 1990s. These advances paved the way for future epidemiological studies that clearly show that mitochondrial disorders are among the most common inherited human diseases.

☐ WHAT ARE MITOCHONDRIAL DISORDERS?

Mitochondria are membrane-bound organelles present within every nucleated cell. They are the principal source of adenosine triphosphate (ATP) – the high energy phosphate molecule needed for all active intracellular processes. Adenosine triphosphate is generated by oxidative phosphorylation, which is carried out by a group of more than 100 proteins situated on the inner mitochondrial membrane and forming the respiratory chain complexes. Reducing equivalents (electrons) are passed from the reduced forms of nicotinamide adenine dinucleotide (NADH) and flavine adenine dinucleotide (FADH2) to complex I and II. They then are passed on to complex III (cytochrome b) and IV (cytochrome c oxidase), pumping protons (H^+) from the mitochondrial matrix into the intermembrane space in the process. This generates an electrochemical gradient that is harnessed by complex V (ATP synthase) to synthesise ATP from adenosine diphosphate (ADP). The term 'mitochondrial disorder' usually means a disorder of oxidative phosphorylation.[1]

Most mitochondrial proteins are synthesised from genes in the cell nucleus, but 13 essential respiratory chain peptides are synthesised within the mitochondria themselves from small circles of DNA – the 16.5 Kb mitochondrial genome or mtDNA (Fig 1).[2] The mtDNA also codes for 24 ribonucleic acids that form part of the protein synthetic machinery within the mitochondrial matrix. Each cell contains many thousands of copies of mtDNA, which are inherited exclusively down the maternal line. The nuclear encoded proteins include:

☐ most of the respiratory chain subunits (including all subunits of complex II, or succinate dehydrogenase)

☐ mitochondrial DNA polymerase (pol γ, encoded by the nuclear gene *POLG1*)

☐ numerous other proteins needed for maintenance of mtDNA, expression of mtDNA, assembly of the respiratory chain, and translocation of nuclear encoded proteins into the mitochondria.

This means that mitochondrial disorders can be autosomal recessive, autosomal dominant, X linked, or inherited maternally (Table 1).

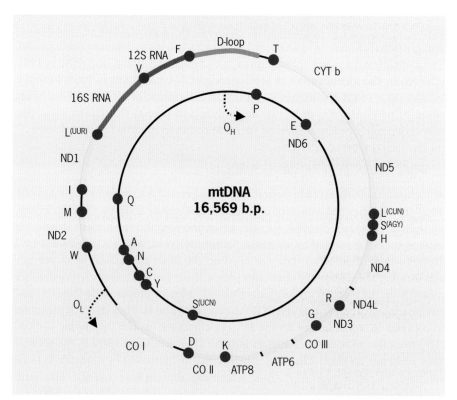

Fig 1 Mitochondrial genome. The human mitochondrial genome (mtDNA) is a small 16,569 kb molecule of double stranded DNA. It encodes for 13 essential components of the respiratory chain. ND1–ND6 and ND4L encode seven subunits of complex I (NADH-ubiquinone oxidoreductase). Cyt b is the only mtDNA encoded complex III subunit (ubiquinol-cytochrome *c* oxidase reductase). COX I to III encode for three of the complex IV (cytochrome *c* oxidase, or COX) subunits, and the ATP 6 and ATP 8 genes encode for two subunits of complex V (ATP synthase). Two ribosomal RNA genes (12S and 16S rRNA) and 22 transfer RNA genes are interspaced between the protein encoding genes. These provide the RNA components needed for intramitochondrial protein synthesis. D-loop is the 1.1 kb non-coding region involved in regulation of transcription and replication of the molecule. It is the only region not involved directly in the synthesis of respiratory chain polypeptides. O_H and O_L are the origins of heavy and light strand mtDNA replication. Adapted from Chinnery et al.[2]

Table 1 Genetic classification of human mitochondrial disorders.

Disorder	Inheritance pattern
Primary mitochondrial DNA disorders*	
Rearrangements (large scale partial deletions and duplications)	
Chronic progressive external ophthalmoplegia	Sporadic or maternal
Kearns-Sayre syndrome	Sporadic or maternal
Diabetes and deafness	Sporadic
Pearson marrow-pancreas syndrome	Sporadic or maternal
Sporadic tubulopathy	Sporadic
Point mutations	
Protein encoding genes	
Leber hereditary optic neuropathy (11778G>A, 14484T>C, and 3460G>A)	Maternal
Neurogenetic weakness with ataxia and retinitis pigmentosa or Leigh syndrome (8993T>G/C)	Maternal
tRNA genes	
Mitochondrial encephalomyopathy with lactic acidosis and stroke like episodes (3243A>G, 3271T>C, and 3251A>G)	Maternal
Myoclonic epilepsy with ragged red fibres (8344A>G and 8356T>C)	Maternal
Chronic progressive external ophthalmoplegia (3243A>G and 4274T>C)	Maternal
Myopathy (14709T>C and 12320A>G)	Maternal
Cardiomyopathy (3243A>G, 4269A>G, and 4300A>G)	Maternal
Diabetes and deafness (3243A>G and 12258C>A)	Maternal
Encephalomyopathy (1606G>A and 10010T>C)	Maternal
rRNA genes	
Non-syndromic sensorineural deafness (7445A>G)	Maternal
Aminoglycoside induced non-syndromic deafness (1555A>G)	Maternal
Nuclear genetic disorders	
Disorders of mtDNA maintenance	
Autosomal dominant progressive external ophthalmoplegia (with secondary multiple mtDNA deletions)	
Mutations in adenine nucleotide translocator (ANT1)	Autosomal dominant
Mutations in DNA polymerase ? (POLG1)	Autosomal dominant or autosomal recessive
Mutations in Twinkle helicase (C10ORF2)	Autosomal dominant
Mitochondrial neurogastrointestinal encephalomyopathy (with secondary multiple mtDNA deletions)	
Mutations in thymidine phosphorylase (TP)	Autosomal recessive
Myopathy with mtDNA depletion Mutations in thymidine kinase (TK2)	Autosomal recessive
Encephalopathy with liver failure Mutations in deoxyguanosine kinase (DGUOK)	Autosomal recessive
Primary disorders of the respiratory chain	
Leigh syndrome	
Complex I deficiency – mutations in complex I subunits (NDUFS2,4,7,8 and NDUFV1)	Autosomal recessive
Complex II deficiency – mutations in complex II flavoprotein subunit (SDHA)	Autosomal recessive

continued over

Table 1 Genetic classification of human mitochondrial disorders – *continued*

Disorder	Inheritance pattern
Nuclear genetic disorders – *continued*	
Leukodystrophy and myoclonic epilepsy	
Complex I deficiency – mutations in complex I subunit (*NDUFV1*)	Autosomal recessive
Cardioencephalomyopathy	
Complex I deficiency – mutations in complex I subunit (*NDUFS2*)	Autosomal recessive
Optic atrophy and ataxia	
Complex II deficiency – mutations in complex II flavoprotein subunit *(SDHA)*	Autosomal dominant
Disorders of mitochondrial protein import	
Dystonia-deafness	
Mutations in deafness-dystonia protein DDP1 (TIMM8A)	X linked recessive
Disorders of assembly of the respiratory chain	
Leigh syndrome	
Complex IV deficiency – mutations in COX assembly protein (SURFI)	Autosomal recessive
Complex IV deficiency – mutations in COX assembly protein (COX10)	Autosomal recessive
Cardioencephalomyopathy	
Complex IV deficiency – mutations in COX assembly protein (SCO2)	Autosomal recessive
Hepatic failure and encephalopathy	
Complex IV deficiency – mutations in COX assembly protein (SCO1)	Autosomal recessive
Complex IV deficiency – mutations in protein affecting COX mRNA stability (LRPPRC)	Autosomal recessive
Tubulopathy, encephalopathy and liver failure	
Complex III deficiency – mutations in complex III assembly (BCS1L)	Autosomal recessive
Encephalopathy	
Complex I deficiency – mutations in the complex I assembly protein (B17.2L)	Autosomal recessive
Disorders of RNA metabolism	
Leigh syndrome	
Complex IV deficiency (LRPPRC)	Autosomal recessive
Multiple complex defects (EFG1)	Autosomal recessive
Disorders of the lipid membrane	
Ataxia, seizures, or myopathy	
Coenzyme Q10 deficiency (COQ2)	Autosomal recessive
Barth syndrome (Taffazzin)	X linked recessive

mtDNA=mitochondrial DNA
*mtDNA nucleotide positions refer to the L chain and are taken from the Cambridge reference sequence

☐ PATHOGENIC MUTATIONS OF MTDNA AND HUMAN DISEASE

Pathogenic mutations of mtDNA fall into two groups: deletions (in which regions of the molecule are absent and often multiple genes are involved) and point mutations (that affect a single base pair).[1] The point mutations directly affect the genes coding for the respiratory chain polypeptides or the RNA genes themselves. Mutations in mtDNA are thought to cause disease primarily because they impair oxidative phosphorylation and thus lead to relative deficiency of ATP. Some mutations of mtDNA affect all of the molecules in a cell or individual and thus are called homoplasmic (for example, the mutations that cause Leber hereditary optic neuropathy (LHON) or maternally inherited non-syndromic deafness). In contrast, many patients with mtDNA mutations have a mixture of normal (wild type) and mutated mtDNA within each mitochondrion and are called heteroplasmic. Heteroplasmic deletions of mtDNA are found in chronic progressive external ophthalmoplegia and Kearns-Sayre syndrome. Heteroplasmic point mutations of mtDNA include:[3]

- the common 3243A>G mtDNA tRNA LeuUUR mutation, which first was described in a patient with mitochondrial encephalomyopathy with lactic acidosis and stroke like episodes

- the 8344A>G mtDNA tRNA Lys mutation, which is found in patients with myoclonic epilepsy with ragged red fibres

- the 8993T>C/G ATPase 6 gene mutation, which is found in patients with neurogenic weakness with retinitis pigmentosa.

In general, human cells can tolerate high levels of mutated mtDNA before a biochemical defect of the respiratory chain occurs. Once a critical threshold is exceeded, however, oxidative phosphorylation is impaired. High proportions of mutated mtDNA are associated with a more severe clinical phenotype, but the relation is complex. The proportion of mutated mtDNA can vary between different organs in the same person and also between cells in the same organ. This contributes to the clinical variability, and changing levels of mutated mtDNA probably contribute to clinical progression. Random and non-random processes change the level of mutated and wild type mtDNA over time, and some evidence shows that this is regulated by nuclear genes that yet have to be identified.

Some nuclear genetic defects cause secondary abnormalities of mtDNA that can be qualitative (secondary deletions or secondary point mutations – for example, the results of mutations in the nuclear genes *POLG1*, *ANT1*, *C10ORF2*, and *TP*) or quantitative (for example, loss of mtDNA – called mtDNA depletion – as a result of mutations in the nuclear genes *DGUOK* and *TK2*). These secondary defects are thought to accumulate with time, contributing to the progressive phenotype of these disorders. As the nuclear defect causes an abnormality in mtDNA, the phenotype can be very similar to primary mtDNA disorders and includes the classic mitochondrial phenotype of chronic progressive external ophthalmoplegia, which can be transmitted as a recessive or dominant trait (see Table 1).[4]

□ EPIDEMIOLOGICAL STUDIES OF MITOCHONDRIAL DISORDERS – DIFFICULTIES

Many patients with mitochondrial disease share features with patients with other inherited conditions and common sporadic disorders. For example, diabetes mellitus, stroke, and cardiomyopathy are common features of mitochondrial disease, which makes it difficult to identify clear cut cases on purely clinical grounds. The second problem is the expanding clinical phenotype. Within the last five years, mitochondrial disorders have been linked to novel clinical phenotypes not previously thought to be relevant. Exercise intolerance is a good example of a phenotype that probably was underrecognised in the past. Invasive clinical tests, such as a muscle biopsy, may be needed to make an accurate assessment of individual cases, and interpretation of the results of laboratory investigations can be difficult. For example, muscle histochemistry and respiratory chain complex analysis may be normal in patients with the 3243A>G mtDNA tRNA Leu(UUR) gene mutation and mtDNA deletions are not present always in limb muscle from patients with autosomal dominant progressive external ophthalmoplegia (ad-PEO). Different centres also may disagree on the precise methods and interpretation of biochemical studies. In addition, genetic studies of mtDNA can be challenging, because the mutation in mtDNA may not be detectable in easily accessible tissues.

☐ PHENOTYPE SPECIFIC STUDIES

The first epidemiological surveys followed the identification of specific mtDNA mutations in patients with specific clinical phenotypes. Studies of the 3243A>G mutation in patients with diabetes mellitus are a good example, although similar work has been carried out in cohorts of deaf patients, young patients with stroke, and patients with other disorders. The reported frequency of 3243A>G in patients with diabetes mellitus ranges from 0.13% to 60% depending upon the specific population under study and the study design. No two studies are comparable, and the reported values reflect only the precise cohort under study, which makes it difficult to draw more general conclusions about mtDNA mutations in the general population. These studies have been reviewed previously.[5]

☐ POPULATION BASED STUDIES

Adults

The first population-based study of a single pathogenic mtDNA mutation was carried out in northern Ostrobothnia in Finland.[6] Majamaa and colleagues took advantage of the structured healthcare system in Finland to examine the medical records and identify a cohort of adults with clinical features suggestive of mitochondrial disease from a population of 245,201. Molecular genetic testing of the probands followed by careful family tracing allowed them to estimate the frequency of the 3243A>G mutation in the general population, giving a minimum point prevalence of 16.3 (95% confidence interval 11.3 to 21.4) per 100,000 or one in 6,135.[6] The frequency of the 3243A>G mutation was particularly high in patients from certain disease groups, including those with deafness and a family history of hearing loss (7.4%), occipital stroke (6.9%), ophthalmoplegia (13%), and hypertrophic cardiomyopathy (14%).

The first population-based study of all mitochondrial disorders was carried out in the northeast of England.[7] This study had a different design and was based on the referral of adults with suspected mitochondrial disease to a single centre in Newcastle upon Tyne, which serves a population of 2,122,290. Thorough clinical, biochemical, and genetic studies were carried out on patients referred over a period of 15 years. Family members were studied, and affected relatives who lived within the study region were included in a minimum point-prevalence figure of 6.57 (5.30 to 7.83) per 100,000 or one in 15,220 for the mid-year period in 1997. Further family tracing in unaffected people enabled an estimation of the unaffected carrier rate on the same prevalence date. When these figures were combined, 12.48 per 100,000, or one in 8,013, people within the region were estimated to have mitochondrial disease or be at risk of developing mitochondrial disease on the basis of the strict diagnostic criteria used at the time.[7] As this was an adult population, most affected people were found to harbour pathogenic mtDNA defects, including point mutations that cause LHON (50%), mtDNA rearrangements (predominantly single deletion disorders, 20%), and other mtDNA point mutations (30%). A more detailed clinical and genetic study of LHON refined the prevalence figures for this disorder to 11.82 (10.38 to 13.27) per 100,000,[8] which confirmed the established predominance of the 11778G>A ND4 mutation as a cause of LHON (56%), followed by the 3460G>A ND4 mutation (31%), and the 14484T>C ND6 mutation (6.3%). Rare primary LHON mutations seem to account for about 5% of families. This work established LHON as a major cause of visual failure in young adults (affecting one in 14,067 men) and showed that about one third of families affected by LHON have at least one member who is heteroplasmic for the causative mtDNA mutation.

Clear discrepancies between the results of these two studies were seen. In the northeast of England, prevalence of the 3243A>G (1.41 (0.83 to 1.20) per 100,000) seemed to be 10-fold lower than the prevalence in Finland (see above). Although it is tempting to suggest that the mutation rate of 3243A>G particularly was high in the Finnish population, obvious differences in the study design precluded any firm conclusions. These issues are only just being resolved with ongoing disease surveillance in the northeast of England. The expanding clinical and molecular spectrum of mitochondrial disease, coupled with the development of new molecular techniques to aid the diagnosis of multiple deletion disorders and non-invasive testing for mtDNA point mutations, confirm that the original prevalence figures were an underestimate. Preliminary data suggest that the 3243A>G mutation is present in at least one in 13,000 of the population in northeast England and that the overall prevalence of mitochondrial disorders in adults is substantially greater than originally thought.

Children

The first published study of paediatric mitochondrial disease was based on a population of 358,616 children in Gothenburg, western Sweden, studied intensively over a period of 15 years.[9] Affected children were defined on clinical, biochemical, and molecular genetic grounds, with a strong emphasis on respiratory chain complex assays given the predominance of nuclear genetic disorders in childhood mitochondrial disease. This approach identified 32 affected children younger than

16 years and gave a minimum point prevalence of 4.7 (2.8 to 7.6) per 100,000, or one in 21,277, on 1 January 1999. In preschool children (born between 1984 and 1992), the incidence of mitochondrial encephalomyopathies was 8.9 (5.3 to 14.0) per 100,000, or one in 11,000, which reflects the median age of onset in this group of children aged three months (range: birth to nine years) and the median survival to 12 years of age.[9]

A similar study was carried out at the same time in south Australia on the basis of referrals to the Melbourne Children's Hospital over a period of 10 years.[10] The study used clinical, biochemical, and molecular genetic criteria to determine the minimum birth prevalence of child respiratory disease in 1,706,694 births as 5.0 (4.0 to 6.2) per 100,000, or one in 20,000. Autosomal recessive respiratory chain disorders were more common in Australian children of Lebanese origin, affecting 58.6 (34.7 to 92.6 per 100,000).[10]

Remarkably, these two studies – carried out at opposite ends of the globe – produced almost identical results. A similar proportion of children had a pathogenic mtDNA mutation in both studies, averaging about 15% of the total. These two concordant studies suggest that the figure of one in 20,000 probably is accurate, which makes respiratory chain disorders among the most common inherited metabolic diseases.

☐ NUCLEAR–GENETIC MITOCHONDRIAL DISORDERS: TIP OF THE ICEBERG?

Until 2005, the role of nuclear gene sequencing was limited in adults and was restricted to families with rare dominant chronic progressive external ophthalmoplegia, which can be the result of mutations in three nuclear genes:

☐ *POLG1*, which codes for the mtDNA polymerase

☐ *C10ORF2*, which codes for the mitochondrial helicase Twinkle

☐ *ANT1*, which codes for adenine nucleotide translocase.[4]

These genes code for proteins that maintain mtDNA, and when mutated they cause secondary mtDNA mutations to accumulate in non-dividing cells, such as skeletal muscle cells and neurons, which leads to the clinical phenotype.

The phenotype associated with *POLG1* mutations currently is being described. Dominant and recessive mutations were described first in families with autosomal dominant or recessive chronic progressive external ophthalmoplegia, some with profound sensory ataxic neuropathy.[11] Some of the dominant families have additional features, including parkinsonism and primary gonadal failure. Children may present with recessive mutations in *POLG1* and encephalopathy and liver failure as a result of depletion of mtDNA (Alper-Huttenlocher syndrome).[12] Recessive *POLG1* mutations also have been found in adults with late onset cerebellar ataxia, particularly in Scandinavia – probably as a result of a founder effect in a geographically isolated population.[13] In some of these patients, epilepsy and headache are the presenting features, and these often persist for many years before the more complex phenotype evolves. This poses a particular diagnostic challenge, because, in the early stages, patients with *POLG1* mutations may have the kind of common neurological problems seen every day in general neurology clinics and no family history, only developing a more complex phenotype after 10 or more years.

☐ CONCLUSIONS

Recent epidemiological studies have shown that, as a group, mitochondrial disorders are among the most common metabolic diseases, affecting at least one in 5,000 of the population. Many mitochondrial disorders present in adult life, with features similar to common general medical disorders. This poses a diagnostic challenge, but it is important to think about mitochondrial disease whenever multiple organ systems are involved or when a relevant family history is present. The treatment of mitochondrial disease remains a challenge. Although a recent Cochrane review failed to identify any clear cut evidence in favour of any particular oral treatment agent, specialist supportive care and genetic counselling can have a major impact and new treatments are under evaluation. Prompt diagnosis therefore is important if we are to minimise the impact of this growing group of multisystem diseases.

ACKNOWLEDGEMENTS

Patrick F Chinnery is a Wellcome Trust Senior Fellow In Clinical Science. He also receives support from the Alzheimer's Research Trust, Ataxia UK, United Mitochondrial Diseases Federation, Association Française contre les Myopathies, and European Union (FP6 EUMITOCOMBAT and Mitocircle).

REFERENCES

1 DiMauro S, Schon EA. Mitochondrial respiratory-chain diseases. *N Engl J Med* 2003;348: 2656–68.

2 Chinnery PF, Schon EA. Neuroscience for neurologists: mitochondria. *J Neurol Neurosurg Psychiatry* 2003;74:1188–99.

3 McFarland R, Taylor RW, Turnbull DM. The neurology of mitochondrial DNA disease. *Lancet Neurol* 2002;1:343–51.

4 Zeviani M, Di Donato S. Mitochondrial disorders. *Brain* 2004;127:2153–72.

5 Chinnery PF, Turnbull DM. Epidemiology and treatment of mitochondrial disorders. *Am J Med Genet* 2001;106:94–101.

6 Majamaa K, Moilanen JS, Uimonen S *et al.* Epidemiology of A3243G, the mutation for mitochondrial encephalomyopathy, lactic acidosis, and strokelike episodes: prevalence of the mutation in an adult population. *Am J Hum Genet* 1998;63:447–54.

7 Chinnery PF, Johnson MA, Wardell TM *et al.* The epidemiology of pathogenic mitochondrial DNA mutations. *Ann Neurol* 2000;48:188–93.

8 Man PY, Griffiths PG, Brown DT *et al.* The epidemiology of Leber hereditary optic neuropathy in the north east of England. *Am J Hum Genet* 2003;72:333–9.

9 Darin N, Oldfors A, Moslemi AR, Holme E, Tulinius M. The incidence of mitochondrial encephalomyopathies in childhood: clinical features and morphological, biochemical, and DNA anbormalities. *Ann Neurol* 2001;49:377–83.

10 Skladal D, Halliday J, Thorburn DR. Minimum birth prevalence of mitochondrial respiratory chain disorders in children. *Brain* 2003;126:1905–12.

11 Van Goethem G, Dermaut B, Lofgren A, Martin JJ, Van Broeckhoven C. Mutation of POLG is associated with progressive external ophthalmoplegia characterized by mtDNA deletions. *Nat Genet* 2001;28:211–2.

12 Naviaux RK, Nguyen KV. POLG mutations associated with Alpers' syndrome and mitochondrial DNA depletion. *Ann Neurol* 2004;55:706–12.

13 Hakonen AH, Heiskanen S, Juvonen V *et al.* Mitochondrial DNA polymerase W748S mutation: a common cause of autosomal recessive ataxia with ancient European origin. *Am J Hum Genet* 2005;77:430–41.

☐ NEUROLOGY SELF ASSESSMENT QUESTIONS

Stroke: advances in acute treatment and secondary prevention

1 The following patients are eligible for thrombolytic therapy with rt-PA within the current licence:
(a) Patients who present to hospital three hours after onset
(b) Patients with a normal computed tomogram
(c) Patients older than 80 years
(d) Patients whose symptoms first are noted on waking from overnight sleep
(e) Patients who are aphasic and arrive at hospital unaccompanied

2 In patients with TIA, the risk of stroke within the next seven days is:
(a) 8%
(b) 2%
(c) 20%
(d) Higher if the TIA affects the brain than if it affects the eye
(e) Lower if the relevant carotid artery shows a smooth stenosis rather than an irregular stenosis

3 For patients with symptomatic carotid stenosis >70%, carotid endarterectomy:
(a) Is inferior to carotid stenting
(b) Gives only modest benefit if surgery is delayed by more than two weeks
(c) Has about similar operative risks among patients at high and low risk of stroke when treated medically
(d) Has about the same risks of stroke, myocardial infarction, and vascular death at 30 days as carotid stenting and angioplasty
(e) Has a likelihood of benefit from surgery that involves cholesterol level as a major determinant

Mitochondrial disorders – more common than you thought?

1 Mitochondrial disorders:
(a) All are inherited maternally
(b) Usually present in childhood
(c) Often cause cardiomyopathy
(d) Can present with stroke
(e) Rarely cause diabetes

2 Mitochondrial DNA:
(a) Is inherited maternally
(b) Codes for most mitochondrial proteins
(c) Is present with many copies in each cell
(d) Mutations are a common cause of mitochondrial disorders in adults
(e) Is deleted in people with Kearns-Sayre syndrome

3   Nuclear-genetic mitochondrial disorders:
   (a) Rarely present in adult life
   (b) Always are familial
   (c) May cause a secondary mtDNA abnormality
   (d) Can be X-linked
   (e) Often cause myopathy

Rehabilitation

Rehabilitation following neurological injury

Lynne Turner-Stokes

☐ WHAT IS REHABILITATION?

Rehabilitation may be defined in terms of concept and service:[1]

- ☐ **Conceptual definition**: a process of active change by which a person who has become disabled acquires the knowledge and skills needs for optimal physical, psychological, and social function

- ☐ **Service definition**: the use of all means to minimise the impact of disabling conditions and to assist disabled people to achieve their desired level of autonomy and participation in society.

In practical terms, it combines three principal approaches, which typically proceed in parallel:

1 **restoration of damaged function** – for example, therapies to restore control of motor activities, such as the ability to stand, walk, speak, etc

2 **compensation for lost function** – for example, provision of equipment and adaptations to the home environment to enable an individual to live independently

3 **adjustment to change** – supporting the individual and their family to come to terms with changes in their lifestyle and aspirations after the onset of acquired disability.

Key texts and initiatives

Until recently, 'rehabilitation' has been considered a 'Cinderella specialty' within medical practice, with poor investment and service provision. In recent years, however, a number of key strategy documents have included rehabilitation as a key component of their recommendations, which has led to greater recognition of its effectiveness. These include:

- ☐ *National clinical guidelines for stroke*[2]

- ☐ *National clinical guidelines for rehabilitation following acquired brain injury*[3]

- ☐ *National service framework for long-term conditions.*[4]

Evidence for effectiveness

A growing body of evidence supports the effectiveness of rehabilitation,[5,6] especially when it is provided in a coordinated fashion by an interdisciplinary team of rehabilitation professionals who are all working towards the same agreed goals.[7] Involvement of the patient and their family in goal-setting and decision-making is a critical part of the process,[7] and hence patient-centred care and individual-care planning was strongly emphasised in the *National service framework for long-term conditions.*

World Health Organization's *International classification of functioning disability and health*

The World Health Organization (WHO) has published a framework for describing the impact of disabling disease on a given individual in terms of their bodily function and their ability to participate in society. The original *International classification of impairments, disabilities and handicaps* (ICIDH) published in 1980 considered illness at four levels (table 1).[8]

Table 1 World Health Organization's ICIDH classification (1980).

Classification	Description
Pathology	The **pathological diagnosis** describes the damage within an organ or organ system – for example, 'cerebrovascular infarct' or 'traumatic brain injury'
Impairment	The **direct physiological consequence** of underlying pathology – the symptoms and signs – for example, hemiparesis, paraparesis, hemianopia, etc
Disability ('activity')	The **functional loss** resulting from impairment – for example, reduced mobility or needing help to get dressed
Handicap ('participation')	The **social disadvantage** imposed by the disability – for example, loss of employment or marital breakdown

Reproduced with permission of the World Health Organization.[8]

Although this classification proved very useful from a clinical perspective, it did not meet with universal approbation from many disabled people themselves. This 'medical model' tends to view disability as a problem of the 'disabled individual', arising from their impairment. The groups who represent disabled people have fought to change the public view to adopt a 'social model' of disability that lays responsibility back on society and the environment, which fail to allow the individual to function to the best of their ability. Instead of focusing on what an individual **cannot** do, this model focuses on what they **can** do. 'Disability' and 'handicap' are replaced with 'activity' and 'participation', respectively. These terms have now been incorporated into the WHO's updated *International classification of functioning disability and health* (ICF).[9] The ICF describes a health condition in terms of its impact on 'body functions and structure', activity, and participation in life situations (Fig 1). In addition, it places the individual's experience in the context of environmental factors (including the physical, social, and attitudinal environment in which the person lives) and personal factors (including their character, beliefs, behaviours, and coping styles).

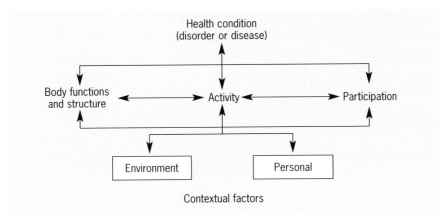

Fig 1 World Health Organization's updated *International classification of functioning disability and health.* Reproduced with permission from the World Health Organization.[9]

☐ THE CHALLENGE OF PROVIDING REHABILITATION IN NEUROLOGICAL CONDITIONS

'Neurological injury' includes any damage to the nervous system that results in injury to the central or peripheral nervous system, including:

- ☐ **trauma** due to accidental injury, assault or post-surgical damage

- ☐ **vascular accident** due to haemorrhage or infarction

- ☐ **infection** (for example, meningitis or encephalitis) or other **inflammation** (for example, vasculitis or demyelination)

- ☐ **toxic or metabolic insult** (for example, anoxia or hypoglycaemia)

- ☐ **degeneration** (for example, motor neurone disease or Parkinson's disease).

Neurological conditions present a number of challenges for rehabilitation service provision:

- ☐ Individuals present with a wide diversity of impairment (including physical, cognitive, communicative, emotional, and behavioural problems) and also with widely varying limitations in terms of activity and societal participation.

- ☐ Neurological conditions affect not just the individual but also their family and friends. They typically last for life, with needs changing over time.

- ☐ A range of different services is needed to support this heterogeneous group of people, but the numbers are relatively small.

- ☐ Neurological conditions are not 'sexy or emotive' in the same way as cancer or heart attacks, yet services are expensive to provide.

Different patients need different types of rehabilitation

Neurological conditions present in a variety of different patterns. The *National service framework for long-term conditions* divided patients into three main groups:

☐ **Sudden onset conditions** – for example, acquired brain or spinal cord injury – start with catastrophic onset of disability followed by recovery to a greater or lesser extent.

☐ **Intermittent conditions** – for example, relapsing–remitting multiple sclerosis – may occur unpredictably, with variable periods of normal function in between.

☐ **Progressive conditions** – for example, motor neurone disease or Parkinson's disease – present with gradual accrual of disability over a time course that again is variable: some conditions progress rapidly to death within a few months while others deteriorate over many years.

Each individual therefore has a unique set of needs and requires different programmes of rehabilitation. Moreover, the same individual will often need different programmes of rehabilitation at different stages in their recovery or progression. Taking acquired brain injury as an example:

☐ Rehabilitation starts as soon as possible, even in the acute stages of intensive care in hospital. Interventions at this stage typically focus on reducing impairment and preventing secondary complications (pathology), such as contractures, malnutrition, pressure sores, pneumonia, etc.

☐ As the patient starts to recover, intensive inpatient rehabilitation may be needed to make the successful transition between hospital and community. Post-acute rehabilitation primarily addresses regaining mobility and independence in self-care to allow the individual to manage safely at home. Interventions tend therefore to focus on improving activity and independence (reducing disability).

☐ Once back in the community, patients need continued input to maximise their ability to function in their environment. In community-based rehabilitation, the emphasis is usually on more extended activities of daily living (EADL), social integration, and return to work or education. Interventions at this stage focus more on enhanced participation, improved quality of life, psychological adjustment, and carer stress.

These main stages are illustrated by the 'Slinky model' of rehabilitation,[10] which summarises the phases of rehabilitation (Fig 2).[3] Patients need to access different services as they progress, but their transition between services should be smoothed by excellent communication and sharing of information between services so that (like a 'slinky' toy) they progress in a seamless continuum of care through the different stages.

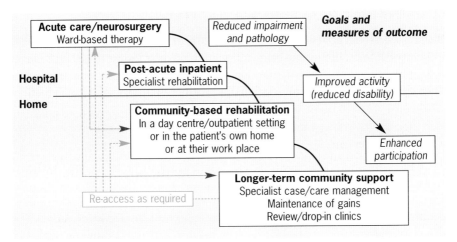

Fig 2 Slinky model of the phases of rehabilitation.[3]

Considerable debate has surrounded whether services should be based in the hospital or community. This is obviously the wrong question – the answer is clearly 'both'. It is not helpful to consider the benefits of one particular service in isolation. The important challenge is to make sure that each patient can access the service most appropriate to their needs at the time they need it.

Although the Slinky model provides a useful illustration of the need for different services at different stages, with seamless continuity of care, the real picture is much more complex and three-dimensional. Within each stage, a range of different service providers, which must somehow be coordinated, are involved, and these services change with the stage of rehabilitation. Fig 3 illustrates some of the different components of community rehabilitation.

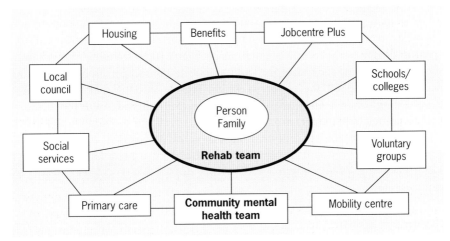

Fig 3 Some components of community rehabilitation.

☐ SOME SPECIFIC AREAS OF MANAGEMENT IN REHABILITATION

Being asked to sum up rehabilitation in the course of a short paper is somewhat akin to Monty Python's 'all England competition to summarise Proust'! The best I can do is to provide a few practical tips for general physicians who find themselves managing patients with neurological disability while awaiting formal rehabilitation. Further information is available in published papers.[3,11]

24-hour management

A 24-hour programme of postural care and management is essential to avoid secondary complications such as pressure sores or soft tissue damage. Regular stretching of joints and muscles will help to maintain muscle length and prevent deformity, but, perhaps even more important, it is the mainstay for management of spasticity. Early intervention with botulinum toxin followed by splints or plaster casting is increasingly being shown to be effective in the prevention of contracture and deformity, and guidelines are now published for the use of botulinum toxin in this context.[12]

Sitting and standing programmes

Neurological injury – especially spinal cord injury – typically leads to loss of cardiovascular and postural reflexes. Gravitational challenge is important to maintain these reflexes, as well as to reduce osteopenia, encourage air entry into lung spaces, and increase awareness and trunk control. As soon as possible, the paralysed patient should be sat out in a wheelchair. It is important, however, that the chair provides an appropriate level of postural support to maintain alignment of the head and trunk and to avoid sheering strains on the skin. Attention should be paid in particular to the position of the pelvis – posterior pelvic tilt, which leads to sheering strains on the sacral and ischial skin, should be avoided. A 'tilt-in-space' seating package is often needed in the early stages – a standard 8L wheelchair rarely being appropriate – but support can then gradually be withdrawn as trunk and head control return.

As soon as possible, the patient should be brought into the standing position. A tilt-table can be used from the early stages, with gradually increasing periods of time spent in progressively vertical orientation. At a later stage, standing frames can be used to support the individual in standing, freeing their upper limbs for function use, but at this point the patient is weight bearing through their feet and it is therefore important to ensure that the feet are properly aligned. Ankle foot orthoses may be needed to maintain correct alignment.

In due course, the patient may then progress to assisted walking – either supported by therapy staff or (increasingly these days) using a harness treadmill. Regular walking practice effectively allows the affected side to relearn a reciprocal gait pattern from the good side.

Bladder management

The bladder and bowel are largely controlled by reflexes, and they usually function automatically to some degree after brain and spinal cord injury. With careful bladder and bowel regimens, it is usually possible to restore bladder and bowel continence, even though they are not under full voluntary control. This process, however, requires an understanding of the underlying physiology and very careful attention to detail.

Urinary control is normally coordinated in the micturition centre in the pons. Neurological damage to pathways above this level may limit awareness and voluntary control over bladder function, but the detrusor and sphincter muscles themselves continue to work automatically in coordinated fashion. Injury below this level, however, for example in the spinal cord, may disrupt coordination, leading to detrusor–sphincter dyssynergia and failure of bladder emptying.

Prolonged indwelling catheterisation should be avoided wherever possible, introducing instead a toileting regimen and, if necessary, intermittent clean (or sterile) catheterisation (ICC). Careful monitoring of bladder function using 24 voided-volume charts and post-micturition bladder scans provides most of the information needed – urodynamics being reserved for the more complex cases. In patients with spinal cord injury, it is important to ensure that the bladder does not fill beyond 500 ml – so the timing of ICC is adjusted accordingly. For persistent residual volumes >50 ml, catheterisation should be undertaken at least once in each 24 hours, even if spontaneous voiding is occurring. Urethral stricture is a not uncommon sequel to prolonged indwelling catheterisation, especially in men and those with larger gauge catheters. This diagnosis should be considered in the presence of recurrent urinary tract infection or persisting dysuria in the absence of infection. The investigation of choice is a retrograde urethrogram.

Bowel management

The rectum is normally empty between evacuations. If this state can be established, faecal continence can usually be maintained, even if the individual does not have voluntary control. The two secrets are avoiding constipation (which is extremely common after neurological injury) and a careful bowel regimen to ensure complete emptying of the rectum.

Constipation should be carefully avoided by:

☐ ensuring adequate fluid and a suitable diet

☐ avoiding constipating drugs

☐ a regular standing/exercise regimen

☐ privacy during evacuation – preferably on a toilet.

Our recommended bowel regimen is shown in box 1.[11]

Autonomic dysreflexia

Autonomic dysreflexia is another important but often poorly understood phenomenon. It occurs as a result of disassociation of the sympathetic and parasympathetic nervous system in patients with spinal cord lesions above the level of

Box 1 Bowel regimen for use in neurological injury.

- **Timing** – find out when the patient usually open their bowels and sit them on the toilet at that time
- **If nothing happens, make it happen** using suppositories, a microenema, or digital stimulation
- **If the rectum is empty**, bring down faeces from above using a bulk or osmotic laxative, such as lactulose
- **If nothing happens for three days running**, use a stimulant laxative (such as senna) on the third night
- **In the case of resistant constipation**, a plain abdominal x-ray is performed to confirm a loaded bowel and exclude other obvious pathology. A vigorous bowel clearing programme of enemas and strong laxatives (such as sodium picosulphate with magnesium citrate (Picolax) or high-dose macrogol (Movicol)) is applied until the constipation clears

T5–6. Painful stimuli (most commonly bladder or bowel distention) pass up the spinal cord to trigger a sympathetic response through the splanchnic plexus (T5–L2). Proximal travel through the spinal cord is blocked, however, so the normal dampening responses are not triggered. Instead, uninhibited sympathetic flow causes intense vasoconstriction below the level of the lesion, with a resulting increase in blood pressure. This in turn stimulates the baroreceptors in the carotid body, which results in a large increase in parasympathetic (vagal) tone, with bradycardia and vasodilatation above the level of the lesion, headache, and sweating. If this is severe and allowed to continue unchecked, it can result in seizures or a risk of cerebrovascular or retinal haemorrhage. Management includes the following:

1   Check for an easily remediable triggering cause – for example, kinked catheter, tight catheter bag, etc.

2   Keep in an upright position and monitor blood pressure.

3   If needed, administer 10 mg nifedipine capsules (chewed for rapid absorption) while a further search is made for the triggering cause.

4   In severe or resistant cases, the patient may need to be managed in an intensive-care or high-dependency care setting to control their blood pressure.

Symptom management

Symptoms such as pain and depression are common in neurological conditions, but patients are often unable to report their symptoms reliably because of cognitive or communication deficits. In this situation, it is important to:

a   **Undertake careful assessment** using adapted tools and recruiting the help of a psychologist, a speech and language therapist, or family members, or their combination, to describe and quantify symptoms as carefully as possible and identify causation b **Consider all treatment options and discuss with the patient and their family**

c **If drugs are used**, such as pain killers and/or anti-depressants, the response should be carefully monitored with serial measurements and reviewed regularly.

The Royal College of Physicians (RCP) has recently published guidelines for the use of antidepressants in the context of acquired brain injury.[13] The guidance is available through the RCP's website (www.rcplondon.ac.uk/pubs/books/antidepressmed-abi/) and includes recommendations for simple scales for the measurement of depression in the presence of profound cognitive and communicative impairments.

☐ SUMMARY

In summary, patients with neurological conditions present many challenges for rehabilitation and the provision of rehabilitation services. A range of services is needed, and programmes must be individualised, with well-coordinated planning and communication as patients move from one service to another in accordance with their changing needs. Although neurological injury frequently presents complex problems to the general physician and rehabilitation team, the keys to successful management are attention to detail and careful monitoring with responsive intervention.

REFERENCES

1 British Society of Rehabilitation Medicine. *Rehabilitation after traumatic brain injury.* London: British Society of Rehabilitation Medicine, 1998.

2 Royal College of Physicians. *National clinical guidelines for stroke.* London: Royal College of Physicians, 2004.

3 Royal College of Physicians and British Society of Rehabilitation Medicine. *National clinical guidelines for rehabilitation following acquired brain injury (working party consensus).* London: Royal College of Physicians and British Society of Rehabilitation Medicine, 2003.

4 Department of Health. *National service framework for long-term conditions.* London: Stationery Office, 2005.

5 Turner-Stokes L, Disler PB, Nair A, Wade DT. Multi-disciplinary rehabilitation for acquired brain injury in adults of working age. *Cochrane Database Syst Rev* 2005;(3):CD004170.

6 Turner-Stokes L, ed. *The effectiveness of rehabilitation: a critical review of the evidence.* London: Arnold Publishers, 1999.

7 Wade DT. Evidence relating to goal-planning in rehabilitation. *Clin Rehabi* 1998;12:273–5.

8 World Health Organization. *International classification of impairments, disabilities and handicaps.* Geneva: World Health Organization, 1980.

9 World Health Organization. *International classification of functioning, disability and health.* Geneva: World Health Organization, 2002.

10 Turner-Stokes L. Head injury rehabilitation – how should it be provided? In: *Head injury rehabilitation – a parliamentary health select committee inquiry.* London: Stationery Office, 2001.

11 Das-Gupta R, Turner-Stokes L. Traumatic brain injury. *Disabil Rehabil* 2002;24:654–65.

12 Turner-Stokes L, Ward A. Botulinum toxin in the management of spasticity in adults. *Clin Med* 2002;2:128–30.

13 Turner-Stokes L, MacWalter R, Guideline Development Group of the British Society of Rehabilitation M; British Geriatrics Society; Royal College of Physicians London. Use of antidepressant medication following acquired brain injury: concise guidance. *Clin Med* 2005;5:268–74.

☐ REHABILITATION SELF ASSESSMENT QUESTIONS

Rehabilitation after neurological injury

1   After neurological injury:
    (a) Sitting out in a wheelchair should be started as soon as possible
    (b) A standard 8L wheelchair will suffice in most cases
    (c) A posteriorly titled pelvic position is maintained to reduce sheering forces
    (d) The use of a tilt-table can help to maintain cardiovascular and postural reflexes
    (e) Patients who do not have head and trunk control require individualised seating assessment

2   The following are important factors in relieving spasticity:
    (a) A regular standing programme
    (b) Injections of botulinum toxin
    (c) Stretching and splinting of affected limbs
    (d) A small dose of β blocker
    (e) Closely fitting underwear

3   After spinal cord injury:
    (a) An indwelling urethral catheter should be used until bladder control has returned
    (b) The bladders should not be allowed to fill more than 250 ml
    (c) As long as the patient is able to void some urine spontaneously, intermittent catheterisation is rarely necessary
    (d) Patients with persistent residual volumes of >50 ml require intermittent catheterisation at least once daily
    (e) Urethral stricture should be considered as a possibility in patients who have persistent frequency and dysuria

4   After severe brain injury, a bowel regimen should be established that includes:
    (a) Adequate fluid and dietary intake
    (b) A bed pan being offered at regular intervals
    (c) Codeine phosphate for overflow diarrhoea
    (d) A daily dose of senna
    (e) Privacy on the toilet

5   Autonomic dysreflexia:
    (a) Commonly occurs in patients with spinal cord lesions below the level of T8
    (b) Can be triggered by bladder or bowel distension
    (c) Is best managed by lying the patient flat
    (d) Usually responds best to a slow-release β blocker
    (e) If severe, can lead to seizures or cerebral haemorrhage, or both

Dermatology

Pigmentation and sunburn

Jonathan L Rees

☐ INTRODUCTION

Of 100 patients referred by their general practitioner to a dermatology outpatient clinic, about half will turn out to have lesions that represent skin cancer or could easily be confused with skin cancer. The other half will have a range of inflammatory rashes, including psoriasis, atopic dermatitis, and, of course, acne. This case mixture is very different from that seen only 40 years ago, when more than 90% of referrals to hospital were for the diagnosis and management of rashes. Now, a range of skin tumours, basal cell carcinomas, squamous cell carcinomas, and, of course, melanomas (or imitators of melanoma) account for half our work.

Most such skin lesions – and here I am referring to lesions such as tumours rather than rashes – can be attributed to two biological factors. The first is sunshine – or, more precisely, exposure to ultraviolet radiation (UVR) – and the second is a relative paucity of melanin in the skin of many in our population. Exposure to UVR is not simply down to the laws of physics but rather, as with so many other topics in modern medicine, a reflection of how we choose to behave. That global warming will affect rates of skin cancer more than changes in the ozone layer seems a paradox: when the weather is hot we change our habits – spending more time outside wearing fewer items of clothing.

The imprint of UVR on clinical practice, however, is not just confined to lesions (rather than rashes). Of the 50 patients with rashes referred by a general practitioner, perhaps 10 will have psoriasis. The main hospital method of treatment for psoriasis is now narrowband ultraviolet B radiation (UVB).[1] We have learned that PUVA therapy, in which the cytotoxic prodrug methoxypsoralen (P) is activated by ultraviolet A (UVA), which was adopted with such enthusiasm 30 years ago, has unacceptable side effects for exactly the patients for whom we thought it most useful.

What of the other rashes and ultraviolet radiation? Atopic dermatitis responds to UVR, but the therapeutic effect is not nearly as consistent or useful as that seen with psoriasis.[2] Then there is perhaps the most curious group of all: patients who are acutely and pathologically sensitive to UVR but who we still treat with UVR – even patients with erythropoietic porphyria (EPP) can be treated with UVR. The time-honoured joke about a dermatologist being a physician who prescribes betamethasone valerate needs updating: for half our patients we mitigate the harmful effects of UVR and for the other half we administer UVR. Even if a patient's rash is caused by UVR, there is a possibility that I will recommend more UVR.

☐ A NEW ROLE FOR PIGMENTATION

Many of the patients I have just described present to medical care – at least in a biological sense – because of two evolutionary decisions made over the last several million years. First, humans have lost most of their body hair, and middle-aged balding professors of dermatology know that hair is a very effective sun block. Without dense body hair, biology had to invent a way to prevent the interfollicular skin from the harmful effects of UVR. In man, the chosen solution, of course, was to move some melanocytes from the follicle to the surrounding interfollicular skin. By contrast, in many mammals, the colour of the skin is irrelevant to protection against UVR, because the overlying hair is a very effective barrier to much of the electromagnetic spectrum. Of course, interesting anomalies exist: some Arctic species have white hair with black skin underneath, and each hair is thought to act like a mini-fibreoptic tube, directing light, and with it heat, down to the universal absorber – a black body – underneath.

We do not know for certain why humans had to lose most of their body hair. The conventional view is that the presence of a dense coat of hair interferes with effective sweating and that the thermoregulatory demands on our ancestors were great. Other alternatives have been suggested. For instance, Pagel and Bodmer recently argued that the parasitic burdens of a dense body of hair outweighed its usefulness.[3] Irrespective of the real reason, the results are all too evident to most of mankind and not just dermatologists. If there is no overlying hair, the interfollicular skin needs a mechanism to protect against the harmful effects of UVR.

Ultraviolet radiation is, of course, the most ubiquitous environmental carcinogen to which humans are exposed. Given this fact, it is not surprising that biology has invested much effort in a series of defence mechanisms that protect against UVR. Rare, but heuristically so important, is xeroderma pigmentosa, in which a focal defect exists in the ability to repair particular types of DNA damage. The defect is not generalised to all forms of DNA-damaging xenobiotics but is focussed on the particular forms of damage induced by short waveband UVR. Although many such patients will die in early childhood without appropriate care, little convincing evidence shows that person-to-person differences in DNA repair explain much of the risk of skin cancer in the otherwise normal population. The same cannot be said of that other method of photoprotection – pigmentation.

The evidence for the crucial role that pigmentation plays in protecting against the harmful effects of UVR is compelling and comes from studies at several different levels of biological organisation. For instance, albinos – individuals who harbour one of a range of mutations that (in an autosomal recessive pattern) confer an inability to synthesise normal levels of melanin – are at a dramatically increased risk of skin cancer. By contrast, a simple clinical experiment with patients with vitiligo also attests to the importance of pigment. If patients are irradiated on the normal and pale areas of skin, a marked difference is seen in the acute erythemal responses. Finally, at the population level, when people with different skin colours are compared, there is a greater than 100-fold variation in rates of skin cancer – differences that are also reflected in the variation in sensitivity to UVR-induced erythema in the short term.

Pigmentation in nature usually serves two diametrically opposing roles: camouflage (the attempt to conceal) and, at the other extreme, a signal to draw attention to particular body parts or behaviours. An example of the latter would be the bright blue colour of the blue vervet monkey scrotum. The colour, in this instance, is the result of the presence of melanin, but it appears blue (rather than brown) for the same reason that the sky is blue: Rayleigh light scattering is inversely related to the magnitude of wavelength. Of course, this pigment is not present as a sunblock.

Colour, by definition, reflects the optical properties of melanin in the visible part of the spectrum. Although these properties are important to those of us with only a modicum of vanity, it is the properties of melanin in the shorter – ultraviolet – wavebands that are so important for DNA protection. Nature's design can be seen with clarity on a simple histological section of skin in which the melanin has been stained. The melanin is concentrated to form a cap – a little sunhat – over the nucleus of the basal keratinocytes. A clear polarity to the anatomy exists: form respects function.

☐ HUMAN VARIATION IN PIGMENTATION

The loss of body hair was not the only evolutionary decision that altered the ecological balance between UVR, skin biology, and human health. The presence of large amounts of skin melanin in populations in areas of the world with high levels of ambient ultraviolet radiation is clearly an advantage. In some parts of the world, however, biology has had to make additional trade-offs. There are (at least) two competing hypotheses to explain this worldwide variation in human pigmentation. First, and most popular, is the theory of positive selection for pale skin since humans moved out of Africa around 25,000 years ago. This positive selection is usually predicated on the basis that individuals with dark skin who eat a cereal-based diet are at risk from vitamin D deficiency and that lighter skin allows more efficient use of whatever ambient ultraviolet radiation is available. An alternative explanation, less popular with most, is that what we see is merely a result of chance. That is, there was no great evolutionary pressure to maintain dark pigmentation in populations outside Africa and that, with the loss of functional constraint seen in African populations, change was tolerated. Biology was, as it were, indifferent to skin and hair colour, as long as there was not too much ambient sunshine.

☐ FROM MOUSE FANCY TO HUMAN DIVERSITY

Melanin is a complex mixture of polymers that to date has resisted precise chemical characterisation with classical biochemical approaches. Instead, insight has largely come from the field of mouse genetics and, more recently, from zebrafish genetics.[4,5] The resource afforded by a range of murine coat-colour mutations largely predates twentieth century genetics. In the Far East as early as the nineteenth century, mice with unusual coat-coloured patterns were collected and traded and crosses performed. This activity was institutionalised in the twentieth century, notably in the Jackson laboratories in the United States. Such animals have afforded pigment biologists a tractable approach to a whole range of human diseases involving the skin and other organ systems.[4,5] Those who think study of animals has not enlightened the study of human disease must have rather bizarre ideas of the nature of scientific evidence.

☐ THE MELANOCORTIN 1 RECEPTOR (MC1R) AND RED HAIR

Until very recently, and despite the identification of many genes that cause a range of rare pigmentary disorders, only one gene – the melanocortin 1 receptor (MC1R) – had been identified that underpinned what I will term normal physiological variation in skin and hair colour.[6] I will say a little bit more about this gene below, as I have worked on it for more than a decade, but it is important to note that a number of studies (one published recently in *Science*[7] and others sure to be published soon) show very clearly that we can explain most human variation in pigmentation – in the normal population – in terms of nucleotide changes in between five and 10 genes. I do not mean to imply that all of the details are worked out, but, in general, one goal of the genetic study of pigmentation – namely to match sequence diversity with phenotypic diversity – has now been achieved. I would also suggest that what we have learned from study of MC1R may be of relevance to those interested in other complex human traits and diseases of man.

☐ MELANOCORTIN 1 RECEPTOR: MORE THAN RED HAIR

A number of animals, not just man, are characterised by two pigmentary phenotypes that can be shown to arise from a relative overproduction of eumelanin over pheomelanin or, alternatively, a relative overproduction of pheomelanin.[6] These pigments can be found in both hair and feathers. Eumelanin is brown or black, whereas pheomelanin is red or yellow. Humans with black hair have a preponderance of eumelanin over pheomelanin, whereas humans with red hair have higher relative levels of pheomelanin, although the molar amount of eumelanin is always greater than that of pheomelanin. Such polymorphism in humans, dogs, foxes, birds, pigs, horses, and cows can all be explained by sequence diversity at the MC1R.

The MC1R encodes a 317 amino acid G-coupled protein receptor. The natural ligand is α-melanocyte-stimulated hormone – itself a cleavage product of pro-opio melanocortin (POMC) (Fig 1). Ten years ago, after Roger Cone cloned the gene in mice, we were able to quickly show that humans with red hair have a different pattern of sequence diversity from those with dark hair.[8] What we have learned subsequently, however, is more than skin deep.

Although the MC1R is a small gene, more than 75 alleles have been identified.[9] Although red hair approximates to a recessive trait, we now know that a large number of these alleles are quantitatively different in functional terms. We know this because of evidence from several different experimental approaches. In family studies, the phenotype was tracked through kindreds and related to sequence diversity. In genetic epidemiological studies, we and others have studied groups with particular phenotypes – freckling, hair colour, melanoma, and sun sensitivity – and related the difference to variation in DNA sequence. We have also been able to take particular alleles and transfect cells or whole animals (via rescue of null mice) to

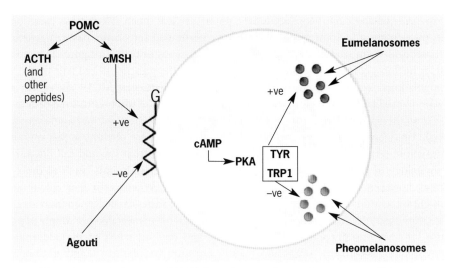

Fig 1 The melanocortin 1 receptor (MC1R) (here shown as the membrane receptor G) is a key control point in the control of eumelanin or pheomelanin. Alpha-melanocyte-stimulating hormone (αMSH) – a cleavage product of pro-opiomelanocortin (POMC) – signals via MC1R and increases in cyclic adenosine monophosphate (cAMP) through protein kinase A (PKA) signalling to increase the relative production of eumelanin over pheomelanin, which results in a darker hair colour. Diminished function mutations at the MC1R act so as to lead to red (pheomelanic) hair. In mice, but not as far as is known in man, agouti acts to antagonise the effects of MC1R. ACTH= adrenocorticotropic hormone; TRP1=tyrosinase related protein 1; TYR=tyrosinase.

define the functional effects of particular alleles in a fashion that is independent of genetic background. The most striking conclusion from all these experiments is that, even with a single locus, it is possible to produce a range of phenotypes on the basis of the combination of two alleles – one from the father and one from the mother. A large number of alleles differ in function quantitatively, so the physiological output acting via the MC1R can literally be varied from 0% to 100% depending on the combination of the two autosomal alleles. It is, pardon the pun, not black or white but all shades of red. Variation in MC1R thus underpins the risk of melanoma, the risk of basal or squamous cell carcinoma, hair colour, the extent of body freckling, and even the risk of what students still refer to as 'senile' lentigines – even when they are on the back of my hands. The exact degree of risk depends on the particular combination of MC1R alleles carried by a person.

☐ THE DISAPPEARING ODDS RATIO

Detailed study of this one particular locus has told us how complex even an apparently straightforward Mendelian trait can be, but a second lesson has been learned – namely, the way variability in the environment curtails the ability to usefully predict relevant phenotypes based on DNA sequence.

Human pigmentation is predominantly genetically determined, or at least that is the sort of sentence people put in grant applications when they are justifying their experimental approach. More accurately, we can say that much, if not most, variation in pigmentation in some populations can be accounted for on the basis of genetic relatedness. Twin studies suggest a heritability in excess of 0.85 – a figure far higher than for most complex diseases of man. If we track the presence of red hair through populations, we find extremely high odds ratios for particular MC1R alleles. If we want to predict the hair colour of a young adult, in terms of whether it is red or non-red, on the basis of DNA from the scene of crime, we can be right perhaps seven or eight times out of 10. Hair colour is still the only gross visible phenotype that we can explain in terms of DNA sequence. Once we move from what I would call the pure physiology of hair colour through to medically relevant endpoints, such as cancer rates, however, our odds ratios come tumbling down. Whereas for hair colour we might see an odds ratio of 30 or 40, depending on the alleles carried by an individual, for skin cancer, the odds ratios are in the region of 3–5[10] – levels that are simply of no use for screening purposes. This is a simple and obvious result of the additional environmental variance – variations in sun exposure and the like – and additional genetic variation at other loci that limit our predictive ability. This observation is perhaps slightly depressing but cannot be considered surprising.

□ FUTURE STUDIES

I suggested above that in broad brushstroke at least, the genetics of normal human pigmentary variation is now understood; however, some interesting biological questions remain. If you look at the pattern of diversity in the MC1R – and I have no reason to believe that other pigment genes will differ – greater diversity exists between continents than within continents.[11] This is, of course, different to what we have expected to see for most loci since Lewontin's classic work on this topic 30 years ago.[12] Lewontin showed, with the markers that were then available, that most diversity was within, rather than between, continents and that the greatest diversity was in African populations – humans have been there far longer than in any other place. As I have just said, however, the MC1R differs, and I would wager that many genes involved in physical appearance and skin biology will differ and that we will see greater diversity between continents. The tectonic plates of genetic diversity in man may therefore show some variation on the basis of clinical discipline. Time will tell if this speculation remains topical.

REFERENCES

1   Gordon PM, Diffey BL, Matthews JN, Farr PM. A randomized comparison of narrow-band TL-01 phototherapy and PUVA photochemotherapy for psoriasis. *J Am Acad Dermatol* 1999;41:728–32.

2   Reynolds NJ, Franklin V, Gray JC, Diffey BL, Farr PM. Narrow-band ultraviolet B and broad-band ultraviolet A phototherapy in adult atopic eczema: a randomised controlled trial. *Lancet* 2001;357:2012–6.

3   Pagel M, Bodmer W. A naked ape would have fewer parasites. *Proc R Soc Lond B Biol Sci* 2003;270 (Suppl 1):S117.

4   Barsh GS. The genetics of pigmentation: from fancy genes to complex traits. *Trends Genet* 1996;12:299–305.

5   Jackson IJ. Mouse coat colour mutations: a molecular genetic resource which spans the centuries. *Bioessays* 1991;13:439–46.

6   Rees JL. Genetics of hair and skin colour. *Annu Rev Genet* 2003;37:67–90.

7   Lamason RL, Mohideen MA, Mest JR *et al.* SLC24A5, a putative cation exchanger, affects pigmentation in zebrafish and humans. *Science* 2005;310:1782–6.

8   Valverde P, Healy E, Jackson I, Rees JL, Thody AJ. Variants of the melanocyte-stimulating hormone receptor gene are associated with red hair and fair skin in humans. *Nat Genet* 1995;11:328–30.

9   Wong TH, Rees JL. The relation between melanocortin 1 receptor (MC1R) variation and the generation of phenotypic diversity in the cutaneous response to ultraviolet radiation. *Peptides* 2005;26:1965–71.

10   Rees JL. The genetics of sun sensitivity in humans. *Am J Hum Genet* 2004;75:739–51.

11   Harding RM, Healy E, Ray AJ *et al.* Evidence for variable selective pressures at MC1R. *Am J Hum Genet* 2000;66:1351–61.

12   Lewontin R. *The triple helix: genes, organisms and environment.* Cambridge, MA: Harvard University Press, 2000.

☐ DERMATOLOGY SELF ASSESSMENT QUESTIONS

Pigmentation and sunburn

1   Phototherapy is a useful treatment for:
    (a) Basal cell carcinoma
    (b) Erythropoietic porphyria
    (c) Psoriasis
    (d) Atopic dermatitis
    (e) Bowen's disease

2   In people with red hair:
    (a) The ratio of eumelanin to pheomelanin is increased
    (b) Mutations in the tyrosinase gene are frequent
    (c) DNA repair in skin is diminished
    (d) The mode of inheritance is autosomal dominant
    (e) Mutations in the melanocortin 1 receptor are common

3   Albinism is:
    (a) The result of a deficiency of melanocyte survival in skin
    (b) The result of diminished production of melanin
    (c) Inherited in a sex-linked manner
    (d) Associated with an increased risk of squamous cell carcinoma
    (e) Unlikely to occur in those with Africa ancestry

Diabetes/endocrinology

New treatments for diabetes mellitus

Jiten Vora

A number of developments, including rapid- and long-acting insulin analogues, thiazolidenediones, 'incretin' analogues/enhancers, and agents specifically aimed at delaying the development of and progression of the microvascular complications of diabetes, will alter the treatment of types 1 and 2 diabetes. In addition, the development of new modes for delivery of insulin, such as inhaled insulin, are well progressed.

☐ RAPID- AND LONG-ACTING INSULIN ANALOGUES

Developments in insulin preparations have been fuelled by results from large-scale clinical trials, such as the Diabetes Control and Complications Trial and the United Kingdom Prospective Diabetes Study, which unequivocally showed the long-term clinical benefits of tight glycaemic control in patients with types 1 and 2 diabetes. These studies also highlighted the limitations of 'conventional' insulin preparations, with periods of hyperglycaemia caused by mismatches between meal intake and exogenous levels of insulin in plasma or by increased frequency of hypoglycaemia with approaching euglycaemia. In an effort to normalise glycaemia in the postprandial and post-absorptive states without hypoglycaemia, more intensive insulin regimens and newer preparations attempt to mimic normal physiological secretion of insulin.[1]

Physiological secretion of insulin

Physiological secretion of insulin in healthy people can be divided into basal and meal-related release of insulin (Fig 1). Basal insulin, secreted throughout the 24-hour period at an approximate rate of 0.5 units/hour, regulates hepatic glucose haemostasis in the fasting and post-absorptive states. Insulin secretion in response to meal ingestion (postprandial) is separated into two phases. The initial phase of insulin secretion occurs within 2–5 minutes and is followed by a more slowly progressive second phase that lasts from 5 to about 60 minutes before returning to basal levels within 2–4 hours of consumption of a meal.[1]

Most patients with type 1 diabetes are entirely dependent on exogenous insulin, while the loss of insulin secretory capacity is more gradual in those with type 2 diabetes. At the time of diagnosis, patients with type 2 diabetes usually have lost 50% of their β-cell function, with a further decline expected over the next 5–10 years. Such progressive β-cell failure results in deficiencies in basal secretion and meal-stimulated release of insulin.

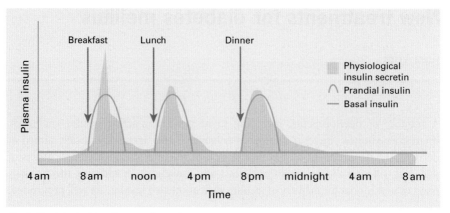

Fig 1 Physiological insulin secretion, with separation into basal and prandial insulin secretion components. Prandial and basal insulin treatment attempts to reproduce basal and prandial insulin requirements.

Clinical insulin replacement therapy

Insulin replacement consists of basal and prandial (bolus) insulin (see Fig 1). Basal insulin is central to achieving glycaemic control in patients with type 1 and type 2 diabetes, and supplementation of basal insulin attempts to mimic basal secretion of insulin. It is used alone or in combination with oral hypoglycaemic agents in patients with type 2 diabetes. Basal insulin is supplemented with multiple prandial boluses of regular soluble insulin or rapid-acting insulin analogues, which attempt to mimic the endogenous insulin secretory response to ingestion of a meal.[1]

Limitations of conventional insulin preparations

In pharmaceutical preparations, human insulin forms zinc-containing hexamers. After subcutaneous injection, these hexamers dissociate into dimers and then monomers and dimers, which are absorbed rapidly through the capillary endothelium. The rate of absorption of soluble insulin formulations from the subcutaneous tissue therefore is determined largely by the rate of dissociation of hexamers. Although plasma levels of glucose peak 30–60 minutes after ingestion of a meal, peak levels of short-acting soluble human insulin are reached 60–180 minutes after subcutaneous injection into the anterior abdominal wall. The resulting mismatch between peak glucose and insulin levels results in early postprandial hyperglycaemia and delayed hypoglycaemia before the next meal.[1]

Preparations should possess a number of specific features to fulfil the requirements of basal insulin. These include an activity profile that allows for a single daily dosage, a lack of pronounced peaks in activity that might result in hypoglycaemia, and a reproducible absorption profile with reduced interpatient and intrapatient variability. The development of 'intermediate-' and 'long-acting' insulin formulations was based on the tendency of insulin to self-aggregate into dimers and hexamers in the presence of zinc at a neutral pH. These preparations included neutral protamine Hagedorn (NPH, or isophane) and the zinc insulin crystalline suspensions Lente (intermediate acting) and Ultralente (long acting).[1]

The 'conventional' intermediate-acting insulin preparations (NPH (stable human insulin protamine suspension) and Lente (crystalline insulin suspension in the presence of excess zinc)) and long-acting preparation (Ultralente insulin) show high interpatient and intrapatient variability in pharmacokinetics, pharmacodynamics, and risk of hypoglycaemia, especially nocturnally, because of the presence of a specific peak in their action profiles. The duration of action of the NPH and Lente insulin preparations is too short to fulfil a 24-hour basal insulin requirement with a single daily dosage, so these formulations of insulin need to be administered twice daily. Although the duration of activity of the Ultralente insulin preparations may be adequate over the 24 hours, its large variability limits its reliability and consequent utility.

Rapid-acting insulin analogues

An increase in the rate of absorption of insulin from the subcutaneous injection site stems from acceleration of the rate of dissociation of insulin hexamers into dimers and monomers for more rapid absorption. Attempts to increase the rate of dissociation have focused on the amino acid residues involved in the interaction between the β chains of adjoining insulin molecules (B8, 9, 12–13, 16, 23–28).[1] Alteration of amino acid residues B12, 16 and 23–25 reduces the biological activity of insulin as they are primarily involved in receptor binding.

Three 'rapid-acting' insulin analogues are now commercially available: insulin lispro, insulin aspart and insulin glulisine. All seem to have very similar pharmacokinetic and pharmacodynamic properties. Insulin lispro (Humalog), in which the amino acid residues of proline and lysine (positions 28 and 29) in the insulin β chain are reversed, provides a more physiological profile of plasma insulin levels compared with regular soluble human insulin. Insulin aspart (in which the proline residue at position B28 is replaced by aspartamine) and insulin glulisine (in which asparagine is replaced with lysine at B3 and lysine with glutamate at B29) show action profiles similar to those of lispro insulin (Fig 2). In comparison with regular human soluble insulin (for which the onset of action is 30–60 minutes after subcutaneous injection, with peak insulin activity at 120–180 minutes), 'rapid-acting' insulin analogues have an onset of action 5–15 minutes after injection, with peak levels achieved 30–60 minutes after injection. When insulin lispro and insulin aspart are compared with regular human soluble insulin in patients with types 1 and 2 diabetes, a distinct reduction in postprandial glycaemic excursions is seen, with minor improvements in levels of haemoglobin A1c (HbA1$_c$) level and a reduction in the overall number of hypoglycaemic episodes.

Long-acting analogues

Long-acting insulin analogues resulted first from analogues of human insulin with an acidic isoelectric point and then from modification of human insulin by fatty acid acylation.[1] An acidic isoelectric point results in a soluble preparation when in an acidic environment but precipitation at the neutral pH of the subcutaneous tissue

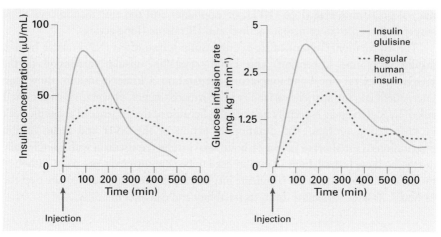

Fig 2 Action profile of rapid-acting insulin analogue glulisine compared with regular human insulin.
(a) Plasma insulin concentrations after administration of insulin glulisine and regular human insulin.
(b) Glucose infusion rates needed to maintain euglycaemia after administration of the two insulin preparations.

and so results in a depot from which insulin is released slowly into the circulation. This was the basis behind the development of insulin glargine.

Fatty acid acylation of human insulin promotes hexamer formation, thus reducing the rate of absorption from the subcutaneous tissue. When injected subcutaneously, the acylated human insulin analogue binds to albumin within the subcutaneous tissue and dissociates from it before it enters the capillary circulation. Further binding to circulating albumin occurs followed by dissociation and then transfer into the extravascular space and interaction with the insulin receptor. These processes result in a reduced rate of absorption from subcutaneous tissue and a prolonged action of duration.[1] Insulin detemir is the first clinically available acylated insulin analogue.

Insulin glargine

In insulin glargine, the α chain contains a glycine substitution for asparagine at position 21 and the β chain is extended by the addition of two arginine residues (B31, 32). This modification of the β chain alters the isoelectric point of the insulin, whereas the α-chain modification conserves stability in the acidic environment of the pharmaceutical formulation. Consequently, insulin glargine is soluble at pH 4.0 but forms stable hexamers that readily precipitate at the neutral pH of subcutaneous tissue after injection.[1]

Insulin detemir

Insulin detemir was developed through the addition of a 14-carbon fatty acid chain to the lysine residue of the β chain (position B29), with the terminal B30 amino acid removed to increase binding to albumin. The pharmaceutical formulation of insulin detemir is a soluble insulin at neutral pH.

Pharmacokinetic and pharmacodynamic properties

Compared with isophane (NPH), Ultralente insulins, and the 'gold standard' continuous subcutaneous insulin infusion (CSII) regimen, the pharmacokinetic and pharmacodynamic properties of insulin glargine show a duration of action of 22 ± 4 hours – longer than that of isophane insulin (14 ± 3 hours). Insulin glargine also showed a flattened action profile with no peaks, similar to that of CSII (Fig 3). Interpatient variability was significantly lower with insulin glargine administration than with NPH or Ultralente preparations and was similar to that seen with CSII. Isoglycaemic clamp studies that compared detemir insulin with NPH insulin in patients with type 1 diabetes have shown a flatter action profile that lasts up to 20 hours for detemir, with reduced variability for the former.

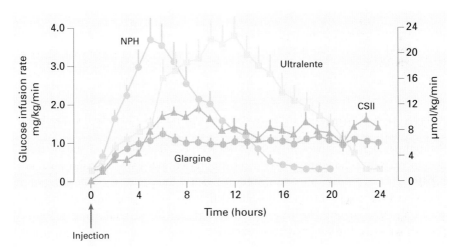

Fig 3 Time action profile of insulin glargine compared with isophane intermediate-acting insulin (NPH), Ultralente long-acting insulin analogue, and continuous subcutaneous insulin infusion (CSII). Activity judged by glucose infusion rates needed to maintain euglycaemia.

☐ INHALED INSULIN

Inhaled delivery of insulin is attractive because of the large surface area, vascular bed, and permeability of the alveoli. The success of inhaled insulin, however, will depend on the development of delivery devices that are able to deliver insulin particles efficiently and reproducibly without significant adverse effects on pulmonary gas transfer. Currently available devices deliver small amounts of preprandial rapid-acting insulin. Patients still need once-daily basal insulin via conventional subcutaneous injection. In healthy people, inhaled insulin has a duration of action between that of the rapid-acting analogue lispro insulin and regular insulin (Fig 4). Inhaled insulin has been shown to be rapidly and reproducibly absorbed. The inhaled insulin Exubera, which delivers rapid-acting dry powder insulin particles, in combination with a single injection of basal insulin, produces similar decreases in HbA$_{1c}$ after six months to those with conventional insulin treatment. Treatment satisfaction was higher with inhaled insulin, and the most common side-effect reported was mild-to-moderate cough. No significant change was noted in pulmonary function, and changes in lung function initially observed remained small and non-progressive.

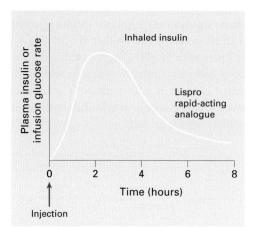

Fig 4 Time action profile of inhaled insulin (Exubera) compared with rapid-acting insulin analogue lispro.

□ ORAL HYPOGLYCAEMIC AGENTS IN THE TREATMENT OF TYPE 2 DIABETES

Pathophysiological changes in patients with type 2 diabetes are characterised by insulin resistance, 'inappropriately' non-suppressed glucagon secretion, increased hepatic glucose production, and insulin deficiency that increases with duration of disease, which results in severe insulin deficiency and the consequent need for insulin therapy in severely hyperglycaemic patients. In patients with established type 2 diabetes, insulin resistance manifests as inadequately restrained hepatic glucose production, impaired insulin-mediated peripheral glucose uptake, and increased lipolysis.

Thiazolidinediones: pioglitazone and rosiglitazone

Peroxisome proliferator-activated receptors (PPARs) are transcription factors that, when activated, bind to specific peroxisome proliferator response elements (PPREs) that modulate transcription activity of target genes involved in carbohydrate and lipid metabolism.[2,3] The thiazolidinediones (TZDs) are represented by pioglitazone and rosiglitazone. They selectively enhance actions of insulin by activating the nuclear peroxisome proliferator-activated receptor-gamma (PPAR-γ), which is expressed mainly in adipose tissue but to a small extent in skeletal muscle, liver and many other tissues (Fig 5).[4] It acts in a complex with the retinoid X receptor to increase the transcription of several insulin-sensitive genes, including lipoprotein lipase, the fatty acid transporter protein, adipocyte fatty acid binding protein, acyl coenzyme A synthetase, glycerol kinase malic enzyme, and the glucose transporter isoform GLUT-4. Thiazolidinediones thus promote adipogenesis and lipogenesis, mainly in subcutaneous adipose depots where new small adipocytes are insulin sensitive and show increased uptake of glucose and fatty acids. They therefore also increase glucose uptake, glycogenesis, and glucose utilisation by muscle tissue and, to a lesser extent, reduce glucose production by the liver. These effects are partly an indirect consequence of altered adipocyte metabolism that reduces circulating free fatty acids. The blood-glucose-lowering effects of TZDs are also partly the result of PPAR-γ-induced reductions in the secretion of adipokines that increase insulin resistance, notably tumour necrosis factor alpha (TNF-α), interleukin (IL)-6, and resistin. In addition, TZDs increase adipocyte secretion of adiponectin, which improves insulin sensitivity.

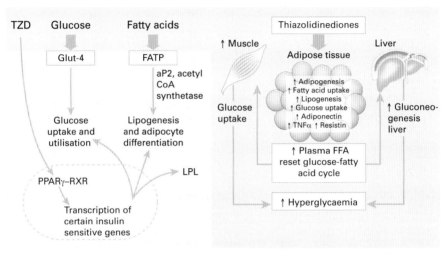

Fig 5 Functional characteristics and activity of thiazolidinediones. TZD=thiazolidinediones; GLUT-4=glucose transporter 4; FATP=fatty acid transporter protein; LPL=lipoprotein lipase. Adapted from Natrass *et al* with permission of Elsevier.[4]

As monotherapy for periods up to one year, TZDs show reductions in levels of HbA$_{1c}$ of up to 1% – similar to those with sulphonylureas and metformin. With the suggestion that insulin resistance *per se* is an independent risk factor for macro-vascular disease, the TZDs are becoming first-line or second-line agents after metformin.[2,3] Indeed, in patients with type 2 diabetes who were receiving usual drugs, treatment with pioglitazone resulted in a significant reduction in cardiovascular endpoints (16%) (Fig 6(a)). In patients with a previous acute coronary syndrome, recurrent fatal and non-fatal cardiovascular events were reduced by 28% and the time to further acute coronary syndrome by 37% (Fig 6(b)). In addition, pioglitazone also reduced the need for permanent insulin usage by about 50% (Fig 6(c)).

Treatment with TZDs often causes weight gain of 2–4 kg, which stabilises by six months, due to accretion of subcutaneous (rather than visceral) adipose tissue. Fluid retention with pitting oedema occurs in about 5% of patients and may be greater if taken with insulin. Possible causes of oedema include increased sodium reabsorption by proximal convoluted tubules, increased capillary permeability as a result of greater production of vascular endothelial growth factor, and altered intestinal ion transport. Oedema can sometimes be managed with a diuretic, but dosage reduction or

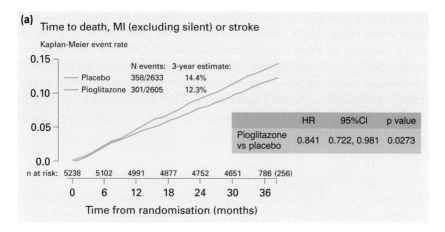

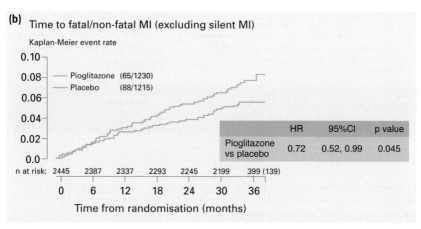

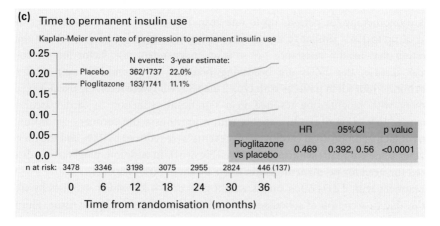

Fig 6 Results from the PROactive study, evaluating the addition of pioglitazone to 'usual' treatment for type 2 diabetes. **(a)** Time to composite primary endpoint of death, myocardial infarction or stroke. **(b)** Time to follow-up fatal/non-fatal myocardial infarction in patients with previous myocardial infarction. **(c)** 50% reduction in permanent insulin usage in patients receiving pioglitazone. HR = hazard ratio. Reproduced with permission of proactive-results.com

discontinuation of the TZD may be needed. In clinical trials with TZDs, congestive heart failure occurred in <1% of patients (similar to placebo). Appropriate monitoring for signs of congestive heart disease is recommended for patients taking a TZD, and these agents are contraindicated in patients with evidence of heart failure. Thiazolidinediones often reduce levels of haemoglobin by up to 1 g/dl, in part because of dilution as a result of fluid retention, although though frank anaemia is uncommon.[2,3,5]

☐ 'INCRETIN' EFFECT

Oral glucose results in a greater increase in pancreatic secretion of insulin than a comparable glucose challenge given intravenously (Fig 7).[6] The search for the responsible gut-derived factors, known as 'incretins' (Box 1), resulted in the identification of glucose-dependent insulinotropic peptide (GIP), which is released from the enteroendocrine cells of the upper gut and stimulates pancreatic secretion of insulin in a glucose-dependent manner, and two glucagon-like peptides, GLP-1 and GLP-2, which are neuroendocrine hormones that originate from intestinal L cells of the distal gut.[7]

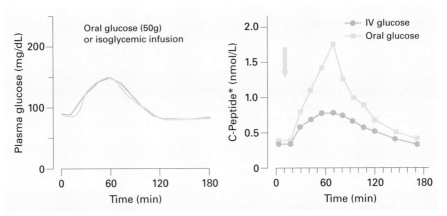

Fig 7 'Incretin' effect in patients with type 2 diabetes. Adapted from McIntyre *et al* with permission of Elsevier.[6]

Box 1 Physiological incretins that enhance glucose-dependent insulin secretion and reduce inadequately suppressed/raised glucagon.

- Secretin
- Glucose-dependent insulinotropic peptide (GIP)*
- VIP
- Glucagon
- Glucagon-like peptides (GLP)
  - GLP-1*
  - GLP-2
  - Glicentin
  - Oxyntomodulin

*Main physiological incretin hormones (50%).

Glucose-lowering and pharmacological properties of GLP-1

Both GLP-1 (7-36) and GLP-1 (7-37) amide exert metabolic actions by stimulating insulin secretion and inhibiting glucagon secretion in a glucose-dependent manner, delaying gastric emptying and reducing gastric motility, thus reducing prandial glucose levels without increasing the risk of hypoglycaemia.[7,8] In addition, GLP-1 has been shown to decrease appetite and energy intake, although the mechanism for this central effect remains unclear. Less weight gain thus occurs with these agents. Infusions of GLP-1 in patients with type 2 diabetes reduces fasting and postprandial glucose levels. The therapeutic potential of GLP-1 is limited by its short plasma half-life (1.5 minutes), as it is rapidly degraded by the enzyme dipeptidyl peptidase 4 (DPP-IV), which cleaves GLP-1 in a process that requires an alanine or proline residue at the second N-terminal position. Research thus has focused on developing GLP-1-like agonists that are resistant to cleavage by DPP-IV and DPP-IV inhibitors.[8]

Exenatide

Exendin-4 is a GLP-1-like molecule (a peptide containing 39 amino acids with 53% structural homology with mammalian GLP-1) that is isolated from the saliva of *Heloderma suspectum* (known as the Gila Monster). Exenatide is a synthetic form of exendin-4. Differences in the penultimate amino acid sequence of exendin-4 and exenatide render these compounds resistant to degradation by DPP-IV.[8]

In patients with type 2 diabetes treated with metformin or sulphonylurea, injected exenatide reduced levels of HbA_{1c} by 1.1% at one year, with a mean weight reduction of 4.5 kg. The glucose-lowering effects of exenatide are mainly attributable to effects on daytime postprandial glucose levels rather than fasting plasma glucose.

GLP-1 agonists

Liraglutide is a long-acting acylated GLP-1 analogue that acts as a full agonist at the GLP-1 receptor. It has a prolonged duration of action (half-life 13 hours) and is suitable for once-daily injection.[8]

DPP-IV inhibitors

The DPP-IV enzyme inactivates GLP-1, so inhibition of DPP-IV prolongs the circulating half-life of endogenous GLP-1, and the DPP-IV inhibitors possess the same physiological properties as GLP-1 analogues. Vildagliptin is an orally active, highly selective DPP-IV inhibitor. Addition of vildagliptin to metformin results in a further reduction in levels of HbA_{1c} of 1.1% at 52 weeks. Vildagliptin is well tolerated, with no significant effects of hypoglycaemia. Other DPP-IV inhibitors at advanced stages of development include sitagliptin. A possible safety concern, however, is that DPP-IV inhibition will prevent the degradation of other bioactive peptides (over 20 peptides are metabolised by DPP-IV) in addition to GLP-1 and GIP.[8]

☐ DUAL-ACTING PEROXISOME PROLIFERATOR ACTIVATED-RECEPTOR AGONISTS

Peroxisome proliferator-activated receptors (PPARs) are members of the nuclear receptor superfamily of ligand-activated transcription factors (see above). The currently available thiazolidinediones (TZDs), rosiglitazone and pioglitazone, are the most well-recognized PPAR-γ ligands. Several new dual-acting PPAR-α and -γ agonists are in clinical development. PPAR-α receptor subtype is specifically involved in lipid metabolism, with the fibric acid derivatives bezafibrate and gemfibrozil being traditional ligands for PPAR-α. Muraglitazar achieved significant reductions in levels of HbA_{1c} and triglycerides and increases in levels of high-density lipoprotein (HDL) cholesterol. Promising data have also emerged with ragaglitazar. Naveglitizar has shown similar reductions in levels of HbA_{1c} and triglycerides. Dual-acting PPAR-α and -γ agonists also seem to cause dose-related oedema and heart failure, and significant problems with liver toxicity have been reported.

□ THE PKC-β-SPECIFIC INHIBITOR RUBOXISTAURIN

Hyperglycaemia promotes *de-novo* synthesis of intracellular diacylglycerol (DAG), which, in turn, results in the activation of protein kinase C (PKC) in the vascular bed.[9] Stimulation of PKC results in increased expression of vascular epidermal growth factor, vascular permeability factor, growth factors (such as transforming growth factor β) and endothelin, which contributes to the structural and functional abnormalities associated with diabetic microangiopathy. Activation of DAG–PKC leads to changes in vascular permeability and expression of pro-inflammatory genes in the retina and kidney (Fig 8).

Several PKC isoforms exist, but high glucose exposure activates $PKC-\beta_I$ and $PKC-\beta_{II}$ to a greater extent than other PKC isoforms. Ruboxistaurin is an orally active PKC inhibitor with considerable selectivity for the PKC-β isoforms. Initial animal

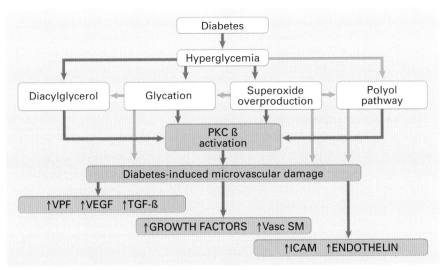

Fig 8 Protein-kinase C system and microvascular complications of diabetes. Stimulation of protein kinase β (PKC β) results in microvascular complications via the stimulation of vascular permeability factor (VPF), growth factors (transforming growth factor-β (TGF-β) and vascular endothelial growth factor (VEGF)), and vasoactive polypeptides (endothelin and intercellular adhesion molecule (ICAM)). Vasc SM = vascular smooth muscle.

studies showed that ruboxistaurin reversed diabetes-induced abnormalities of blood flow, especially retinal blood flow, glomerular filtration rate, and albuminuria. Intravitreal and oral administration of ruboxistaurin significantly reduced (by >95%) the increase in retinal fluorescein leakage induced by vascular endothelial growth factor injected into the vitreous cavity. Large-scale human trials with ruboxistaurin have shown reductions of 40% in progression of severe retinopathy and 40% in sustained visual loss and a twofold higher gain in visual acuity. Progression of macular oedema was significantly reduced. In patients with established proteinuria, ruboxistaurin reduced albuminuria by 50%, as well as significantly reducing progression of microalbuminuria to established nephropathy.[10] Pharmacological blockade of PKC-β activation offers a novel approach to reducing diabetic microvascular complications as an adjunct to existing glucose- and blood-pressure-lowering treatments.

REFERENCES

1   Vora JP, Owens DR. Insulin analogues. In: Barnett AH (ed), *Diabetes: best practice and research compendium.* London: Elsevier, 2006:223–3.

2   Simonson GD, Kendall DM. Different actions of peroxisome proliferator-activated receptors: molecular mechanisms and clinical importance. *Curr Opin Endocrinol Diabetes* 2006;13:162–70.

3   Kendall DM. Thiazolidinediones: the case for early use. *Diabetes Care* 2006;29:154–7.

4   Natrass M, Bailey CJ. New oral agents for type 2 diabetes. In: Barnett AH (ed), *Diabetes: best practice and research compendium.* London: Elsevier, 2006:209–22

5   Dormandy JA, Charbonnel B, Eckland DJ *et al.* Secondary prevention of macrovascular events in patients with type 2 diabetes in the PROactive study (PROspective pioglitAzone Clinical Trial In macroVascular Events): a randomised controlled trial. *Lancet* 2005:366;1279–89. See also proactive-results.com, accessed 2 August 2006.

6   McIntyre N, Holdsworth CD, Turner DS. New interpretation of oral glucose tolerance. *Lancet* 1964:41:20–1.

7   Ahren B. Incretins and islet function. *Curr Opin Endocrinol Diabetes* 2006:13;154–61.

8   Sinclair EM, Drucker DJ. Glucagon-like peptide 1 receptor agonists and dipeptidyl peptidase IV inhibitors: new therapeutic agents for the treatment of type 2 diabetes. *Curr Opin Endocrinol Diabetes* 2005;12:146–51.

9   He Z, King GL. Can protein kinase C beta-selective inhibitor, ruboxistaurin, stop vascular complications in diabetic patients? *Diabetes Care* 2005;28:2803–5.

10 Tuttle KR, Bakris GL, Toto RD *et al.* The effect of ruboxistaurin on nephropathy in Type 2 diabetes. *Diabetes Care* 2005;28:2686–90.

Understanding glucocorticoids

David William Ray, Rachelle Donn and Midori Kayahara

□ INTRODUCTION

Glucocorticoid hormones are essential for human survival. Their effects are mediated by the ubiquitously expressed glucocorticoid receptor, and they exert diverse effects on virtually all tissues and organs. Early physiological experiments showed two broad functional groups of actions. At low, or non-stress, concentrations of cortisol, major effects are seen on enzymes involved in metabolism – for example, maintenance of euglycaemia. In contrast, at high, or stress, concentrations of cortisol, a network of anti-inflammatory and stress-coping mechanisms becomes activated. A common exemplar of this dichotomous relation between non-stress and stress levels of circulating glucocorticoids is that patients with structural damage to the pituitary adrenal axis cope well with the demands of everyday life but are particularly vulnerable to intercurrent stress, such as surgical intervention or development of febrile illness.

Production of glucocorticoids by the adrenal cortex is tightly controlled by the brain via activation of hypothalamic neurones that secrete corticotropin-releasing factor (CRF) into the hypophyseal portal system; this, in turn, induces secretion of adrenocorticotropic hormone (ACTH) from pituitary corticotroph cells. Adrenocorticotropic hormone is involved in the final common pathway that results in adrenal hyperplasia and augmented production of hormones – principally cortisol in humans and corticosterone in rodents. This axis is under negative feedback from glucocorticoids at the levels of the pituitary, hypothalamus, and higher centre. Clinical manifestations of altered glucocorticoid sensitivity typically arise because isolated tissues or organs acquire a differential sensitivity threshold to the central glucocorticoid sensors or because, in the face of generalised resistance to glucocorticoid action, the increased tone of the hypothalamic–pituitary–adrenal (HPA) axis gives rise to production of abnormal quantities of other adrenal steroids with a discrete pattern of effects.

Glucocorticoid action

Glucocorticoids, natural (cortisol in humans and corticosterone in rodents) and synthetic (such as prednisolone and dexamethasone), are lipophilic and gain access to cells by diffusion across the plasma membrane. Within target cells, glucocorticoids are subject to metabolism by 11β-hydroxysteroid dehydrogenase (HSD), an enzyme that exists in two principal isoforms. The type 1 enzyme acts primarily to generate the active glucocorticoid cortisol from inactive cortisone. It is predominantly expressed in liver and adipose tissue and so acts not only to increase the circulating concentration of active glucocorticoid but also, in a tissue-specific manner, to amplify the action of glucocorticoids. The type 2 enzyme predominantly acts in the opposite direction and results in inactivation of cortisol by oxidation to inactive cortisone. The tissue distribution of the type 2 enzyme is restricted to mineralocorticoid target tissues, notably the renal tubule. Defects in the type 2 enzyme cause apparent mineralocorticoid excess by allowing cortisol unrestricted access to the mineralocorticoid receptor in the kidney, which allows unrestrained mineralocorticoid bioactivity. This results in hypertension and hypokalaemia but with suppression of serum levels of renin and aldosterone.[1]

Cortisone reductase deficiency

A series of patients with a genetic deficiency in the peripheral enzymatic conversion of cortisone to cortisol has now been described[2] and represents an example of pre-receptor glucocorticoid resistance. The causative mutations have been identified in the 11β HSD type 1 gene and the gene that encodes hexose 6 phosphate dehydrogenase – a critical enzyme that is responsible for generating the reduced nicotinamide adenine dinucleotide phosphate (NADPH)[2] that 11β HSD type 1 needs to catalyse regeneration of active cortisol from cortisone. The phenotype of the predominantly female patients includes a number of features typically associated with metabolic syndrome and polycystic ovary syndrome.[1] Most women presented with hirsutism in association with high levels of serum testosterone and adrenal androgen. Investigation revealed increased urinary clearance of cortisone metabolites compared with cortisol metabolites.

☐ GLUCOCORTICOID RECEPTOR FUNCTION

The glucocorticoid receptor in its inactive state is predominantly found in the cytoplasm of target cells. After ligand binding, the receptor becomes transformed and rapidly translocates to the cell nucleus. Within the nucleus, the receptor exhibits highly dynamic behaviour and binds to target sequences within the genome by:[3]

☐ forming a homodimer and binding to conserved DNA sequences

☐ acting as a monomer and binding to other transcription factors on their cognate DNA response elements – eg NFκB or activator protein-1 (AP-1).

Glucocorticoid receptors and other transcription factors

A further important example of crosstalk between glucocorticoid receptor function and other signalling cascades is direct physical interaction between the glucocorticoid receptor and other transcription factors. The best characterised examples of these are NFκB and AP-1. NFκB is a heterodimeric complex of transcription factors that share the Rel homology domain. The p65 component, otherwise known as Rel A, has been shown to be capable of binding directly to the glucocorticoid receptor. This physical interaction results in mutual inhibition of transcriptional activation of the two factors. For example, the glucocorticoid receptor will inhibit p65-dependent gene transcription, and, equally, p65 overexpression inhibits gene activation by the glucocorticoid receptor. As NFκB is activated downstream of the proinflammatory cytokines tumour necrosis factor alpha (TNFα) and interleukin (IL)-1 and forms an important part of the innate immune response, its activation may act to prevent the anti-inflammatory activities of glucocorticoids within foci of active inflammation (Fig 1).[3,4]

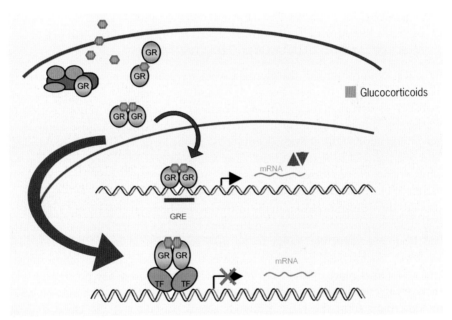

Fig 1 Glucocorticoids diffuse into target cells and activate the cytosolic glucocorticoid receptor (GR), which then translocates to the nucleus. In the nucleus the glucocorticoid receptor can form homodimers, and bind to a specific recognition motif in gene regulatory DNA termed a glucocorticoid response element (GRE). The activated glucocorticoid receptor can also bind to other transcription factors (TF), including AP-1, and NKfB to inhibit their activity to upregulate target genes.

A further example of transcription factor crosstalk is seen between the glucocorticoid receptor and AP-1. The AP-1 transcription factor is activated as a consequence of mitogen-activated protein (MAP) kinase pathways and was the first documented example of transcription factor crosstalk that involves the glucocorticoid receptor. The mode of action is complex, with mutual inhibition of glucocorticoid receptor and AP-1 activity or, certainly in the case of the well-studied proliferin gene, a rather complex interaction with particular heterodimeric complexes of AP-1 inhibiting transactivation by the glucocorticoid receptor and others augmenting such transcriptional activity.[3]

Interleukin-2 has been well recognised to cause a glucocorticoid-resistant state within its target cells. More recently, the basis for this interaction has been defined as the result of interaction between the glucocorticoid receptor and signal transducer and activator of transcription (STAT) 5 transcription factor, which is activated downstream of IL-2 receptor activation. This transcription factor is capable of productive synergy with the glucocorticoid receptor on some target genes, particularly milk protein genes, and gene expression in the liver, where it is activated by prolactin or growth hormone, but in a cell type and target gene-specific way it is also capable of inhibiting glucocorticoid actions in response to IL-2, as shown within cells of the lymphoid lineage.[5] In addition, IL-4 is also capable of inducing glucocorticoid resistance in target cells by activation of the related transcription factor STAT 6.

☐ GENETIC VARIATIONS IN GLUCOCORTICOID RECEPTOR GENE AND THEIR ASSOCIATION WITH GLUCOCORTICOID SENSITIVITY

Several polymorphisms in the glucocorticoid receptor gene have been described. Three of these have been studied in detail and have been found to associate with increased or decreased glucocorticoid sensitivity, as well as with various surrogate markers of potential glucocorticoid activity.[6] A more comprehensive analysis of genetic variation of the glucocorticoid receptor gene locus has also been performed. This analysis lead to the identification of four common haplotypes that span the entire region. One of these haplotypes was found to be significantly associated with increased glucocorticoid sensitivity to dexamethasone suppression. This haplotype contains three polymorphisms in the intron located between exons 2 and 3. Notably, one of the polymorphic variants was the same BCL 1 polymorphism that previously had been independently found to be associated with increased glucocorticoid sensitivity. Such haplotype analysis increases the power of gene association studies and also allows more efficient use of resources, as relatively few polymorphisms subsequently need to be typed to confidently identify all of the common haplotypes in Caucasians from the UK.[7] Although genetic variation at the glucocorticoid receptor gene locus undoubtedly affects glucocorticoid sensitivity and a considerable effect can be found in epidemiological studies in large cohorts, this only explains a proportion of the observed variability in glucocorticoid sensitivity. Most interindividual variation, therefore, is the result of genetic variation not related to the glucocorticoid receptor or possibly other changes acquired as a result of exposure in the intrauterine environment or the early postnatal period.

☐ METABOLIC PROGRAMMING

Seminal observations by Barker *et al* identified previously unsuspected links between the intrauterine environment and the subsequent long-term risk of acquired disease. The central tenet of this is that an adverse intrauterine environment, as manifested by low birth weight, powerfully predicts the development of obesity in later life, with attendant hypertension, dyslipidaemia, and a greatly increased risk of cardiovascular mortality. Because a number of features of metabolic syndrome were also seen in patients with glucocorticoid excess or Cushing's syndrome, a mediating role of glucocorticoid production or sensitivity was advanced. Animal studies of maternal protein restriction and early postnatal maternal behaviour confirm the impact and importance of insults at certain critical developmental stages for long-term metabolic programming. Strikingly, these effects seemed to be transmissible not only to the first generation born but also to the offspring of these animals. This long-term change cannot be the result of changes in DNA sequence but clearly needs some long-term change in RNA expression from the conserved genomic DNA of these individual animals. Analysis of glucocorticoid receptor expression in the brains of animals showed a striking change in the pattern of expression seen in adult offspring after early life manipulations. This altered pattern of glucocorticoid receptor expression seemed to stem from differential methylation of the promoter. The resultant altered glucocorticoid sensitivity in key brain regions was thought to explain the long-term changes in basal tone of the HPA axis and thereby the chronic increased production of glucocorticoid from the adrenal cortex. This relatively subtle overproduction of glucocorticoids that act on the key metabolic tissues of liver and adipose may give rise to local, tissue-specific manifestations of Cushing's syndrome and thereby explain the observed metabolic association.[8]

☐ ACQUIRED GLUCOCORTICOID RESISTANCE IN INFLAMMATORY DISEASE

The characteristic response to any inflammatory focus is augmented production of glucocorticoids. Despite these endogenous glucocorticoids having potent anti-inflammatory activity, the inflammatory process tends to continue, and pharmacological doses of glucocorticoid are usually needed to suppress it. For this reason, locally released mediators of inflammation have been proposed to induce a privileged glucocorticoid-resistant state within the focus of inflammation. As discussed above, the glucocorticoid receptor is capable of forming direct protein contacts with components of the AP-1 and NFκB transcription factors. As AP-1 and NFκB are activated in response to proinflammatory cytokines and other stress-induced pathways, they will be found in an activated state in most cells within a focus of inflammation. Indeed, a recent study importantly identified differential expression of NFκB, p65 as a powerful predictor of glucocorticoid responsiveness in patients with asthma.[9] Activation of members of the MAP kinase family may also lead to alterations in glucocorticoid sensitivity – notably, activation of Jun N-terminal kinase (JNK) gives rise to N-terminal glucocorticoid receptor phosphorylation and impaired function, whereas evidence shows that activation of cyclic adenosine monophosphate pathways and protein kinase A may result in augmentation of glucocorticoid sensitivity. This latter mechanism may be relevant in terms of the clinical observation that long-acting β_2 agonists function as steroid-sparing or steroid-potentiating agents in the treatment of patients with bronchial asthma.[10] In the future it may be possible to design glucocorticoid molecules that retain effective anti-inflammatory potency, but lack metabolic side-effects.

Role of macrophage migration inhibitory factor

Although most proinflammatory cytokines are implicated in impairment of glucocorticoid sensitivity and, in turn, are repressed by exposure to glucocorticoids, an unusual cytokine – macrophage migration inhibitory factor (MIF) – was originally described as being paradoxically induced by low concentrations of glucocorticoid. More recently, this observation and a number of the other earlier descriptions of MIF bioactivity have been called into question, but undoubtedly MIF expression is found to be augmented within foci of inflammation and, importantly, genetic studies have not only associated but also linked the MIF gene with development of chronic inflammatory autoimmune disease. Importantly, the MIF genotype also predicts the steroid response to intra-articular administration of glucocorticoid. The precise molecular mechanism by which MIF opposes glucocorticoid bioactivity remains mysterious, but it is also a topic of enduring clinical relevance.[11,12]

Glucocorticoid resistance in chronic obstructive pulmonary disease

An important paradox exists between bronchial asthma, which is characteristically very sensitive to glucocorticoids, and chronic obstructive pulmonary disease (COPD), a syndrome of chronic airway inflammation strongly associated with cigarette smoking, which is characteristically resistant to glucocorticoid inhibition. Chronic obstructive pulmonary disease imposes a huge burden of morbidity and mortality on the world's population, and treatment is currently restricted to symptomatic management and smoking cessation. Unfortunately, even in patients who stop smoking cigarettes, the disease may persist or even progress. *In vitro* studies confirm that airway-derived cells from cigarette smokers with this disease are resistant to the cytokine inhibitory actions of glucocorticoids. The precise mechanism is still under investigation, but the role of histone deacetalyse enzymes has been implicated.[13] These enzymes act to regulate accessibility of target DNA to not only the glucocorticoid receptor but to other transcription factors and there seems to be abnormal activity of histone deacetylases in cells derived from patients with COPD.

REFERENCES

1   Draper N, Stewart PM. 11beta-hydroxysteroid dehydrogenase and the pre-receptor regulation of corticosteroid hormone action. *J Endocrinol* 2005;186:251–71.

2   Draper N, Walker EA, Bujalska IJ *et al.* Mutations in the genes encoding 11beta-hydroxysteroid dehydrogenase type 1 and hexose-6-phosphate dehydrogenase interact to cause cortisone reductase deficiency. *Nat Genet* 2003;34:434–9.

3   Rhen T, Cidlowski JA. Antiinflammatory action of glucocorticoids – new mechanisms for old drugs. *N Engl J Med* 2005;353:1711–23.

4   Garside H, Stevens A, Farrow S *et al.* Glucocorticoid ligands specify different interactions with NF-kappaB by allosteric effects on the glucocorticoid receptor DNA binding domain. *J Biol Chem* 2004;279:50050–9.

5   Biola A, Lefebvre P, Perrin-Wolff M *et al.* Interleukin-2 inhibits glucocorticoid receptor transcriptional activity through a mechanism involving STAT5 (signal transducer and activator of transcription 5) but not AP-1. *Mol Endocrinol* 2001;15:1062–76.

6   van Rossum EF, Russcher H, Lamberts SW. Genetic polymorphisms and multifactorial diseases: facts and fallacies revealed by the glucocorticoid receptor gene. *Trends Endocrinol Metab* 2005;16:445–50.

7   Stevens A, Ray DW, Zeggini E *et al.* Glucocorticoid sensitivity is determined by a specific glucocorticoid receptor haplotype. *J Clin Endocrinol Metab* 2004;89:892–7.

8   Seckl JR, Meaney MJ. Glucocorticoid programming. *Ann N Y Acad Sci* 2004;1032:63–84.

9   Hakonarson H, Bjornsdottir US, Halapi E *et al.* Profiling of genes expressed in peripheral blood mononuclear cells predicts glucocorticoid sensitivity in asthma patients. *Proc Natl Acad Sci USA* 2005;102:14789–94.

10 Barnes PJ. Scientific rationale for inhaled combination therapy with long-acting beta2-agonists and corticosteroids. *Eur Respir J* 2002;19:182–91.

11 De Benedetti F, Meazza C, Vivarelli M *et al.* Functional and prognostic relevance of the −173 polymorphism of the macrophage migration inhibitory factor gene in systemic-onset juvenile idiopathic arthritis. *Arthritis Rheum* 2003;48:1398–407.

12 Donn R, Alourfi Z, Zeggini E *et al.* A functional promoter haplotype of macrophage migration inhibitory factor is linked and associated with juvenile idiopathic arthritis. *Arthritis Rheum* 2004;50:1604–10.

13 Ito K, Lim S, Caramori G *et al.* Cigarette smoking reduces histone deacetylase 2 expression, enhances cytokine expression, and inhibits glucocorticoid actions in alveolar macrophages. *FASEB J* 2001;15:1110–2.

Cushing's syndrome

John Newell-Price

☐ INTRODUCTION

Cushing's syndrome results from prolonged and inappropriate exposure to excessive levels of circulating free glucocorticoids. The use of supraphysiological amounts of exogenous glucocorticoids is the most common cause of Cushing's syndrome, and an adequate drug history is essential. This article will focus on endogenous Cushing's syndrome.

Diagnosis is usually straightforward when presentation is florid. In contrast, diagnosis in the context of more subtle disease, especially when associated with common conditions such as type 2 diabetes and obesity, is a considerable challenge. Diagnosis of hypercortisolism must be established before searching for the underlying cause.

☐ EPIDEMIOLOGY AND PROGNOSIS

Patients with incompletely controlled severe Cushing's syndrome have a five-fold excess mortality. The reported prevalence ranges from 0.7 per million population per year to 2.4 per million population per year. Recent studies, however, indicate that Cushing's syndrome with a subtle phenotype is present in 2–5% of obese patients with type 2 diabetes, poor metabolic control, and hypertension and that metabolic control improved after intervention for Cushing's syndrome. If confirmed, these data suggest that widespread screening for Cushing's syndrome may be warranted, but control of mild cortisol excess still needs to be shown to be of benefit.[1]

☐ CAUSES OF CUSHING'S SYNDROME

Endogenous Cushing's syndrome is divided into adrenocorticotrophin (ACTH)-dependent and -independent causes and is more common in women than men (Table 1). Cushing's disease (pituitary adenoma) accounts for most cases. The most common sites of ectopic secretion of ACTH are small cell carcinomas of the lung and bronchial carcinoid tumours. Ectopic ACTH syndrome may have a rapid onset and severe features, although, in some patients, wasting may mask hyper-cortisolism, and hypokalaemia may be a clue to diagnosis (see below). In contrast, the clinical phenotype of carcinoid tumours may be very similar to that of Cushing's disease.[2]

Table 1 Aetiology of Cushing's syndrome.

Cause	Cases (%)	Female:male ratio	Female cases (%)	Male cases (%)
ACTH-dependent				
Cushing's disease	70	3.5:1	90	60–70
Ectopic ACTH syndrome	10	1:1	10	30
Unknown source of ACTH*	5	5:1		
ACTH-independent				
Adrenal adenoma	10	4:1		
Adrenal carcinoma	5	1:1		
ACTH-independent macronodular adrenal hyperplasia (AIMAH)	<2			
Primary pigmented nodular adrenal disease (PPNAD)	<2			
McCune-Albright syndrome	<2			

ACTH=adrenocorticotrophin
*Patients may ultimately prove to have Cushing's disease.

In most cases, ACTH-independent Cushing's syndrome is the result of a unilateral tumour: adrenal carcinoma in 40% and adenoma in 60% of cases. Other very rare adrenal causes of Cushing's syndrome include ACTH-independent macronodular adrenal hyperplasia (AIMAH), primary pigmented nodular adrenal disease (PPNAD), and McCune-Albright syndrome.

In many cases, patients with AIMAH have, in both adrenal glands, aberrant expression of receptors that are not normally present or increased expression of receptors that are usually present. In cases where receptors are coupled to increased cyclic adenosine monophosphate (cAMP), activation is thought to cause adrenal hyperplasia over many years. The cause of abnormal expression of these receptors is not known. Less commonly, aberrant receptors also occur in unilateral adenomas.[3]

Primary pigmented nodular adrenal disease can be sporadic or part of the Carney complex, and most cases occur in late childhood or in young adults, with small, often radiologically invisible, nodules on the adrenal gland. Mild cyclical features make diagnosis difficult. Germline mutations of the regulatory subunit R1A of PKA (*PRKAR1A*) are present in about 45% of patients with Carney complex and also in patients with sporadic PPNAD.[1]

In McCune-Albright syndrome, a postzygotic-activating mutation in the *GNAS1* gene causes hyperactivity in the affected tissues. The resulting tissue mosaicism results in a varied phenotype, and the disease may present in the first few weeks of life.

☐ CLINICAL FEATURES OF CUSHING'S SYNDROME

Clinical features are variably present in any given patient (Table 2) and may vary in a 'cyclical fashion', which causes diagnostic difficulty. The signs that most reliably distinguish Cushing's syndrome from simple obesity are thin skin in the young, easy bruising, and proximal myopathy.[4] In children, obesity and decreased linear growth are particularly common. More than 70% of patients with Cushing's syndrome present with psychiatric symptoms ranging from anxiety to frank psychosis. Some degree of psychiatric disturbance often persists after cure of Cushing's syndrome.[5]

Table 2 Clinical features of Cushing's syndrome (most discriminating features shown in bold).

Feature	Cases (%)	Feature	Cases (%)
Obesity or weight gain	95*	Hirsutism	75
Facial plethora	90	Depression/emotional lability	70
Rounded face	90	**Easy bruising**	65
Decreased libido	90	Glucose intolerance	60
Thin skin	85	**Proximal myopathy**	60
Decrease linear growth in children	70–80	Osteopaenia or fracture	50
Menstrual irregularity	80	Nephrolithiasis	50
Hypertension	75		

*100% in children.

☐ BIOCHEMICAL DIAGNOSIS OF HYPERCORTISOLAEMIA

Diagnostic evaluation is usually prompted by clinical suspicion, but screening may be warranted in certain patient groups without classical clinical features, such as patients with poorly controlled diabetes and hypertension and men with unexplained osteoporosis. Biochemical confirmation of the hypercortisolaemic state must be established before any attempt at differential diagnosis: failure to do so will result in misdiagnosis and inappropriate treatment and management (Fig 1). Hypercortisolaemia is also found in some patients with depression, alcoholism, anorexia nervosa, and late pregnancy; in contrast with true endogenous Cushing's syndrome, however, the biochemistry improves when the underlying condition has resolved.

Several tests are usually needed. Investigation should be performed when there is no acute concurrent illness, as this may cause false positive results. If in doubt, tests should be repeated or further opinion sought. The three main tests in use are the 'low-dose' dexamethasone suppression test, 24-hour urinary free cortisol, and assessment of midnight plasma or late-night salivary cortisol.[1,4]

Low-dose dexamethasone suppression tests

Two low-dose dexamethasone suppression tests are in common use. In the overnight test, 1 mg of dexamethasone is administered at 2300, and levels of cortisol in serum are measured the next day at 0800–0900. In the 48-hour dexamethasone suppression test, dexamethasone is administered at a dose of 0.5 mg every six hours for two days at 0900, 1500, 2100, and 0300 hours, with levels of cortisol in serum measured at 0900 at the start and end of the test. The 48-hour test is more specific and with adequate

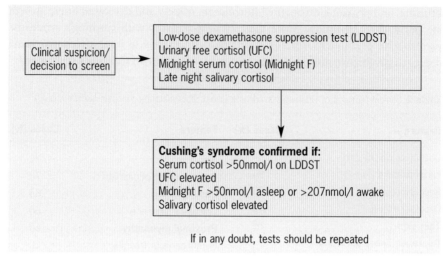

Fig 1 Biochemical diagnosis of Cushing's syndrome.

written instructions can be performed by outpatients. Moreover, a 30% decrease in levels of cortisol in serum with the 48-hour test is suggestive of a pituitary origin of disease.[6] After either test, the serum level of cortisol should be <50 nmol/l to exclude Cushing's syndrome, but, importantly, 3–8% of patients with Cushing's disease (pituitary) show suppression of serum levels of cortisol to <50 nmol/l on either test (false negative). If clinical suspicion remains high, therefore, repeated tests and other investigations are indicated. False positive responses may result from malabsorption of dexamethasone, drugs that increase hepatic clearance of dexamethasone (including carbamazepine, phenytoin, phenobarbital, and rifampicin), and oestrogen treatment or pregnancy, which increase cortisol-binding globulin (CBG) and thus the total cortisol as measured by most assays. Oral oestrogens need to be stopped for a period of 4–6 weeks so that levels of CBG can return to basal values.

Urinary free cortisol

Excess circulating cortisol is excreted in urine as free cortisol (urinary free cortisol, UFC). Levels of UFC fourfold greater than the upper limit of normal are rare except in patients with Cushing's syndrome. Three collections are needed to avoid mild or cyclical disease being missed. Levels of UFC frequently overlap with those seen in patients with other causes of hypercortisolaemia. The use of high-performance liquid chromatography and tandem mass spectrometry improves diagnostic accuracy. Moreover, if renal impairment is present or collection is incomplete, the level of UFC may be falsely low.

Midnight plasma cortisol or late night salivary cortisol

The normal circadian rhythm of cortisol secretion is lost in patients with Cushing's syndrome, and a single sleeping midnight level of cortisol in plasma <50 nmol/l effectively excludes Cushing's syndrome at the time of the test.[7] This may be particularly helpful when incomplete suppression was seen with dexamethasone testing. Values >50 nmol/l are found in patients with Cushing's syndrome, but this lacks specificity, as patients with acute illness also have values higher than this level. An awake midnight plasma level of cortisol >207 nmol/l (7.5 μg/dl) differentiates between Cushing's syndrome and other causes of hypercortisolaemia, but it may miss mild disease in about 7% of cases.[8]

Late-night salivary cortisol

Salivary levels of cortisol reflect levels of free circulating cortisol, are easy to collect, and are stable at room temperature, which makes them a highly suitable screening tool for outpatient assessment.[1,9] The test has a sensitivity and specificity of 95–98% and is particularly useful in the assessment of cyclical Cushing's syndrome and in children. Currently, access to salivary cortisol assays in the United Kingdom is not widespread, and as the levels of salivary cortisol are an order of magnitude lower than serum levels, it is essential that the performance of any assay is known and that the appropriate cut-off point is used.

☐ DIFFERENTIAL DIAGNOSIS – DETERMINING THE CAUSE OF CUSHING'S SYNDROME

Once a diagnosis of Cushing's syndrome is established, the next step is to determine the cause, and this is best done in major referral centres. The first step is to measure levels of ACTH in plasma (Fig 2). The plasma should be separated rapidly and stored at –40°C to avoid degradation and a falsely low result. Levels of ACTH consistently <5 pg/ml indicate ACTH-independent Cushing's syndrome, while levels persistently >15 pg/ml almost always reflect ACTH-dependent pathologies and require investigation, as detailed below. Levels between these two values need cautious interpretation, as, occasionally, patients with Cushing's disease and adrenal pathologies may have intermediate values: in patients with low baseline levels of ACTH in plasma, a positive test for corticotrophin-releasing hormone (see below) may show pituitary ACTH dependency.

Adrenocorticotrophin-independent Cushing's syndrome

In ACTH-independent Cushing's syndrome caused by an adrenal adenoma, carcinoma, or AIMAH, the anatomical cause is invariably visible on imaging with computed tomography (CT). In PPNAD, the adrenal glands may appear normal. Thus, in an established diagnosis of ACTH-independent Cushing's syndrome with normal appearances of the adrenal glands on imaging, exogenous glucocorticoid ingestion should be reconsidered, and genetic testing for mutations of *PRKAR1A* or assessment of other features of Carney complex (lentigines and myxoma) may be of benefit as a diagnostic procedure.

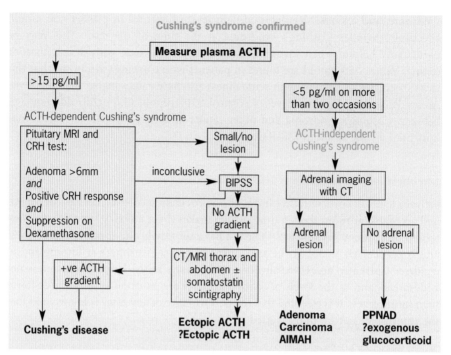

Fig 2 Diagnosis of cause of Cushing's syndrome. CRH=corticotrophin-releasing hormone; AIMAH=adrenocorticotrophin (ACTH)-independent macronodular hyperplasia; PPNAD=primary pigmented nodular adrenal disease; BIPSS=bilateral inferior petrosal sinus sampling; SCLC=small-cell lung cancer.

Adrenocorticotrophin-dependent Cushing's syndrome

Biochemical evaluation, rather than imaging, is the key to differentiating between pituitary and non-pituitary sources. If a patient has ACTH-dependent Cushing's syndrome with responses on dexamethasone suppression and CRH testing that both suggest pituitary disease and a pituitary magnetic resonance image that shows an isolated lesion of ≥6 mm, most doctors will regard a diagnosis of Cushing's disease to have been made. In all other circumstances, bilateral inferior petrosal sinus sampling (BIPSS) is recommended (see Fig 2 and below). Ectopic ACTH syndrome is usually associated with higher circulating levels of cortisol. These high levels overcome the activity of the 11β-hydroxysteroid dehydrogenase type II enzyme, which allows cortisol to act as a mineralocorticoid in the kidney. Consequently, hypokalaemia is more frequent in ectopic ACTH syndrome, but it is also present in 10% of cases of Cushing's disease.[4]

Corticotrophin-releasing hormone test

Recombinant human or ovine-sequence CRH is administered as an intravenous bolus dose of 1 µg/kg or, more usually, 100 µg intravenously. This stimulates corticotroph tumour cells in the pituitary to release ACTH and hence increase serum levels of cortisol, while responses in patients with ectopic ACTH syndrome are uncommon.

Bilateral inferior petrosal sinus sampling (BIPSS)

Sampling of the gradient of ACTH from the pituitary to the periphery is the most reliable means for discriminating between pituitary and non-pituitary sources of ACTH. Bilateral inferior petrosal sinus sampling is a highly skilled and invasive technique that requires placement of catheters in both inferior petrosal sinuses. A basal central:peripheral ratio of >2:1 or a CRH-stimulated ratio of >3:1 is consistent with Cushing's disease, with a sensitivity and a specificity of 94%.[10]

□ RADIOLOGY

Pituitary

Magnetic resonance imaging (MRI) is the investigation of choice for imaging of the pituitary gland. With standard MRI protocols, 40% of corticotroph microadenomas are not visualised, while in the normal population, the rate of 'incidentalomas' is 10%, which emphasises the importance of biochemical assessment.

Adrenal

In 30% of cases of Cushing's disease, the adrenal glands appear normal. In patients with ectopic ACTH syndrome, the adrenals are almost always homogeneously enlarged.

Imaging in ectopic ACTH syndrome

Axial imaging with thin-cut, multi-slice CT of the thorax and abdomen or MRI of the thorax, or both, has the highest detection rate for ectopic ACTH syndrome. Most patients harbour small neuroendocrine tumours that may express somatostatin receptors and also may be disclosed on somatostatin receptor scintigraphy, but this approach has only rarely been shown to disclose truly 'occult' tumours that are not visible on CT. Positron emission tomography (PET) with 18-flurodeoxyglucose (FDG) is of little benefit, as such tumours are usually of low metabolic activity. The use of ^{11}C-5-hydroxytryptophan has been proposed as a universal imaging technique for neuroendocrine tumours, but few patients have been studied. Despite extensive investigation, the cause of ACTH may remain 'occult' in 5–15% of patients, and these patients need continued follow up.

□ TREATMENT

Surgery for Cushing's syndrome

Transsphenoidal surgery

Transsphenoidal selective microadenomectomy by an experienced surgeon is the treatment of choice for the vast majority of patients with Cushing's disease, but it produces long-lasting remission in only 50–60% of cases. This emphasises the continued need for other effective treatments to reduce levels of ACTH in patients with Cushing's disease.

Adrenal surgery

Laparoscopic unilateral adrenalectomy is the treatment of choice for patients with an isolated adrenal adenoma. The prognosis after removal of adrenocortical cortisol-secreting adenomas is good. In contrast, the prognosis is almost uniformly very poor in patients with adrenocortical carcinomas.

With ACTH-dependent Cushing's syndrome of any cause, bilateral adrenalectomy may be needed to achieve adequate control of the circulating levels of cortisol. A major concern after bilateral adrenalectomy in patients with refractory Cushing's disease is the development of Nelson's syndrome – a potentially locally aggressive pituitary tumour that secretes high levels of ACTH, which result in pigmentation. This can be monitored by measurement of plasma levels of ACTH and MRI of the pituitary, and the tumour itself can be treated with further surgery and radiotherapy if needed.

Ectopic ACTH

Complete excision of an ACTH tumour usually results in long-lasting remission.

Medical treatment to reduce levels of cortisol

Treatment to reduce levels of cortisol may be used as preparation for surgery after unsuccessful surgery. It is rarely a good long-term solution and is mainly used as adjunctive treatment to other methods such as surgery and pituitary radiotherapy.[1]

Metyrapone (500–1000 mg three or four times daily, with dose increments every 72 hours) and ketoconazole (200–400 mg three times daily, with dose increments at 2–3 weekly intervals) are frequently used to inhibit synthesis of cortisol, with the aim of a mean level of plasma cortisol of 150–300 mmol/l. Metyrapone causes an increase in steroid androgenic precursors, and hirsutism is a major adverse effect in women; this does not occur with ketoconazole. In the United Kingdom, o,p'-dichloro-diphenyldichloroethane (o,p'DDD, mitotane), an adrenolytic agent, is usually reserved for the treatment of adrenocortical carcinoma. Recent studies on the use of rosiglitazone and cabergoline to reduce levels of ACTH in plasma and hence cortisol in patients with Cushing's disease have had disappointing results.

Pituitary radiotherapy

After transsphenoidal surgery, persisting hypercortisolaemia may be treated with pituitary radiotherapy. Progressive anterior pituitary failure is the major side effect, and, in particular, growth hormone deficiency is virtually uniform 10 years after treatment, while gonadotrophin deficiency is present in about 15% of cases.

□ CONCLUSIONS

The diagnosis and management of Cushing's syndrome remains a considerable challenge and warrants referral to major centres. Cushing's syndrome may be present in a significant minority of patients with poorly controlled type 2 diabetes, and this has considerable implications for screening of this at-risk population. Salivary cortisol is a promising screening tool and may be particularly suited for this purpose. The outcome of treatment for Cushing's disease remains disappointing in many patients, and further developments are needed in this area.

REFERENCES

1   Newell-Price J, Bertagna X, Grossman AB, Nieman LK. Cushing's syndrome. *Lancet* 2006;367: 1605–17.

2   Nieman LK. *Cushing's syndrome.* Philadephia: WB Saunders, 2001.

3   Bertagna X, Groussin L, Luton JP, Bertherat J. Aberrant receptor-mediated Cushing's syndrome. *Horm Res* 2003;59 (Suppl 1):99–103.

4   Newell-Price J, Trainer P, Besser M, Grossman A. The diagnosis and differential diagnosis of Cushing's syndrome and pseudo-Cushing's states. *Endocr Rev* 1998;19:647–72.

5   Arnaldi G, Angeli A, Atkinson AB *et al.* Diagnosis and complications of Cushing's syndrome: a consensus statement. *J Clin Endocrinol Metab* 2003;88:5593–602.

6   Isidori AM, Kaltsas GA, Mohammed S *et al.* Discriminatory value of the low-dose dexamethasone suppression test in establishing the diagnosis and differential diagnosis of Cushing's syndrome. *J Clin Endocrinol Metab* 2003;88:5299–306.

7   Newell-Price J, Trainer P, Perry L *et al.* A single sleeping midnight cortisol has 100% sensitivity for the diagnosis of Cushing's syndrome. *Clin Endocrinol (Oxf)* 1995;43:545–50.

8   Papanicolaou DA, Yanovski JA, Cutler GB Jr, Chrousos GP, Nieman LK. A single midnight serum cortisol measurement distinguishes Cushing's syndrome from pseudo-Cushing states. *J Clin Endocrinol Metab* 1998;83:1163–7.

9   Findling JW, Raff H. Diagnosis and differential diagnosis of Cushing's syndrome. *Endocrinol Metab Clin North Am* 2001;30:729–47.

10 Lindsay JR, Nieman LK. Differential diagnosis and imaging in Cushing's syndrome. *Endocrinol Metab Clin North Am* 2005;34:403–21, x.

☐ DIABETES/ENDOCRINOLOGY SELF ASSESSMENT QUESTIONS

Understanding glucocorticoids

1   Glucocorticoids act through the glucocorticoid receptor, which:
   (a) Is a member of the nuclear receptor superfamily
   (b) Translocates to the nucleus in response to ligand
   (c) Works exclusively by binding to DNA
   (d) Is the only receptor capable of binding cortisol in humans
   (e) Potentiates NFkB function

2   11β hydroxysteroid dehydrogenases:
   (a) Are extracellular enzymes
   (b) Act on aldosterone
   (c) Exclusively inactivate cortisol
   (d) Can potentiate the action of cortisol
   (e) Are unidirectional

3   Glucocorticoid resistance in inflammation may be the result of:
   (a) The action of NFkB
   (b) Modification of the structure of chromatin
   (c) The action of 11β hydroxysteroid dehydrogenase type I
   (d) Local production of macrophage migration inhibitory factor
   (e) Genetic variation in the glucocorticoid receptor gene

Cushing's syndrome

1   The most discriminating clinical signs for Cushing's syndrome are:
   (a) Hirsutism
   (b) Proximal myopathy
   (c) Thin skin
   (d) 'Buffalo hump'
   (e) Easy bruising

2   The following are used to make a diagnosis of Cushing's syndrome:
   (a) Urinary free cortisol
   (b) Low-dose dexamethasone-suppression test
   (c) 0900 levels of cortisol in serum
   (d) Levels of ACTH in plasma
   (e) Glucagon stimulation test

3   Cushing's syndrome is caused by:
   (a) Pituitary adenoma in 40% of cases
   (b) Ectopic ACTH in 30% of cases
   (c) Adrenal adenoma in 20% of cases
   (d) Aberrant receptor expression in 5% of cases
   (e) Primary pigmented nodular adrenal disease in 5% of cases

Geriatrics

Advances in Parkinson's disease

Jeremy R Playfer

Parkinson's disease affects around four million people worldwide and 120,000 in the United Kingdom. It is a major cause of physical and psychiatric disability in old age and is almost the perfect example of an age-related disease. Unique among neurogenerative diseases, effective drug treatment with dopaminergic therapy has now been available for more than 40 years. Advances in the past 10 years have greatly increased the understanding of the pathophysiology and pathogenesis of the disease. The hope is that this greater understanding will identify new therapeutic interventions, including methods for disease modification and prevention.

☐ LEWY BODIES

The definitive pathological finding in patients with idiopathic Parkinson's disease is the Lewy body,[1] a hyaline eosinophilic neuronal inclusion body first described by Frederick Lewy in 1907. Lewy was a student of Alzheimer, and just as plaques and tangles described by Alzheimer characterised Alzheimer's disease, so the Lewy body is pathognomonic of Parkinson's disease, being present in all cases. This pathological marker is not exclusive to Parkinson's disease, however, occurring in a number of juvenile neuro-genetic neurodegenerative conditions – most notably Hallervordan-Spatz disease. Lewy bodies are also identified in about 10% of all post-mortem examinations of people who died after the age of 60 years (incidental Lewy body disease), and this may represent a preclinical phase before development of the full disease. Lewy bodies also occur with a slightly different morphology in the cerebral cortex in patients with Lewy body dementia.

The classic Lewy body occurs in monoaminergic and cholinergic neurones in the brain stem, mid-brain, basal forebrain, cerebral cortex, and autonomic ganglia. Lewy bodies are around 5–25 μm in diameter and have a spherical, dense, hyaline core surrounded by a paler staining halo. The electron microscopic ultrastructure shows an aggregated filamentous structure that radiates from a dark, osmiophilic, granular core. The development of immunohistochemical techniques that use anti-ubiquitin and anti-α-synuclein stains has led to recognition that Lewy bodies are widespread and that their morphology differs from location to location. The classic Lewy body contrasts with non-spherical shapes that appear in sympathetic ganglia, basal forebrain, and brainstem nuclei, including the dorsal motor nucleus of the vagus.

Although the ultrastructure of Lewy bodies is complex, our increasing understanding of the aetiology and pathophysiology of Parkinson's disease makes sense of a number of these elements. The filamental structures derive from cytoskeletal elements. Ubiquitin and protease enzymes are derived from elements of the proteosome system. The bodies are rich in phosphate because of the presence of enzymes of phosphorylation and dephosphorylation. A number of other epitopes seem to be fairly large proteins that are passively attracted to the aggregation. They are generally tau-negative – unlike in the pathology of Alzheimer's disease.

Clues from the pathology indicate failures in the information- and energy-support systems of cells, which mirror the presence of genetic and environmental factors in the pathogenesis of Parkinson's disease. Hallmarks of an accumulative process are also present. The informational system that fails is proteonomic and centres on the proteosome, a structure found universally in eukaryotic cells. This system is likened to an office shredder: misfolded or damaged proteins are labelled by ubiquitin in a series of adenosine triphosphate (ATP)-dependent steps catalysed by ubiquitin ligases. An ubiquitinated protein has a tail of polymerised ubiquitin that allows it to be unfolded and to pass into the cylindrically structured 26S proteosome complex, which comprises four cylindrical subunits. As the protein enters the complex and is broken down to amino acids, the ubiquitin chain is cleaved and broken down into monomers, which are recycled.

In patients with Parkinson's disease, the ubiquitin proteosome system fails at several different levels.[2] Understanding of this has been achieved through the discovery of rare Mendelian variants of Parkinson's disease, in which the causal mutations affect a variety of steps involving protease activity and ubiquitination. The mutation coding for α-synuclein causes the protein to misfold and resist clearance by the ubiquitin proteosome system, which leads to the accumulation of α-synuclein that is so characteristic with the Lewy body. How the accumulation of large amounts of α-synuclein affects normal cellular function is uncertain, and the Lewy body may be a protective mechanism to sequester large amounts of abnormal protein.[3] The mitochondria seem particularly vulnerable and lose membrane potential, which triggers a bioenergetic crisis, as well as a caspase cascade that leads to apoptotic death of the neuromelanin-containing cells of the pars compacta of the substantia nigra. Why these cells are especially susceptible is not known.

☐ GENETICS OF PARKINSON'S DISEASE

One of the questions most frequently asked by patients with newly diagnosed Parkinson's disease is whether their children will have an increased risk of developing the disease. Any index case will have about a 17% chance of having at least one first-degree relative affected by the condition. A twin study by Chris Ward showed that Parkinson's disease had the lowest heritability of any disease in which a twin study had been undertaken.[4] Estimates of heritability increased when studies were followed up with functional neuroimaging, as many unaffected co-twins were found to have subclinical dopaminergic abnormalities that, if taken as evidence of preclinical disease, raised the concordance rate to as high as 45% between monozygotic twins.

The past decade has seen identification of various Parkinson's disease-related mutations (Table 1).[5] All are rare, and single gene mutations account for around 3% of all cases of sporadic Parkinson's disease. Mutations are named 'PARK', followed by a

Table 1 Genetics of Parkinson's disease.

Locus	Designation	Transmission	Gene/linkage
4q21-23	PARK 1	AD	α-synuclein
6q25-27	PARK 2	AR	Parkin
4q21	PARK 4(1)*	AD	α-synuclein
4p14	PARK 5	AD	UCHL1
1p36	PARK 6	AR	PINK1
1p36	PARK 7	AR	DJ1
12p11.2-q13.1	PARK 8	AD	LRRK2
2p13	PARK 3	AD	Unknown
1p36	PARK 9	AR	Unknown
1P32	PARK 10	Unknown	Unknown
2q36-37	PARK 11	Unknown	Unknown

AD = autosomal dominant; AR=autosomal recessive
* Mitochondrial mutations.

number signifying the order of their discovery. PARK 4 was subsequently discovered to be a triplication of the PARK 1 *α-synuclein* gene. The gene in which PARK 1 occurs was first discovered in a kindred comprising 50 members from four generations of a family that originated in Conturski, Italy, with latter generations who had migrated to America. This mutation first drew attention to α-synuclein, which had already been recognised as a component of Lewy bodies. Mutations in *α-synuclein* result in a misfolded protein that aggregates as protofibrils. These can cause a failure of mitochondrial function. PARK 1 is a very rare variant that is autosomal dominant and gives rise to an atypical phenotype of Parkinson's disease with young onset and a benign course but associations with premature mortality from other causes.

PARK 2 (*parkin*) is an autosomal recessive mutation first found in Japan. Although Lewy bodies are not a feature of this variant, the *Parkin* gene encodes from an enzyme in the ubiquitin protease system. Mutations in other recessive genes, Park 6 (*Pink 1*) and Park 7 (*DJI*), are associated with atypical juvenile forms. The *DJI* gene seems to be linked with cells' capability to withstand oxidative stress, and *Pink 1* codes for a mitochondrial protein kinase.

PARK 8 is an autosomal dominant mutation of the enzyme leucine-rich repeat kinase (LRRK2), which encodes for the protein dardarin – a tyrosine kinase that affects the phosphorylation of key proteins involved in ubiquitation. This variant produces a phenotype of Parkinson's disease that is fairly typical, although it has variable underlying pathology and a benign prognosis.

Mitochondria

Recent studies of mitochondrial DNA have linked mutations that encode for mitochondrial complex I with cases of Parkinson's disease. Mitochondria play an important part in movement disorders. Their role in Parkinson's disease first became apparent when the neurotoxin 1-methyl-4-phenyl-1,2,3,6-tetrahydropyridine (MPTP) was shown to be taken up in the form of the free radical 1-methyl-4-phenylpyridinium (MPP+) through the dopamine transporter system and to inhibit mitochondrial complex 1 in the mitochondria of dopaminergic cells. Professor Schapira at the Royal Free Hospital showed that mitochondria in patients with Parkinson's disease lose their membrane potential and that this is one of the initial steps that lead to cell death.[6] The same defect in mitochondrial complex 1 is seen in patient with sporadic Parkinson's disease, and Professor Schapira showed that this anomaly could also be detected in mitochondrial complex 1 in the platelets of patients with Parkinson's disease.

When mitochondrial dysfunction sets in, an increase in free radical production results from oxidative stress, which damages proteins that cannot be cleared if proteosomal dysfunction is present.[7] This therefore leads to aggregated proteins, cell damage, and cell death. The rare monogenic disorders affect distinct steps in this pathway, but some environmental insults are also liable to increase free radical damage or are toxic to mitochondria, which can lead to the same common pathway. In most sporadic cases, a combination of increased susceptibility because of a number of genes plus an environmental factor is likely. For a person to develop clinical Parkinson's disease, they need to have lost more than 50% of their dopaminergic cells, which is largely because of apoptosis. This seems to be triggered by mitochondrial depolarisation, which prompts activation of the caspase cascade.[8]

As gliosis is present in the area of the basal ganglia, a number of other mechanisms may be involved, and inflammatory change may be a factor. In addition, compensatory neuronal changes can lead to excessive release of excitatory neurotransmitters and death of cells by exitotoxicity. Parkinson's disease seems likely to prove to be a heterogeneous disease characterised by a common final pathway that leads to excessive cell death of dopaminergic cells. Increasing understanding of these mechanisms is opening up targets for intervention and the possibility, in the long term, of halting the disease process and achieving neuroprotection.

☐ BRAAK'S HYPOTHESIS

The type of advances I have described so far depend on advanced molecular biological techniques, but the improved ability to recognise Lewy bodies led to the classic work of Professor Heiko Braak, a German professor of anatomy.[9] He initially surveyed brains for Lewy bodies using the haematoxylin and eosin technique, but he subsequently repeated the work with a modern immunostaining method. He described the geographical distribution of Lewy bodies in a series of anatomical sections of brains and, analysing these statistically, he hypothesised that the evolution of Parkinson's disease has six stages. He found that the earliest evidence of Lewy bodies was not in the substantia nigra but in the dorsal motor nucleus of the vagus nerve in the brainstem. After the work of Chris Hawks described the loss of smell as an early feature of Parkinson's disease, Braak also showed an early presence of Lewy bodies in the olfactory bulb. As the disease progresses, the Lewy bodies seem to progress retrogradely up the brain – from the brainstem to the mid-brain and basal ganglia and towards the frontal cortex from the olfactory bulb.

In the late stages of the disease, cortical involvement is extensive, and patients develop cognitive impairment. Braak's study described the presence of Lewy bodies, which do not necessarily correlate with cell death. The neuropigmented neurones of the ventral-lateral region of the substantia nigra seem to be particularly vulnerable to cell death once Lewy bodies appear. Although Parkinson's disease is an age-related disease, the pattern of neuronal death associated purely with old age has a different geographical distribution that affects the dorsal rather than ventral region of the pars compacta of the substantia nigra, with the vulnerability conferred by age probably a combination of natural ageing of the dopaminergic system and added pathological insult. Age confers an increased risk of psychiatric side effects.

Braak's hypothesis explains why Parkinson's disease is not just a movement disorder but is always associated with a variety of non-motor features (Box 1). The neuropsychiatric features are particularly important, as they have a disproportionate effect on quality of life (Box 2). Debate about the relation between dementia with Lewy bodies (DLB) and Parkinson's disease dementia (PDD) is active. Many regard DLB as a syndronomic variation of Lewy body (α-synuclein) pathology, in which cortical involvement becomes apparent before that of the basal ganglia. The clinical picture is complicated by the frequently associated neuropathological changes of Alzheimer's disease, which is more common in patients with Parkinson's disease. Aarsland, Meara and McKeith all have shown that the burden of psychiatric disease in patients with Parkinson's disease is greater than previously recognised.[10–12] Aarsland's recent epidemiological work showed that more than 80% of patients with Parkinson's disease will eventually develop dementia.

Mood disturbance and depression affect about one third of patients with Parkinson's disease at any one time.[13] The evidence base on treatment of psychiatric

Box 1 Non-motor features of Parkinson's disease.

Autonomic	**Sensory**
• Orthostatic hypotension	• Pain
• Impaired thermoregulation	
• Disorders of sweating	**Sleep disorders**
• Sexual dysfunction	
• Urinary dysfunction	
• Gastro-intestinal motility	
• Dysphagia	

Box 2 Neuropsychiatric features in Parkinson's disease.

• Cognitive impairment	• Hallucinations
• Dementia	• Anxiety
• Depression	• Hedonistic dysregulation syndrome
• Drug-induced psychosis	

illness in Parkinson's disease is inadequate, and this is an area that requires much more clinical research.[14]

□ MANAGEMENT

The management of Parkinson's disease is defined by a clinical pathway paradigm developed by MacMahon *et al*[15] (Box 3). Parkinson's disease is a complex, multi-faceted disorder, and patients need a comprehensive service that is flexible through the key stages of management, diagnosis, maintenance, complex management, and palliation. Diagnosis always should be confirmed by a neurologist or geriatrician with expertise in the field. Patients require education and support from a variety of specialists. Support from specialist nurses, physiotherapists, occupational therapists, and speech and language therapists working in a multi-disciplinary team has been shown to reduce disability, and the evidence base for treatments in patients with Parkinson's disease is rapidly developing and supported by recent guidelines from the National Institute for Health and Clinical Excellence.

Medical management of Parkinson's disease aims to achieve optimum control of symptoms while reducing potential side effects.[16] Levodopa (L-dopa), although remaining the gold standard of treatment, is beset by complications of long-term treatment (Box 4). Controlled trials that compared L-dopa with dopamine agonists have shown the potential of dopamine agonists to reduce long-term motor fluctuations. The trials, however, suffer from selection bias, particularly with regard to age. Agonists not as effective as L-dopa have more psychiatric side effects, particularly in the older patient. The concept of continuous dopaminergic stimulation as an explanation of agonists having fewer motor complications has led to the use of adjunct therapy with L-dopa. Both catechol-O-methyltransferase (COMT) and monoamine oxidase (MAO) inhibitors increase the half-life of L-dopa and, as a consequence, reduce wearing off. The COMT inhibitor entacapone in fixed combination with L-dopa (combined L-dopa, carbidopa and entacapone) is well established as a safe and effective treatment and the outcome of the ongoing STRIDE trial may change its indication to initial use. Safety concerns have reduced the use of the MAO inhibitor selegiline, but the recently licensed rasagiline overcomes these difficulties. A number of drugs with novel actions are in phase I and II clinical trials, including possible neuroprotective agents such as caffeine, coenzyme Q_{10}, nicotine, minocycline, GM1 ganglioside, rasagaline, and creatinine.

Box 3 Clinical paradigm of Parkinson's disease. Reproduced from MacMahon *et al*, with permission of Springer Science and Business Media.[15]

Clinical stages

Diagnosis
Maintenance
Complex management
Palliative

Box 4 Complications of treatment with levodopa.

Intermediate
- Gastrointestinal tract upset
- Postural hypotension

Motor
- Wearing off
- End-of-dose deterioration
- On–off syndrome
- Dose failure
- Freezing
- Dyskinesias
- Dystonia

Non-motor
- Muscle pain
- Excess swelling
- Hypersomnolence

Neuropsychiatric
- Hallucinations
- Psychosis
- Hypersexuality

Age, frailty, and comorbidity remain dominant factors in the management of patients with Parkinson's disease.

REFERENCES

1 Gibb WR, Lees AJ. The relevance of the Lewy body to the pathogenesis of idiopathic Parkinson's disease. *J Neurol Neurosurg Psychiatry* 1988;51:745–52.

2 McNaught KS, Olanow CW. Proteolytic stress: a unifying concept for the etiopathogenesis of Parkinson's disease. *Ann Neurol* 2003;53(Suppl 3):S73–84.

3 Halliday GM, Ophof A, Broe M *et al.* Alpha-synuclein redistributes to neuromelanin lipid in the substantia nigra early in Parkinson's disease. *Brain* 2005;128:2654–64.

4 Ward CD, Duvoisin RC, Ince SE *et al.* Parkinson's disease in 65 pairs of twins and in a set of quadruplets. *Neurology* 1983:33:815–24.

5 Mouraduian MM. Recent advances in the genetics and pathogenesis of Parkinson disease. *Neurology* 2002;58:179–85.

6 Schapira AH. Causes of neuronal death in Parkinson's disease. *Adv Neurol* 2001;86:155–62.

7 Gu M, Owen AD, Toffa SE *et al.* Mitochondrial function, GSH and iron in neurodegeneration and Lewy body diseases. *J Neurol Sci* 1998;158:24–9.

8 Love R. Mitochondria back in the spotlight in Parkinson's disease. *Lancet Neurol* 2004;3:326.

9 Braak H, Del Tredici K, Rub U *et al.* Staging of brain pathology related to sporadic Parkinson's disease. *Neurobiol Aging* 2003;24:197–211.

10 Aarsland D, Zaccai J, Brayne C. A systematic review of prevalence studies of dementia in Parkinson's disease. *Mov Disord* 2005;20:1255–63.

11 Hobson P, Gallacher J, Meara J. Cross-sectional survey of Parkinson's disease and parkinsonism in a rural area of the United Kingdom. *Mov Disord* 2005;20:995–8.

12 McKeith I, Mintzer J, Aaarsland D *et al.* Dementia with Lewy bodies. *Lancet Neurol* 2004;3:19–28.

13 Ehrt U, Bronnick K, Leentjens AF, Larsen JP, Aarsland D. Depressive symptom profile in Parkinson's disease: a comparison with depression in elderly patients without Parkinson's disease. *Int J Geriatr Psychiatry* 2006;21:252–8.

14 Hindle JV. Neuropsychiatry. In: Playfer JR, Hindle J, eds. *Parkinson's disease in the older patient.* London: Arnold, 2001.

15 MacMahon DG, Thomas S. Practical approach to quality of life in Parkinson's disease: the nurse's role. *J Neurol* 1998;245 (Suppl 1):S19–22.

16 Bhatia K, Brooks DJ, Burn DJ *et al.* Updated guidelines for the management of Parkinson's disease. *Hosp Med* 2001;62:456–70.

☐ GERIATRICS SELF ASSESSMENT QUESTIONS

Advances in Parkinson's disease

1   Mitochondria:
   (a) Patients with Parkinson's disease have a disorder of mitochondrial complex I
   (b) Mutations in mitochondrial DNA are associated with Parkinson's disease
   (c) Once affected by oxidative stress, mitochondria trigger apoptosis through the caspase cascade
   (d) Synuclein is associated with loss of mitochondrial membrane potential
   (e) Mitochondrial mutations are inherited from the male parent

2   Management of Parkinson's disease:
   (a) Choice of treatment is unaffected by the age of patient
   (b) Dopamine agonists are the most effective type of treatment
   (c) Levodopa causes dyskinesias but not dystonias
   (d) Dopamine agonists have been clearly shown to be neuroprotective
   (e) Long-acting drugs are less likely to cause motor fluctuations

3   Psychiatry of Parkinson's disease
   (a) Most patients with Parkinson's disease eventually develop dementia
   (b) Depression affects about 10% of patients with Parkinson's disease at any given time
   (c) Cognitive impairment can be detected before motor symptoms
   (d) Clinical trials of selective serotonin reuptake inhibitors have been undertaken in patients with Parkinson's disease
   (e) Dopaminergic drugs can cause hypersexuality

4   Lewy bodies:
   (a) Occur only in idiopathic Parkinson's disease
   (b) Occur exclusively in pigmented neurones
   (c) Contain the protein α-synuclein
   (d) Are tau-negative
   (e) Occur in glial cells in multi-symptom atrophy

5   Genetics of Parkinson's disease
   (a) Most cases of Parkinson's disease are explained by simple Mendelian genetics
   (b) Twin studies indicate that the environment is more important than genetics in the aetiology of Parkinson's disease
   (c) The PARK 2 gene gives rise to a juvenile form of Parkinson's disease in which Lewy bodies are scarce
   (d) Mutations in the mitochondrial DNA can give rise to parkinsonism
   (e) PARK 8 (LRRK2) is the most common mutation to cause Parkinson's disease

Nephrology

IgA nephropathy and Henoch–Schönlein purpura

John Feehally

☐ INTRODUCTION AND DEFINITIONS

IgA nephropathy

IgA nephropathy (IgAN) is a mesangial proliferative glomerulonephritis (GN) characterised by diffuse mesangial deposition of IgA. Although its most common clinical presentation is visible haematuria provoked by mucosal infection, this is neither universal nor necessary for the diagnosis. IgA nephropathy is the most prevalent pattern of glomerular disease seen in most Western and Asian countries in which renal biopsy is widely practised, and it is an important cause of end-stage renal disease (ESRD). IgA nephropathy is likely not to be a single entity but rather to be a common response to various injurious mechanisms. Most typically, IgAN is a slowly progressive disease, in which the mesangial proliferative GN is followed relentlessly by glomerulosclerosis and tubulo-interstitial fibrosis, although spontaneous resolution can occur.

Henoch–Schönlein purpura

Henoch–Schönlein purpura (HSP) is a small-vessel vasculitis that affects the skin, joints, gut, and kidney, predominantly in children. It is defined by tissue deposition of IgA. The nephritis associated with HSP is also characterised by mesangial IgA deposition, and the histological features of Henoch–Schönlein (HS) nephritis can be indistinguishable from those of IgAN. IgA nephropathy has sometimes been called 'HSP without the rash'.

☐ CLINICAL MANIFESTATIONS

IgA nephropathy

The wide range of clinical presentations of IgAN varies in frequency with age. No clinical presentation is pathognomonic of IgAN.

Macroscopic haematuria

In 40–50% of cases, the clinical presentation is episodic macroscopic haematuria, most frequently in the second and third decades of life. The urine is usually brown rather than red, and clots are unusual. Haematuria usually follows intercurrent mucosal infection in the upper respiratory tract or, occasionally, in the gastrointestinal tract. Haematuria is usually visible within 24 hours of the onset of the symptoms of infection, which differentiates it from the 2–3-week delay typically seen between infection and subsequent haematuria in post-infectious (for example post-streptococcal) GN. The macroscopic haematuria resolves spontaneously in the course of a few days. Microscopic haematuria is persistent between attacks. The episodes become less frequent and resolve over a few years at most.

Microscopic haematuria and proteinuria

Asymptomatic urine testing identifies 30–40% of patients with IgAN in most reported series. Microscopic haematuria is present with or without proteinuria. The number of patients identified in this way will depend on local attitudes to urine screening, as well as the use of renal biopsy in patients with isolated microscopic haematuria. Most cases of IgAN are completely asymptomatic and would be detected only if population-based urine screening were in place. For proteinuria to occur without microscopic haematuria is rare. Nephrotic syndrome occurs in only 5% of all patients with IgAN.

Acute renal failure

Acute renal failure is very uncommon in patients with IgAN (<5% of all cases) and develops by two distinct mechanisms. Acute severe immune injury with necrotising GN and crescent formation, 'crescentic IgA nephropathy', may be present; this may be the first presentation of IgAN or may develop superimposed on established less-aggressive disease. Alternatively, acute renal failure can occur with mild glomerular injury when heavy glomerular haematuria leads to tubular occlusion and injury by red cells.

Chronic renal failure

Some patients already have renal impairment and hypertension when first diagnosed. These patients tend to be older, and it is probable that they have long-standing disease that previously remained undiagnosed because the patient neither had frank hematuria nor underwent routine urinalysis. Hypertension is common, as in other chronic glomerular disease, and accelerated hypertension occurs in 5% of patients.

Clinical associations with IgAN

Although IgAN is clinically restricted to the kidney in most cases, associations with other conditions, particularly a number of immune and inflammatory diseases including coeliac disease, ankylosing spondylitis, and dermatitis herpetiformis, are known. Mesangial IgA deposition is a frequent finding in autopsy studies of patients with chronic liver disease, particularly those with alcoholic cirrhosis, and is thought to be a consequence of impaired hepatic clearance of IgA. Only a small minority of patients have any clinical evidence of renal disease other than microscopic haematuria, although occasionally patients will develop ESRD.[1]

Henoch-Schönlein purpura

Henoch-Schönlein purpura is most prevalent in the first decade of life but may occur at any age. A palpable purpuric rash, which may be recurrent, occurs on extensor surfaces. Polyarthralgia (usually without joint swelling) and abdominal pain caused by gut vasculitis may be present. Abdominal pain may be severe, with bloody diarrhoea if intussusception develops. In practice, the diagnosis is made by clinical criteria in most children, in whom HSP is a self-limiting illness, but a precise diagnosis requires tissue confirmation of IgA deposition in renal or skin biopsies. Adults have similar clinical features, and much renal involvement in patients with HSP is transient. Urine abnormalities are noted during the acute presentation but may disappear. In cases referred to a nephrologist, asymptomatic urine abnormality is still the most frequent clinical manifestation. Nephrotic syndrome occurs in 20–30% of patients. Acute renal failure may develop as a result of crescentic GN.

☐ EPIDEMIOLOGY

Geographical and racial variation in the prevalence of IgAN is striking (Fig 1).[2] It represents up to 50% of primary glomerular disease in Japan and Southeast Asia compared with 20–25% in Europe, and it is very uncommon in Africa (<5%) and in African-Americans (2%). No information is available on geographical variations in HSP.

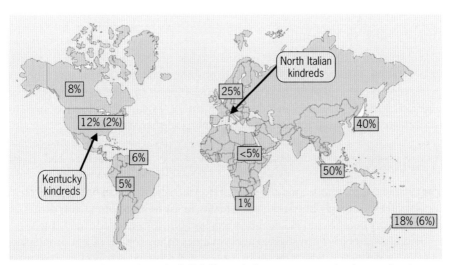

Fig 1 Epidemiology of IgA nephropathy (IgAN). Figures indicate percentage of patients undergoing renal biopsy to investigate primary glomerular disease who have IgAN. Figures in parentheses indicate the prevalence of IgAN in minority populations (African-Americans in United States and Maoris and Pacific Islanders in New Zealand). More than 90% of cases are sporadic, but large kindreds have been reported in the United States and Italy. Adapted from Feehally with permission of Elsevier.[2]

Genetic variations may be important in explaining geographical differences, but thus far, case-control studies of candidate polymorphic genes marking susceptibility to IgAN or HS nephritis or its risk of progression have been unfruitful.[3] Urine abnormalities increase in frequency among the relatives of those with IgAN, although only in a few pedigrees is IgAN found in multiple generations. One very large pedigree has been described in Kentucky, US, and other large families have been found in Italy; however, more than 90% of all cases of IgAN seem to be sporadic.

☐ DIFFERENTIAL DIAGNOSIS

IgA nephropathy

In its most characteristic clinical setting (recurrent macroscopic haematuria coinciding with mucosal infection in a male in the second or third decade of life), the diagnosis can be strongly suspected. Such a diagnosis cannot be made without a biopsy, however, as recurrent macroscopic haematuria also occurs in other glomerular diseases, particularly in children and young adults. Levels of IgA in serum may be increased in patients with IgAN, but this is not a diagnostic discriminator. When IgAN presents with hypertension, proteinuria, and chronic renal impairment, it is clinically indistinguishable from many forms of chronic renal disease. The renal biopsy may be diagnostic by identifying mesangial IgA, even when structural damage is so advanced on light microscopy that it has the non-specific features of 'end-stage kidney'.

In patients with acute renal failure, urgent renal biopsy may be needed to differentiate the acute tubular injury that occasionally follows heavy glomerular haematuria from crescentic IgAN or other coincidental causes of acute renal failure.

Henoch–Schönlein purpura

In children, the diagnosis of HSP is usually made on the basis of clinical criteria. Confirmatory evidence of tissue IgA deposition will not be obtained unless persistence of renal disease results in a renal biopsy. In adults, the differential diagnosis is much wider and includes other forms of systemic vasculitis that need to be diagnosed by clinical, serological, and histological characteristics.

☐ PATHOGENESIS

The frequent recurrence of IgAN and Henoch–Schönlein nephritis after renal transplantation strongly implies an abnormality in the host IgA immune system. The mesangial IgA in IgAN and HS nephritis is predominantly polymeric IgA1 (pIgA1).

Recent studies have investigated abnormalities of the control of IgA production in patients with IgAN, which results in exaggerated systemic IgA immune responses to mucosal antigen challenge. Abnormalities of O-glycosylation of pIgIA1, which are associated with mesangial IgA deposition in IgAN and HSP, have also been described.[4] As yet, these insights have had no direct impact on clinical management. Why some patients develop IgAN and others a systemic form of the illness, HSP, is not clear.[5] Although processes that result in glomerular deposition of IgA and the induction of glomerular inflammation are likely to be specific to IgAN and HS nephritis, the 'downstream' mechanisms of renal injury are generic to other progressive renal diseases (Fig 2).

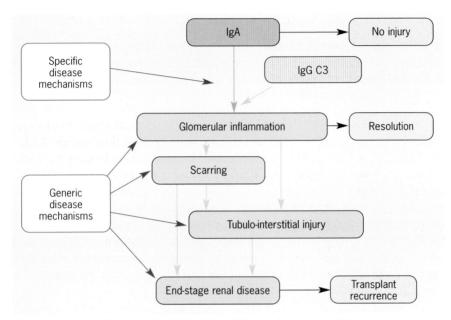

Fig 2 Mechanisms of injury in IgA nephropathy and Henoch–Schönlein nephritis.

☐ NATURAL HISTORY

Natural history of IgA nephropathy

Although clinical remission (disappearance of haematuria and proteinuria) occurs in up to one third of patients with mild disease, large studies with prolonged follow up indicate a slow attrition.[6] By 20 years after diagnosis, one quarter of patients will have ESRD and a further 20% will have impaired renal function and hence are also at high risk of eventual ESRD. It is important, however, to appreciate that these data on natural history are based on studies initiated more than 20 years ago; it is possible that long-term prognosis has improved significantly since the introduction of more active and widespread supportive therapy.

Episodes of macroscopic haematuria seem to confer a good prognosis, probably as a result of lead-time bias, as such episodes usually result in early diagnosis.[6] The risk of renal failure is not uniform. As in any chronic glomerular disease, the presence of hypertension, proteinuria, and renal impairment at presentation and histological evidence of glomerular and interstitial fibrosis identify those with a poor prognosis at the time of diagnosis.[1,5] During follow up, only hypertension and proteinuria are reliable predictors of the risk of progression. A Canadian study indicated that the risk of progression is negligible when proteinuria remains

<0.2 g/24 hours with normal blood pressure.[7] In contrast, however, data from Hong Kong suggest that among those who present with isolated microscopic haematuria, as many as 44% may subsequently develop proteinuria, hypertension, or renal impairment over a seven-year follow-up period.

Natural history of Henoch–Schönlein nephritis

Available data are restricted to patients referred for renal biopsy, which therefore excludes most patients with minor transient renal involvement, who have an excellent prognosis. The renal prognosis is worse in adults than in children.[8,9] Up to 10% of adults will have ESRD 10 years after biopsy. One series reports an increased mortality in adults with HSP because of lung and gastrointestinal malignancies.[9]

☐ TRANSPLANT RECURRENCE

Mesangial IgA deposits recur in the donor transplant kidney in up to 60% of patients with IgAN.[10] They may occur within days or weeks, but the risk increases with the duration of the transplant. The deposits seem benign in the short term and are not often associated initially with light microscopic evidence of nephritis. Graft failure because of recurrent IgAN associated with proteinuria and hypertension occurs in about 5% of cases within five years, but it significantly worsens the prognosis of grafts from 10 years onwards and for patients who have repeated transplantation.[10]

Henoch–Schönlein nephritis can recur as isolated IgA deposits in the graft (about 50% of transplants), full-blown yet isolated IgAN, or, rarely, as a full recurrence of systemic involvement, including a rash. Renal recurrence apparently exhibits characteristics similar to those of recurrent primary IgAN. Delay of transplantation once ESRD is reached does not reduce the risk of recurrence.

☐ TREATMENT

The ideal specific treatment for IgAN would remove IgA from the glomerulus and prevent further IgA deposition. This remains a remote prospect while the pathogenesis remains incompletely understood.

Mechanisms of chronic disease progression in IgAN are unlikely to be unique; it is probable, therefore, that treatment trials will provide information applicable to other forms of chronic GN. It is disappointing that, despite the prevalence of IgAN and consensus about its definition and natural history, few randomised controlled trials have adequate power (available trials are reviewed in Feehally[11]). Patients with HSP have been excluded from almost all treatment trials, but little evidence indicates that treatment strategies should differ from those used in patients with IgAN. Table 1 summarises the treatment recommendations.

Macroscopic haematuria

Episodes of macroscopic haematuria are usually self-limiting. The provoking infection should be treated conventionally; prophylactic antibiotics have no role.

Table 1 Treatment recommendations for patients with IgA nephropathy and Henoch-Schönlein nephritis. Adapted from Feehally[11] and Barratt.[12]

Symptom	Treatment
Recurrent macroscopic haematuria (preserved renal function)	Aggressive hydration (no role for antibiotics or tonsillectomy)
Macroscopic haematuria with acute renal failure	Renal biopsy mandatory if acute renal failure is persistent
Acute tubular necrosis	Supportive measures only

Crescentic IgA nephropathy	Induction
	    Prednisolone 0.5–1 mg/kg/day for up to eight weeks
	    Cyclophosphamide 2 mg/kg/day for up to eight weeks
	    No evidence favours oral or intravenous route (follow local practice)
	Maintenance
	    Prednisolone in reducing dosage
	    Azathioprine 2.5 mg/kg/day

Proteinuria <1 g/24 hours (with or without microscopic hematuria)	No specific treatment
Nephrotic syndrome, with minimal change on light microscopy	Prednisolone 0.5–1 mg/kg/day (children, 60 mg/m^2/day) for up to eight weeks
Non-nephrotic proteinuria >1 g/24 hours (with or without microscopic haematuria)	Angiotensin-converting enzyme inhibitor and/or angiotensin receptor blocker (maximise dosage or combine to achieve target blood pressure and proteinuria <0.5 g/day) If proteinuria remains >1 g/24 hours on maximal supportive treatment, consider fish oil or corticosteroids (controversial)

Hypertension	Angiotensin-converting enzyme inhibitors and/or angiotensin receptor blockers are agents of first choice to achieve target blood pressure:
	    130/80 mmHg if proteinuria < 1 g/24 hours
	    125/75 mmHg if proteinuria > 1 g/24 hours

Transplantation	No special measures required

Tonsillectomy reduces the frequency of episodic haematuria when tonsillitis is the provoking infection and has been popular in Japan and France, but no evidence is available from randomised controlled trials, and retrospective data do not convincingly show benefit.

Acute renal failure and crescentic IgAN

Uncommonly, acute renal failure may accompany macroscopic haematuria. Unless renal function improves in a few days, renal biopsy is mandatory to distinguish between acute tubular injury caused by heavy haematuria, which will settle with supportive measures, and crescentic IgAN, for which immunosuppressive therapy – typically with prednisolone and cyclophosphamide followed by azathioprine – may be indicated as long as there is not histological evidence of substantial pre-existing chronic renal damage (which makes a useful response to immunosuppression much less likely).

Slowly progressive IgAN and HS nephritis

Little evidence indicates that the events of progressive glomerular injury are unique to patients with IgAN. Treatments that have been assessed are non-specific approaches for chronic glomerular diseases, of which IgAN is the most common and most easily defined. Trials of corticosteroids and immunosuppressive agents are inconclusive in patients with IgAN.

Corticosteroids

A randomised controlled trial suggested that six months of intravenous 'pulse' methylprednisolone plus alternate-day corticosteroids in adults with low-grade proteinuria may protect renal function during long-term follow-up. Another controlled trial with smaller doses of corticosteroids, however, showed some reduction in protein excretion but no protection of renal function.

Cyclophosphamide

Cyclophosphamide followed by azathioprine combined with prednisolone preserved renal function in a controlled trial in patients with a poor prognosis. Other trials of cyclophosphamide showed no definite benefit, and many doctors regard the toxicity of cyclophosphamide in young adults with IgAN as unacceptable.

Mycophenolate mofetil

Mycophenolate mofetil has been used in three controlled trials in high-risk patients. Two trials in Caucasian patients failed to show any benefit, whereas a short-term study in Chinese patients noted reduced proteinuria. Whether racial effects underlie these discrepant results remains to be clarified.[13]

Fish oil

A randomised controlled trial provided convincing evidence of protection from two years' treatment with fish oil in patients with proteinuria and increasing levels of serum creatinine, although treatment with fish oil did not significantly reduce proteinuria – a major risk factor for progression. Other smaller controlled trials of fish oil have shown no benefit. Treatment with fish oil is safe, apart from a decrease in blood coagulability, which is not usually a practical problem, and an unpleasant taste and flatulence, which may make compliance difficult.

Hypertension

Compelling evidence shows the benefit of decreasing blood pressure in the treatment of patients with chronic progressive glomerular diseases such as IgAN. Two prospective controlled trials strongly support the use of angiotensin-converting enzyme (ACE) inhibitors and particularly the combination of ACE inhibitors with angiotensin receptor blockers (ARB) as first-choice hypotensive agents to minimise proteinuria, as well as control blood pressure, in patients with IgAN. Low target levels for blood pressure (<130/80 mmHg if proteinuria <1 g/24 hours, 125/75 mmHg if proteinuria >1 g/24 hours) are recommended from a number of large studies of patients with chronic progressive renal disease. In a randomised study in patients with IgAN, achieving a mean blood pressure of 129/70 mmHg prevented the fall in renal function over three years seen in those who achieved mean levels of blood pressure of 136/76 mmHg.

Unfortunately, available randomised controlled trials of corticosteroids, immunosuppressive agents, and fish oil in patients with IgAN have not always controlled blood pressure rigorously to these low targets and have not uniformly used ACE inhibitors and ARBs. It is therefore not possible to be certain whether the apparent benefits in these trials would be sustained if tight blood pressure control with renin-angiotensin blockade is maintained. Inconsistencies in the outcomes of the immunosuppressive trials in part may be explained by differences in achieved blood pressure and the variable use of renin-angiotensin blockade.

Recommendation

Tight control of blood pressure with ACE inhibitors and ARBs should be the first line of treatment. Fish oil, or other immunosuppressives, should be considered only if proteinuria >1 g/24 h persists on maximal treatment with ACE inhibitors or ARB inhibitors, or both, with blood pressure <125/75 mmHg. In this author's opinion, however, the case has not been made in this context for fish oil, corticosteroids, or any other immunosuppressive regimen.

Transplant recurrence

No evidence has shown that newer immunosuppressive agents used in renal transplantation have modified the frequency of recurrent IgA deposits or are of value in patients with recurrent disease.[10] Recurrence should otherwise be managed in the same manner as IgAN in native kidneys, with an emphasis on control of blood pressure and proteinuria.

REFERENCES

1　Pouria S, Feehally J. Glomerular IgA deposition in liver disease. *Nephrol Dial Transplant* 1999;14:2279–82.

2　Feehally J. IgA nephropathy and Henoch-Schönlein nephritis. In: *Comprehensive clinical nephrology.* Johnson RJ, Feehally J (eds). St Louis, MI: Mosby, 2003.

3　Hsu SI, Ramirez SB, Winn MP *et al.* Evidence for genetic factors in the development and progression of IgA nephropathy. *Kidney Int* 2000;57:1818–35.

4　Barratt J, Feehally J, Smith AC. Pathogenesis of IgA nephropathy. *Semin Nephrol* 2004;24: 197–217.

5   Davin JC, Ten Berge IJ, Weening JJ. What is the difference between IgA nephropathy and Henoch- Schönlein purpua nephritis. *Kidney Int* 2001;59:823–34.

6   D'Amico G. Natural history of idiopathic IgA nephropathy and factors predictive of disease outcome. *Semin Nephrol* 2004;24:179–96.

7   Bartosik L, Lajoie G, Sugar L, Cattran DC Predicting prognosis in IgA nephropathy. *Am J Kidney Dis* 2001:38:728–35.

8   Ronkainen J, Nuuiten M, Koskimies O. The adult kidney 24 years after childhood Henoch-Schönlein purpura: a retrospective cohort study. *Lancet* 2002;360:666–70

9   Pillebout E, Thervet E, Hill G *et al.* Henoch-Schonlein purpura in adults: outcome and prognostic factors. *J Am Soc Nephrol* 2002;13:1271–8.

10 Floege J. Recurrent IgA nephropathy after renal transplantation. *Semin Nephro* 2004;24: 287–91.

11 Feehally J. IgA nephropathy and Henoch-Schonlein purpura. In: *Therapy in nephrology and hypertension.* Brady HR, Wilcox CS (eds). Philadelphia, PA: WB Saunders, 2002.

12 Barratt J, Feehally J. Treatment of IgA nephropathy. *Kidney Int* 2006;69:1934–8.

13 Floege J. Is mycophenolate mofetil an effective treatment for persistent proteinuria in patients with IgA nephropathy? *Nature Clin Pract Nephrol* 2006;2:16–7.

Haemolytic uraemic syndrome

David Kavanagh and Timothy HJ Goodship

Haemolytic uraemic syndrome (HUS) is characterised by the triad of a microangiopathic haemolytic anaemia (Coombs' test negative), thrombocytopenia, and acute renal failure.[1,2] It can be further divided into diarrhoeal (D+) and non-diarrhoeal-associated (D–) disease (also known as atypical HUS, aHUS). The latter, in turn, is classified further as sporadic or, if more than one member of a family is affected, familial. Sporadic aHUS can be associated with pregnancy, systemic lupus erythematosus (SLE), human immunodeficiency virus (HIV), and various drugs, including the oral contraceptive pill and cyclosporin. Haemolytic uraemic syndrome belongs to a wider group of conditions, all of which are characterised by a thrombotic microangiopathy. These include antiphospholipid antibody syndrome, malignant hypertension, pre-eclampsia, HELLP (haemolysis, elevated liver enzymes, and low platelet count) syndrome, acute fatty liver of pregnancy, scleroderma, and acute renal allograft vascular rejection. In all of these conditions, the mechanism that underlies the microangiopathy is thought to involve endothelial cell activation. A variety of factors – including anti-endothelial cell antibodies, immune complexes, toxins, lipopolysaccharide, and complement – are known to activate the endothelial cell, thus causing it to change from its normal anticoagulant to a procoagulant phenotype.

☐ DIARRHOEAL HUS

Overall, 95% of cases of HUS are (D+), and most are associated with a preceding infection with *Escherichia coli* O157.[3] Haemorrhagic colitis and HUS associated with *E. coli* O157 were first described in 1983. The incidence of cases of *E. coli* O157 reported in England and Wales (Public Health Laboratory Service) and Scotland (Scottish Centre for Infection and Environmental Health) increased steadily in the 1980s and early 1990s, which culminated in an outbreak in central Scotland in 1996. Since then, the incidence has shown a gradual decline, although it still remains about twice as great in Scotland as in England and Wales.

The main reservoir of *E. coli* O157 is healthy cattle, but the organism can be transmitted to humans through a variety of contaminated food sources. Those reported include minced meat (especially hamburgers), cooked meats, salami, radish sprouts, and lettuce. Transmission through drinking fluids, including tap water and cider, as well as ingestion of water during bathing and swimming, has been reported. A very small inoculum of bacteria can cause infection. Within days of ingestion, gastrointestinal symptoms including bloody diarrhoea develop. In most patients, these symptoms resolve, but about 10% of patients will go on to develop HUS within a matter of days.

The virulence of *E. coli* O157 is related to its ability to tightly adhere to colonocytes via intimin and the cytotoxity of the toxins it produces.[4,5] *E. coli* O157 produces two verocytotoxins (VT-1 and VT-2), which are also known as shiga toxins. They consist of an A unit and 5 B units. The B units bind to a glycosphingolipid globotriaosyl ceramide (Gb3) receptor on endothelial cells. The A unit is subsequently internalised and inhibits protein synthesis. Until recently, the mode of transport of VT from the gastrointestinal tract to the renal endothelium has not been known. Recent studies show that it binds exclusively to polymorphonuclear cells (PMNs) but with a lower affinity than for the Gb3 receptor. It also has been established that VT bound to PMNs can be detected in asymptomatic family members of patients with (D+) HUS.

Recent studies suggest that coexposure to endotoxin may significantly increase the risk of HUS developing in patients infected with *E. coli* O157. Evidence of thrombogenesis can be seen early in those patients who later go on to develop HUS. Whether this is causal or reflects the changes associated with endothelial activation, particularly increased expression of tissue factor, remains to be determined.

The improvement in the morbidity and mortality of patients with (D+) HUS is mainly the result of supportive care, including maintenance of fluid and electrolyte balance, antihypertensive treatment, control of seizures, nutritional support, and dialysis. Little evidence supports the use of plasmapheresis in patients with (D+) HUS. Recent interest has centred on the potential of binding VT in the gastrointestinal tract or systemic circulation. This led to the development of Synsorb Pk – a synthetic trisaccharide VT receptor bound to an inert silica-like substrate. Although the results of phase I trials were promising, development of the product was discontinued before the onset of phase III trials. A new water-soluble carbohydrate ligand (named Starfish) is under development and has been shown to have a high *in vitro* inhibitory activity. The possibility of using anti-VT antibodies is also currently being examined. Use of antibiotics and antimotility drugs to treat the gastrointestinal symptoms is not recommended, as they may increase the risk of developing HUS. To reduce the current prevalence of *E. coli* O157 infections will require assiduous application of the recommendations of the Pennington group, which examined the circumstances of the 1996 *E. coli* O157 outbreak in central Scotland. These recommendations targeted all levels at which *E. coli* O157 might enter the food chain.

The prognosis for patients who develop HUS after infection with *E. coli* O157 is better than in atypical HUS, but it is not always favourable: about 5% die within the acute episode, 5% develop chronic renal failure, and 30% show evidence of chronic renal damage with persistent proteinuria. The remaining 60% have no adverse sequelae.

☐ ATYPICAL HUS (AHUS)

Mutations in three complement regulators have been described in patients with atypical HUS. About 30% of patients have a mutation in factor H (*CFH*),[6,7] about

10% a mutation in membrane cofactor protein (*MCP*),[8] and about 10% a mutation in factor I (*IF*).[9] Factor H, a soluble protein produced by the liver, is one of the most important regulators of the alternative complement pathway. *CFH* is located on chromosome 1q32 in a region that harbours a cluster of complement regulatory genes (the RCA cluster). These proteins all share a common basic structure consisting of multiple (contiguous) homologous modules called complement control protein modules (CCPs). Factor H has 20 CCPs. Mutations in *CFH* in patients with aHUS have now been described by several groups. Most are heterozygous missense mutations that cluster in the C-terminal exons and are associated with normal levels of factor H. A minority are deletions or missense mutations that result in a severely truncated protein or impaired secretion. This leads to systemic deficiency in factor H, usually heterozygous. The clustering of missense mutations in the C-terminal region of the molecule is remarkable. The alternative pathway is activated by 'foreign' surfaces. It exhibits spontaneous activity that is regulated by factor H in four ways: factor H acts as a cofactor for factor I-mediated cleavage of C3b (cofactor activity), accelerates the decay of the C3 convertase C3bBb (decay-accelerating activity), competes with factor B for binding to C3b, and binds to polyanions on cell surfaces. The C terminal region of factor H where mutations cluster is known to be important in the latter two functions. Structural models of the mutants suggest that interference with binding to polyanions is particularly important, and functional studies have confirmed this.

Two animal models of factor H deficiency now exist: the Norwegian Yorkshire pig and a murine model. In both models, homozygous animals develop mesangio-capillary (membranoproliferative) glomerulonephritis rather than HUS. This form of glomerulonephritis has also been reported in humans with homozygous deficiency of factor H and N-terminal heterozygous *CFH* missense mutations.

Our current knowledge suggests, therefore, that factor H deficiency is more commonly, although not exclusively, associated with mesangiocapillary glomerulo-nephritis rather than with HUS. Missense mutations that cluster in the C-terminal exons of *CFH* are usually associated with aHUS, while those found in the N-terminal exons are associated with mesangiocapillary glomerulonephritis.

Membrane cofactor protein (MCP, CD46) is a transmembrane regulator of both the alternative and classic pathways. It is expressed widely and is particularly found on endothelial cells. It has cofactor activity (but not decay-accelerating activity) for the alternative and classic pathways. Mutations in patients with aHUS that lead to deficiency of MCP (lack of expression at the cell surface) and impaired function of an expressed protein have been described.

Factor I is a serine protease that cleaves C3b and renders it inactive. Factor H and MCP act as cofactors for this factor. The gene for factor I is at 4q32, and it is synthesised by the liver. Homozygous deficiency of factor I had been reported previously only in association with recurrent pyogenic infections as a result of functional C3 and factor B deficiency. Recently, several reports have been made of heterozygous factor I deficiency in association with aHUS. In addition, reports have also been made of factor I mutations that are associated with normal secretion; whether these are functionally significant remains to be determined.

How does overactivity of the alternative complement pathway result in a thrombotic microangiopathy? An initial insult may result in endothelial cell activation with ensuing complement activation. Dysregulation of the alternative pathway means that the procoagulant phenotype of the activated endothelium is maintained, with the formation of platelet-rich microthrombi.

Is it possible to explain why the microangiopathy particularly affects the kidney? The plasma from patients with HUS has been shown to induce apoptosis of renal and cerebral endothelial cells but not cells of the lung or large-vessel endothelia. This may be related to differential expression of pro- and anti-apoptotic genes.

These recent findings have implications for the management of patients with aHUS. Plasma exchange has long been known to be of benefit in these patients, and the rationale for this is now apparent. Removal of mutant protein (factor H and factor I) and replacement with wild-type soluble complement regulators in fresh frozen plasma will be beneficial. Despite treatment with plasma exchange, most patients do not recover renal function and need renal replacement treatment. Transplantation is associated with a significant recurrence rate in the allograft. Several series suggest that the recurrence rate approaches 50% in all patients with aHUS.[10] In patients known to have a mutation of *CFH* or *IF*, the recurrence rate is higher, with an 80% risk of the graft being lost to recurrent HUS. Conversely, in patients known to have a mutation of *MCP*, no reports of recurrent disease after transplantation have been made. This is expected, because MCP is a transmembrane regulator. All patients with aHUS to be considered for transplantation thus are now recommended to undergo screening for mutations of *CFH*, *MCP*, and *IF*. Live, related transplantation is not recommended unless the donors themselves have been screened, because donors may be asymptomatic carriers and *de-novo* disease has been reported in donors within a short period of donation.

Are these findings of relevance to the pathogenesis of (D+) HUS?

Low levels of C3 (indicative of activation of the alternative complement pathway) have been reported in about 50% of patients with (D+) HUS, and the level of C3 is inversely related to the outcome. Complement components thus may be acting as susceptibility factors for the development of (D+) HUS.

Are these findings of relevance to other diseases?

Landmark publications in 2005 showed that a polymorphism in CCP 7 of factor H (*Y402H*) was associated with a substantially increased risk of developing age-related macular degeneration.[11] The retina and glomerulus both have exposed basement membranes that rely on factor H to prevent complement-mediated host injury.

☐ CONCLUSIONS

In recent years, substantial advances have been made in our understanding of the molecular mechanisms responsible for HUS. The elucidation of the transport and cytotoxicity of verotocytotoxin has provided further avenues for therapy of (D+) HUS. The association of atypical HUS with mutations of *CFH, MCP,* and *IF* has raised the possibility of logical targeted treatment with complement inhibitors. By understanding the molecular pathophysiology of these diseases, logical treatment can be developed.

REFERENCES

1   Warwicker P, Goodship THJ. Haemolytic uraemic syndrome. In: Warrell DA, Cox TM, Firth JD, Benz EJJ (eds), *Oxford Textbook of Medicine.* Oxford: Oxford University Press, 2003:407–10.

2   Moake JL. Thrombotic microangiopathies. *N Engl J Med* 2002;347:589–600.

3   Mead PS, Griffin PM. Escherichia coli O157:H7. *Lancet* 1998;352:1207–12.

4   Frankel G, Phillips AD, Rosenshine I *et al.* Enteropathogenic and enterohaemorrhagic Escherichia coli: more subversive elements. *Mol Microbiol* 1998;30:911–21.

5   Law D. Virulence factors of *Escherichia coli* O157 and other Shiga toxin-producing E. coli. *J Appl Microbiol* 2000;88:729–45.

6   Warwicker P, Goodship THJ, Donne RL *et al.* Genetic studies into inherited and sporadic haemolytic uraemic syndrome. *Kidney Int* 1998;53:836–44.

7   Richards A, Buddles MR, Donne RL *et al.* Factor H mutations in hemolytic uremic syndrome cluster in exons 18-20, a domain important for host cell recognition. *Am J Hum Genet* 2001;68:485–90.

8   Richards A, Kemp EJ, Liszewski MK *et al.* Mutations in human complement regulator, membrane cofactor protein (CD46), predispose to development of familial hemolytic uremic syndrome. *Proc Natl Acad Sci U S A* 2003;100(22):12966–71.

9   Kavanagh D, Kemp EJ, Mayland E *et al.* Mutations in complement factor I predispose to development of atypical hemolytic uremic syndrome. *J Am Soc Nephrol* 2005;16(7):2150–5.

10 Bresin E, Daina E, Noris M *et al.* Outcome of renal transplantation in patients with non–shiga toxin–associated hemolytic uremic syndrome: prognostic significance of genetic background. *Clin J Am Soc Nephrol* 2006;1:88–99.

11 Hageman GS, Anderson DH, Johnson LV *et al.* A common haplotype in the complement regulatory gene factor H (HF1/CFH) predisposes individuals to age-related macular degeneration. *Proc Natl Acad Sci U S A* 2005;102:7227–32.

☐ NEPHROLOGY SELF ASSESSMENT QUESTIONS

IgA nephropathy and Henoch-Schönlein purpura

1   Macroscopic haematuria in IgA nephropathy:
   (a) Usually results in acute renal failure
   (b) Requires early treatment with penicillin
   (c) Is associated with normal C3 complement in the serum
   (d) Rarely occurs after the age of 40 years
   (e) Occurs within 24 hours of symptoms of upper respiratory infection

2   The following features at the time of diagnosis indicate a poor prognosis in IgA nephropathy:
   (a) Hypertension
   (b) Levels of IgA in serum
   (c) Glomerular sclerosis on renal biopsy
   (d) History of recurrent macroscopic haematuria
   (e) Reduced glomerular filtration rate

3   In patients with IgA nephropathy:
   (a) A diagnosis can be made only by renal biopsy
   (b) Nephrotic syndrome is usually an indication for treatment with corticosteroids
   (c) Choice of immunosuppression does not alter the risk of transplant recurrence
   (d) Treatment with fish oil is proved to delay renal failure
   (e) Tonsillectomy has not been proved to prevent renal failure in patients with recurrent macroscopic haematuria

4   In patients with Henoch-Schönlein purpura:
   (a) Nephritis is always present in the first month after presentation
   (b) A clinical diagnosis can be made in adults
   (c) Only a minority of people have persistent nephritis
   (d) Corticosteroids are indicated for all patients with persistent nephritis
   (e) Nephrotic syndrome is more common than in patients with immunoglobulin A nephropathy

Haemolytic uraemic syndrome

1   Diarrhoeal associated (D+) HUS:
   (a) Should always be treated with plasmapheresis
   (b) Usually leads to irreversible renal failure
   (c) Is most common in middle age
   (d) Has a 5% mortality
   (e) Is the most common form of HUS

2   Familial atypical HUS:
    (a) Can be both autosomal dominant and recessive
    (b) Is completely penetrant
    (c) May be associated with mutations of factor H
    (d) Always presents in childhood
    (e) Is associated with a high rate of recurrence after transplantation

3   Sporadic atypical HUS:
    (a) Frequently leads to irreversible renal failure
    (b) Can be associated with pregnancy
    (c) May be associated with mutations of factor H
    (d) Can be treated with cyclosporin
    (e) Can be associated with HIV infection

4   Infection with *E. coli* 0157:
    (a) Always causes HUS
    (b) Can result only from eating meat products
    (c) Can cause haemorrhagic colitis
    (d) Is associated with the production of a verotoxin
    (e) Should always be treated with antibiotics

Rheumatology

Understanding osteoarthritis

Michael Doherty

☐ INTRODUCTION

Osteoarthritis (OA) is traditionally regarded as an inevitable consequence of ageing that largely reflects 'wear and tear' and age-related decline in joint function. This has led to the pessimistic beliefs that symptomatic OA is inevitably progressive, that palliation is the sole aim of medical management, and that only surgical joint replacement is truly effective.

This review first examines general observations about the nature of OA, which all support the view of OA as the repair process of synovial joints. Recognised risk factors for development and progression of OA, which confirm that OA is a common complex disorder with several modifiable risk factors that relate to lifestyle, are then reviewed. Finally, the positive implications for primary and secondary prevention that come from this better understanding of OA are presented.

☐ GENERAL OBSERVATIONS ON THE NATURE OF OSTEOARTHRITIS

Evolutionary and phylogenetic preservation

Studies of ancient skeletal remains confirm that OA has accompanied man throughout our evolution.[1] This is in contrast to other arthropathies, such as rheumatoid arthritis, which apparently appeared only a few centuries ago. Osteo-arthritis also occurs in other animals with synovial joints, and palaeopathological evidence supports its antiquity in many species, including dinosaurs. Such evolutionary and phylogenetic preservation suggests a possible biological advantage to OA.

Osteoarthritis is a metabolically dynamic process

Although focal loss of hyaline cartilage is a cardinal feature of osteoarthritis (Fig 1), chondrocytes throughout the cartilage of patients with osteoarthritis multiply to form 'nests' of cells and increase their production of matrix components. Subchondral osteocytes also increase their activity, and new fibrocartilage develops at the joint margins and undergoes endochondral ossification to form osteophytes. The synovium undergoes hyperplasia, and its outer layer, the capsule, thickens. Synoviocytes frequently undergo metaplasia to form cartilaginous 'loose bodies' embedded in the synovium; these may ossify to form osteochondral bodies that are visible on an X-ray.

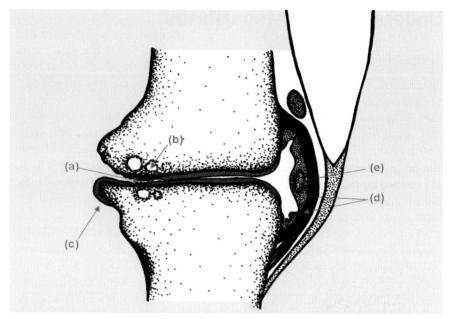

Fig 1 Pathology of osteoarthritis. Key pathological features include **(a)** focal loss of hyaline cartilage; **(b)** subchondral sclerosis (maximal under the site of cartilage thinning), bone cysts; **(c)** ossification of new fibrocartilage at the margin to form osteophytes, remodelling of bone ends; **(d)** synovial hyperplasia and capsular thickening; **(e)** synovial osteochondral bodies.

It thus seems that all tissues that make up the organ of the joint sense the joint is in trouble and try to produce new tissue, especially cartilage. Bony remodelling and marginal osteophytes increase the articulating surface area and help dissipate force transmission across the joint. Capsular thickening and osteophytes splint the joint and minimise instability resulting from cartilage loss (surgical removal of knee osteophytes increases instability). The osteoarthritic process therefore shows a combination of tissue attrition (especially cartilage) and increased metabolic activity of all joint tissues. The biophysiological changes that accompany OA are distinct from those of ageing alone, confirming that the term 'degenerative joint disease' is inappropriate – OA is a potentially regenerative joint condition.

Most osteoarthritis is clinically occult

Many studies confirm that OA commonly exists in joints without causing symptoms or disability.[2] Even in patients with symptoms that relate to OA, pain is often intermittent and non-progressive and has a good prognosis. This is exemplified by nodal OA of the hand, which often causes intermittent symptoms in middle age, as Heberden's and Bouchard's nodes and interphalangeal OA slowly develop. Once fully established, however, symptoms often abate, leaving the person with anatomically abnormal fingers but no more symptoms or disability than similarly aged people without OA of the hand.

Osteoarthritis as inherent repair

The above observations support OA as the inherent repair process of synovial joints.[1,2] A wide variety of insults may injure a joint and trigger the need for repair. This slow repair process involves all joint tissues. In general, it is an efficient repair process that rectifies the adverse effects of the insult ('compensated OA', Fig 2). In some cases, however, because of overwhelming insult or poor tissue response, the joint cannot compensate and has to continue attempted repair and remodelling. This may result in 'decompensated OA' ('joint failure'), which more commonly associates with symptoms and disability. This scenario readily explains the observed clinical heterogeneity of OA in terms of number of joints involved, age of onset, rate of progression, and clinical outcome. It also suggests that OA is not a single disease but a process with diverse triggers and outcomes.

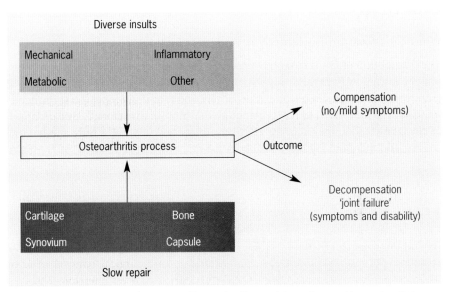

Fig 2 Osteoarthritis is a repair process. Diverse insults may trigger the need to repair, which involves all joint tissues and has a variable outcome.

Further observations that support OA as a repair process include the changes in joint biology during growth and maturation (Fig 3). Hyaline cartilage during growth displays epitopes characteristic of immature cartilage, a rich subchondral vasculature, and a tendency to calcify (allowing ossification of cartilage and growth at bone ends). At maturity, the vasculature recedes, cartilage no longer calcifies, and immature epitopes are replaced by those of mature cartilage. If an adult joint is injured and develops OA, however, the vasculature again increases through angiogenesis and neovascularisation, immature cartilage epitopes reappear ('neo-epitopes'), and the cartilage again shows a tendency to calcify with basic calcium phosphates and calcium pyrophosphate. The OA joint thus seems to revert to the immature situation, which, of course, is geared to produce new tissue.

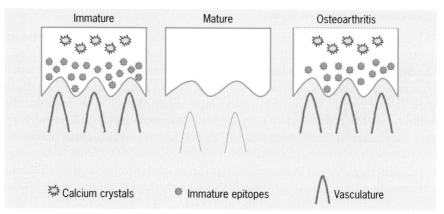

Fig 3 Characteristics of immature, mature, and osteoarthritic cartilage with respect to vascularity, neo-epitopes, and tendency to calcify.

Why does osteoarthritis selectively target certain joints?

The distribution of OA is strikingly selective (Fig 4). The cause for this is uncertain, but one intriguing hypothesis suggests an evolutionary design fault.[1,3] Man has only recently assumed upright posture, bipedal gait, and multifunctional use of the hand. Joints that have changed in recent evolution may not yet, therefore, be fully adapted to their new tasks; they may be relatively underdesigned, have little mechanical reserve, and therefore fail more readily in the face of insult. The distribution of OA

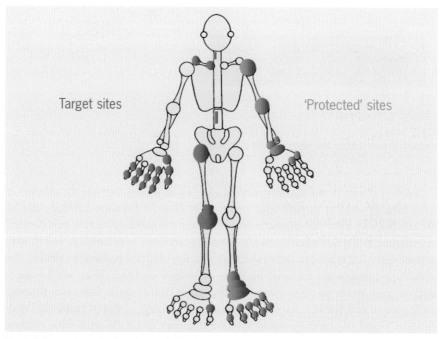

Fig 4 Selective targeting by osteoarthritis. Joints shown on the left have a much higher prevalence of osteoarthritis than those on the right.

in man is consistent with this hypothesis. Other animals have their own characteristic distributions of OA, which also fit their recent evolution.

☐ RISK FACTORS FOR OSTEOARTHRITIS

Osteoarthritis is a common complex disorder with multiple risk factors that are broadly divisible into genetic, constitutional, and local factors (Fig 5).[2,4]

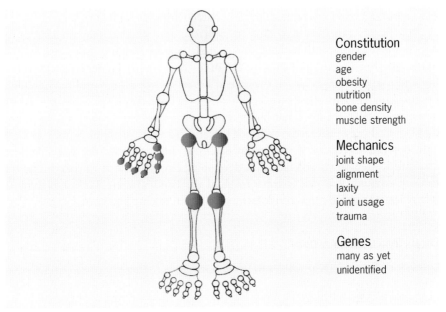

Constitution
gender
age
obesity
nutrition
bone density
muscle strength

Mechanics
joint shape
alignment
laxity
joint usage
trauma

Genes
many as yet
unidentified

Fig 5 Recognised risk factors for osteoarthritis. These can vary according to joint site (hand, knee, and hip) and whether they predispose to development or progression of osteoarthritis.

Genetic predisposition

Strong genetic predisposition to OA of the hand, knee, and hip is evident from classic twin, sibling, and segregation studies.[5] The heritability of OA is 40–60%, which means that about half the variance in the community relates to genetic rather than environmental factors. Associations are reported with several candidate genes – for example, COL2A1 (a structural gene for type II collagen), vitamin D receptor gene, asporin, calmodulin, and frizzled related protein 3 – as well as with chromosomal locations where the candidate is unknown. At present, however:

☐ No genetic associations have been replicated with confidence in other populations.

☐ Different associations are reported for different joint sites (hands, hips, and knees) and for multiple-site versus single-site OA.

☐ It is likely that multiple genes are involved and that these are common polymorphisms not rare mutations.

☐   Although structural genes for joint tissues are favourite candidates, genes that relate to generalised metabolic or inflammatory processes (such as interleukins) may also be involved.

Generalised constitutional risk factors

Ageing is a strong risk factor for OA at all sites. In addition, being a woman increases the risk at all sites other than the hip and also increases the likelihood of having symptoms and more severe disability associated with structural OA.

Risk factors can vary according to joint site and whether they predispose to development or progression of OA. For example, obesity is an important risk for OA of the knee but a weak risk factor for OA of the hip. If a person develops OA of the hip and is also obese, however, they are at higher risk of more rapid radiographic progression than non-obese people. Similarly, high bone density increases the risk of developing OA of the knee and hip, but low bone density is a risk factor for more rapid clinical progression of established OA at these sites. The same factor can even have opposite effects on development of OA at different sites. For example, low quadriceps strength is a risk factor for developing OA of the knee, whereas increased forearm strength is a risk factor for OA of the hand in men. Table 1 highlights differences and similarities in risk factors for OA of the hip and knee.

Local biomechanical factors

Local constitutional factors include:

☐   Dysplasia, which alters the shape and biomechanics of a joint and is a recognised risk factor for OA of the hip and knee

Table 1 Some key risk factors for osteoarthritis of the knee and hip.

Risk factor	Osteoarthritis	
	Knee	**Hip**
Heredity	+++	+++
Dysplasia	+	+++
Increasing age	+++	++
Female gender	+++	−
Obesity	+++	+
High bone density	++	++
Muscle weakness	+++	+
Laxity	++	−
Malalignment	++	−
Injury	+++	+
Occupation	Mining Professional football	Farming

□ Malalignment – varus–valgus alignment increases the risk of OA of the knee

□ Increased joint laxity, which is a risk factor for OA of the knee and possibly thumb base but a protective factor for interphalangeal OA.

Certain occupations are recognised to increase the risk of OA through adverse mechanical insult. For example, farmers have more than a twofold increased risk of OA of the hip and miners a twofold increased risk of OA of the knee – sufficient risk to permit the award of industrial compensation. The specific activities that cause risk within such occupations are less studied, although repetitive knee bending while carrying heavy loads has been identified as a risk factor for OA of the knee in several occupations.

Data on recreational use of the joints is conflicting and controversial.[6] In general, recreational use shows a U-shaped rather than linear relation (Fig 6). Joint tissues are built to move and require regular activity to maintain health. Relative underuse causes joint tissue atrophy and is detrimental. Moderate sporting activity may encourage osteophyte formation but may not be a risk for OA, whereas marked overuse associates with injury and can cause damage and OA through repetitive impact and tortional loading. Although regular sensible activity is considered beneficial, debate continues about the exact dose and frequency to recommend. Certain sports clearly have a high risk of injury (for example, meniscal and ligament tears from football and skiing), and such overt trauma is an important risk factor, especially for monoarticular OA.

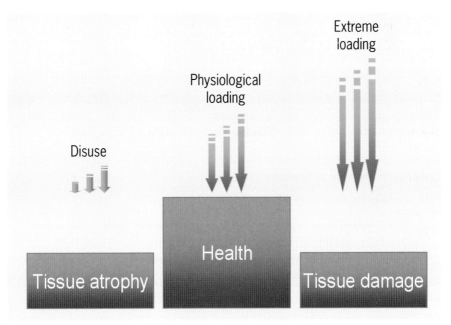

Fig 6 Use of joints and osteoarthritis. Regular sensible use within a 'physiological' range is essential for joint health. Underuse encourages tissue atrophy, and overuse can result in tissue damage.

Interaction between risk factors

Variable interactions can occur between risk factors for OA. For example, a person who is obese and has normal knee alignment has a relatively small risk of OA of the knee through obesity, but if that person also has mild varus–valgus malalignment, obesity becomes a major attributable risk factor for OA of the knee. Similarly, meniscectomy is a recognised risk factor for subsequent OA of the knee, but if a person undergoes meniscectomy in their twenties and then develops nodal OA of the hand in middle age (a marker for systemic predisposition to polyarticular OA), the risk and severity of post-meniscectomy OA of the knee greatly increases – blurring any distinction between 'primary' and 'secondary' OA.

Osteoarthritis is different at each joint site

Knee and hip joints clearly differ anatomically and functionally. The hip is a deep seated, very stable, ball-and-socket joint with movement in several planes, whereas the knee has three compartments, moves in one plane only, and is prone to destabilising injury. Unsurprisingly, therefore, joint failure affects these two sites differently (Fig 7). For example:

☐ Osteoarthritis of the knee is much more prevalent than that of the hip and shows female predominance at all ages; OA of the hip predominates in men in younger age groups but shows female predominance in elderly people.

☐ Osteoarthritis of the knee is predominantly bilateral, whereas OA of the hip is often unilateral.

☐ Osteoarthritis is more prevalent and severe in right knees, but no such asymmetry is seen with OA of the hip.

☐ Osteoarthritis of the knee has a better prognosis than osteoarthritis of the hip.

Osteoarthritis of the hip and knee therefore behave as two different conditions with respect to prevalence, risk factors, and outcome. Whatever is learnt about OA at one joint cannot necessarily, therefore, be extrapolated to other joints.

Factors that associate with osteoarthritic pain

Pain associated with OA has three main sites (Fig 8):

☐ Bone – local intra-osseous hypertension consequent upon subchondral bone remodelling and microfracture and abnormal bone signal on magnetic resonance imaging (so-called 'bone oedema') associate with pain.

☐ Synovium or capsule – intra-articular hypertension with synovial hyperplasia, inflammation, and effusion can all cause pain.

☐ Peri-articlar tissues – secondary bursitis and enthesopathy of the capsule, ligaments, and tendons are painful lesions that result from the altered biomechanics of a remodelled osteoarthritic joint.

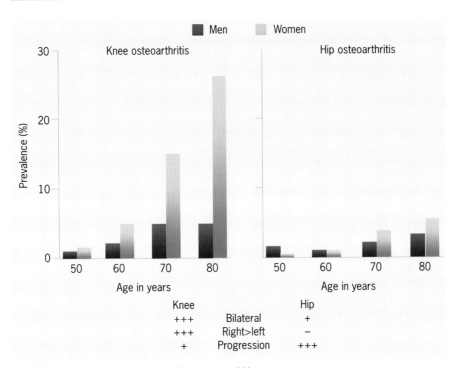

Fig 7 Comparison of osteoarthritis of the knee and hip.

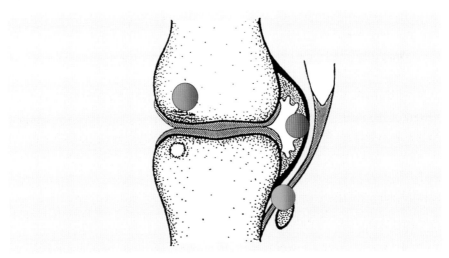

Fig 8 Pain from osteoarthritis may arise from the bone (blue), synovium and capsule (red) or from secondary bursitis and enthesopathy (green).

The correlation between structural OA and pain and disability varies between joints, being strongest at the hip, only moderate at the knee, and poor at small joints. Interestingly, the epidemiological associations of pain and disability can differ from those for structural OA. For example, obesity and reduced muscle strength are risk factors for the presence and severity of knee pain as well as for structural OA of the knee, but anxiety and depression associate with knee pain and disability but not structural OA. If muscle weakness, obesity, anxiety, and depression are successfully addressed, pain and disability can be reduced irrespective of any alteration in structure. Although the natural focus of interest is on structural OA, successful intervention in these modifiable factors can considerably impact on clinical outcomes.

Physiological correlates of osteoarthritis

A number of physiological abnormalities are known to accompany osteoarthritis of the knee and possibly hip, including:

- □ weakness of muscles acting across the joint (especially the quadriceps for OA of the knee)

- □ reduced proprioception – muscle is a key proprioceptive organ, so quadriceps dysfunction is probably the main mechanism for this

- □ subtle incoordination ('microclutziness') of gait

- □ varus–valgus instability

- □ increased sway when standing

- □ increased incidence of falling.

With the exception of instability, all of these can be reversed by quadriceps strengthening exercises. Again, therefore, even though structural OA cannot be reversed, the accompanying physiological abnormalities can.

□ STRATEGIES FOR MANAGING AND PREVENTING OSTEOARTHRITIS

Review of the nature of OA and its risk factors suggests a number of interventions and lifestyle changes for secondary and primary prevention.

Exercise

Strengthening exercises improve the muscle weakness, reduced proprioception, impaired balance, and tendency to fall in people with OA of the knee. Long-term trials (two years in duration) confirm that strengthening exercise also reduces pain and disability in people with symptomatic OA of the knee.[7] Virtually no contraindications exist to this simple, safe intervention. It should be prescribed to people with symptomatic OA of the knee and to people at obvious high risk of developing OA of the knee (for example, patients who present with symptomatic OA of the hand in midlife, who are at high risk of subsequently developing OA of the knee).

The second type of beneficial exercise that reduces pain and disability in long-term trials is aerobic fitness training. This also improves wellbeing and sleep and is beneficial for common comorbidities such as obesity, diabetes, and cardiovascular disease. Again, few contraindications exist.

Strengthening exercises and aerobic fitness training offer benefits through different mechanisms and both should be prescribed.[7,8] Osteoarthritis thus is yet another rationale for programmes that aim to increase aerobic fitness at the population level.

Reduction in adverse mechanical factors

Obese and overweight people should be advised and encouraged to lose weight. This can reduce pain and disability in patients with symptomatic OA of the knee.[8,9] Furthermore, in population studies, weight loss reduced the risk of incident structural OA at the knee.[2,4] Aerobic exercise, which carries its own benefits, is often a component of effective weight-loss programmes.

Modification of occupational and recreational activities can greatly reduce the incidence of structural and symptomatic OA. Obvious primary prevention strategies include:

- avoidance of repetitive knee bending while carrying weights

- avoidance of high-impact and tortional-loading sports, especially in those with established risk factors for OA

- avoidance of overt trauma through the use of protective devices during contact sports and at work

- regular activity and exercise to maintain musculoskeletal health

- widespread use of appropriate footwear (with a thick but soft sole and no raised heel) to reduce impact loading through knees and hips.

In the United States, the combined effects of a successful weight-loss programme in obese and overweight people, successful adaptation of the workplace to reduce repetitive knee bending, and avoidance of major knee injury during sport and at work have been estimated to potentially have major benefits in reducing the incidence of OA of the knee and hip – by as much as 30%.[10]

REFERENCES

1   Brandt K, Doherty M, Lohmander S. Introduction: the concept of osteoarthritis as failure of the diarthrodial joint. In: *Osteoarthritis*. Oxford: Oxford University Press, 2003:69–71.

2   Arden N, Nevitt MC. Osteoarthritis: epidemiology. *Best Pract Res Clin Rheumatol* 2006;20: 3–26.

3   Hutton CW. Generalised osteoarthritis: an evolutionary problem? *Lancet* 1987;1:1463–5.

4   Felson DT, Lawrence RC, Dieppe PA *et al*. Osteoarthritis: new insights. Part I: the disease and its risk factors. *Ann Intern Med* 2000;133:635–46

5   Zhang W, Doherty M. How important are genetic factors in osteoarthritis? Contributions from family studies. *J Rheumatol* 2005;32:1139–42.

6   Buckwalter JA, Martin JA. Sports and osteoarthritis. *Curr Opin Rheumatol* 2004;16:634–9.

7   Roddy E, Zhang W, Doherty M. Aerobic walking or strengthening exercise for osteoarthritis of the knee? A systematic review. *Ann Rheum Dis* 2005;64:544–8.

8   Roddy E, Doherty M. Changing life-styles and osteoarthritis: what is the evidence? *Best Pract Res Clin Rheumatol* 2006;20:81–97.

9   Messier SP, Loeser RF, Miller GD *et al.* Exercise and dietary weight loss in overweight and obese older adults with knee osteoarthritis: the Arthritis, Diet, and Activity Promotion Trial. *Arthritis Rheum* 2004;50:1501–10.

10   Felson DT, Zhang Y. An update on the epidemiology of knee and hip osteoarthritis with a view to prevention. *Arthritis Rheum* 1998;41:1343–55.

FURTHER READING AND GENERAL REFERENCES FOR OSTEOARTHRITIS

Arden N, Nevitt MC (eds). Osteoarthritis. *Best Pract Res Clin Rheumatol* 2006;20:1–176.

Brandt K, Doherty M, Lohmander S (eds). *Osteoarthritis.* Oxford: Oxford University Press, 2003.

Developments in rheumatoid arthritis

Deborah PM Symmons

☐ INTRODUCTION

Rheumatoid arthritis (RA) exhibits a very dynamic epidemiology. The first definite description in the European literature appeared in 1800. After this, a very rapid increase in the incidence, prevalence, and severity of this disease must have occurred. By the 1950s, when John Lawrence (the founder of the Arthritis Research Campaign (arc) Epidemiology Unit), conducted his landmark prevalence study in Leigh and Wensleydale, RA affected around 1% of the adult population. Since then the prevalence has decreased, although this is still the most common inflammatory musculoskeletal disease and now affects around 0.8% of the adult population.[1] Rheumatologists who practised in the 1950s and 1960s would describe how their clinics and wards were full of patients – bedridden or in wheelchairs – with severe extra-articular features such as systemic vasculitis, Felty's syndrome, and peripheral neuropathy. The recent decline in occurrence of rheumatoid vasculitis has been documented clearly in the Norfolk population. Many other extra-articular features are becoming increasingly rare. Whether this is the result of the natural history of RA (perhaps there has been an epidemic that is now in the decline) or the result of advances in treatment is not entirely clear. Both have probably played a role.

Interesting developments have also occurred with regard to our understanding of the aetiology of RA. A number of environmental and dietary factors have been identified. In addition, major advances have been made in terms of the types of treatment available and the way in which existing treatments are used. This now means that genuine opportunities exist for primary and secondary prevention of this unpleasant disabling disease.

☐ GENETIC SUSCEPTIBILITY TO RHEUMATOID ARTHRITIS

Rheumatoid arthritis is a complex genetic disease. The aetiology involves genetic susceptibility and environmental triggers. Two genetic susceptibility factors have now been identified, although neither is specific for RA. These genes are involved in immune regulation and associated with the development of autoimmunity. The HLA-DRBI genes that carry the shared epitope (a conserved nucleotide sequence in the third hypervariable region) were first hypothesised to be associated with RA in 1987.[2] The part of the molecule coded by the shared epitope folds into a recognition structure that contains a peptide-binding groove. More recently, the association with a particular polymorphism of PTPN22 – a gene that codes for intracellular tyrosine phosphatase and is associated with T cell-mediated immune regulation – has been confirmed in a number of cohorts of patients with RA.[3] Other susceptibility genes that have not yet been identified are likely.

☐ EARLY DIAGNOSIS

Traditionally, patients have been required to satisfy the Arthritis Research Campaign's 1987 criteria for RA[4] in order to be enrolled in clinical trials or longitudinal observational studies. These criteria include the presence of rheumatoid factor and radiological erosions. Many patients who ultimately are diagnosed with RA do not satisfy these criteria in the early months of disease, and more sensitive tests are needed.

Anti-cyclic citrullinated peptides antibodies

Rheumatoid factor is an autoantibody directed against the Fc component of immunoglobulin G (IgG). Although present in around 80% of patients with established RA, it is also present in up to 10–20% of healthy people (especially elderly people). Rheumatoid arthritis is also associated with a number of other autoantibodies, including anti-perinuclear and anti-keratin antibodies (first described in 1964). The antigenic targets of these antibodies are now recognised to be citrulline residues. Citrullination is the post-translational conversion of arginine to citrulline by the enzyme peptidylarginine deiminase (PADI) – of which there are five isoforms. Anti-cyclic citrullinated peptides (CCP) antibodies are found in the serum of around 75% of patients with established RA and 55% of patients with early RA. Studies in blood donors show that they may precede the development of RA by up to 14 years. They are much more specific for RA than rheumatoid factor and have proved useful in distinguishing, for example, erosive systemic lupus erythematosus and the arthropathy of chronic hepatitis C from rheumatoid arthritis in patients who are positive for rheumatoid factor.[5] The conversion of arginine to citrulline increases the affinity of the peptide for binding to HLA-DRB1. Citrullination occurs during apoptosis, cellular terminal differentiation, and inflammation within the joint. Smoking causes citrullination of proteins within the lung.

Anti-CCP antibodies are strongly associated with the shared epitope. They predict the development and progression of erosions but not of extra-articular disease. They convey no additional prognostic information in the presence of rheumatoid factor, but around 40% of patients with RA negative for rheumatoid factor have anti CCP antibodies. Notably, the absence of anti-CCP antibodies does not predict remission. The prognosis in patients with RA negative for anti-CCP antibodies is unknown. The suggestion by some manufacturers that enzyme-linked immunosorbent assays for anti-CCP antibodies can be used as a screening tool to decide which patients with inflammatory polyarthritis should be referred to secondary care should be resisted.

Imaging

Conventional radiography shows only bony erosion and joint space narrowing, which may take some years to develop and are irreversible. On the other hand, magnetic resonance imaging (MRI) can also visualise bone marrow, synovium, articular cartilage, ligaments, and tendons. Bony erosions may be visible on magnetic resonance images up to two years before they can be seen on a conventional radiogram. Magnetic resonance imaging thus offers the potential to identify patients with RA who are most likely to have rapid disease progression and could be used as an outcome measure in clinical trials – thus enabling smaller studies of shorter duration to show treatment efficacy. Some of the earliest changes seen on magnetic resonance images – bone marrow oedema and inflammation – may be reversible. Recent reports suggest that low field MRI (0.2 Tesla), which is quicker and thus cheaper, can be used with intravenously administered gadolinium enhancement to measure synovial volume in individual joints.

Ultrasound is more sensitive than conventional radiography, but less sensitive than MRI, at detecting erosions. It can also be used to visualise joint effusions, synovial tissue, tendons, and articular cartilage.[6] Both MRI and ultrasound thus have the potential to aid early diagnosis of RA and target treatment to those with the worse prognosis.

□ PRIMARY PREVENTION OF RHEUMATOID ARTHRITIS

As well as genetic factors, environmental triggers are also needed for the development of (or protection against) RA.[7] A decline in the incidence of RA in women, noted in many countries including the US and UK, coincides with the widespread use of the oral contraceptive pill (OCP). A large number of epidemiological studies have shown an approximate halving of the incidence of RA in women currently taking the OCP compared with those who have never taken the OCP. The use of the OCP thus seems likely to postpone the onset of RA rather than prevent it altogether. This would be in keeping with the observed increase in the peak age at onset of RA in women over recent years. A marked increase in the incidence of RA in women older than 55 years may be seen as the first cohort of women to have taken the OCP for long periods of time passes through the menopause. By contrast, the incidence and prevalence of RA in men has risen in recent years.

A number of lifestyle risk factors for the development of RA have also been identified. Current smokers have an approximately twofold risk of developing RA compared with non-smokers. Smoking is well recognised, at a population level, to be associated with production of rheumatoid factor. Smoking is particularly important for the development of RA positive for rheumatoid factor and, more particularly still, for RA positive for anti-CCP antibodies. The gene–environment interaction is apparent, in that smoking increases the risk of RA positive for anti-CCP antibodies around 21-fold in people who have two copies of the shared epitope compared with non-smokers who are negative for the shared epitope. By contrast, smoking carries no risk for RA negative for anti-CCP antibodies in those who are negative or positive for the shared epitope.[8]

Rheumatoid arthritis is also associated with obesity and consumption of a diet high in red meat and low in fruit and vegetables. The relative risk of the highest tertile of intake of red meat is 2.3 (95% confidence interval 1.1 to 4.9) compared with the lowest tertile. The protective effective of coloured fruits and vegetables high in β-cryptoxanthin and zeanxanthin is particularly marked. Moderate amounts of alcohol have been noted to be protective in some studies. That these lifestyle risk factors for RA are shared with a number of other diseases, particularly coronary heart disease, is probably no coincidence. Adoption of a more healthy lifestyle with respect to smoking, diet, and physical exercise might reasonably be expected to further reduce the incidence of RA.

☐ SECONDARY PREVENTION

Improving outcomes

Non-steroidal anti-inflammatory drugs (NSAIDs) in those without specific contra-indications have long been the first-line treatment in patients with RA. Although NSAIDs improve the pain and stiffness of RA, however, no evidence shows that they influence disease progression. The first so-called second-line or disease-modifying antirheumatic drug (DMARD) – intramuscular gold – was introduced in the 1920s. Other DMARDs include the antimalarials, D-penicillamine, and sulfasalazine. Disease-modifying antirheumatic drugs have a direct influence on the inflammatory process and are able to suppress levels of C-reactive protein (CRP), the erythrocyte sedimentation rate, and the degree of synovial swelling and proliferation and to slow the progression of radiological erosions.[9]

Disease-modifying antirheumatic drugs are slow to produce any beneficial effect, however, and share a poor side-effect profile. By 2–3 years after starting a traditional DMARD, most patients with RA have discontinued the drug because of inefficacy or adverse events. Methotrexate – in widespread use as a DMARD in patients with RA since the early 1990s – has a better discontinuation profile, with more than 50% of patients who start the drug still taking it at five years. During the 1990s, ciclosporin and leflunomide were licensed as DMARDs for the treatment of RA and were the first in this class to be introduced on the basis of their known mode of action.

At the same time, it was becoming clear that the proinflammatory cytokine tumour necrosis factor alpha (TNFα) played a central role in the pathogenesis of RA.[10] Tumour necrosis factor α acts on macrophages to produce proinflammatory cytokines and chemokines (which leads to increased inflammation), on endothelial cells to produce adhesion molecules and vascular endothelial growth factor (which promotes cellular infiltration and increased angiogenesis), on hepatocytes to produce acute phase reactants such as CRP, and on synoviocytes to synthesise metalloproteinases and so enhance the degradation of articular cartilage.

The development and introduction of drugs that block TNFα has proved a major revolution in the treatment of RA. Three drugs are currently licensed in this class:

☐ Two monoclonal antibodies – infliximab (a chimeric antibody) and adalimumab (a human sequence antibody)

☐ One soluble recombinant TNF-α receptor fusion protein – etanercept.

Randomised controlled trials showed that these agents lead to impressive response rates in patients who failed to respond to other DMARDs, including methotrexate.[11] The response rates of all the anti-TNFα agents are substantially higher if they are administered with methotrexate or another DMARD. The Tight Control of Rheumatoid Arthritis (TICORA) trial from Glasgow suggested that it could be possible to achieve the same degree of suppression of disease activity with aggressive use of conventional DMARDs as with anti-TNF treatment, but the anti-TNF agents seem to be uniquely good at slowing or halting radiographic progression.

Other biologic agents are on the horizon for patients who fail to respond to treatment with anti-TNFα agents. These include rituximab, which is a monoclonal antibody that is directed against CD20 on B cells and leads to depletion of B cells. This seems to have a role in the management of patients with RA positive for rheumatoid factor. Another agent is CTLA4IG (abatacept), which inhibits co-stimulation of T cells.

Treatment strategies

The goals of treatment in patients with RA are to reduce the symptoms of pain, stiffness, and fatigue and to limit structural damage, thus optimising physical function. Until recently, when treatment options were limited, this was achieved by progressing slowly up the treatment pyramid of NSAIDs, DMARDs, and steroids, with each change made reluctantly and only when absolutely necessary. Treatment with DMARDs was generally initiated only when radiological erosions were apparent. It then became increasingly clear that treatment should be more aggressive and should be started earlier to try to prevent the development of erosions. Many patients have an acute – often post-viral – inflammatory polyarthritis that resolves spontaneously within a few weeks, and the 'cusp' between arthritis being more likely to resolve and more likely to persist comes at around 12 weeks. The presence of rheumatoid factor and the involvement of large joints, however, points to a poor prognosis. All patients with an inflammatory polyarthritis that persists beyond 12 weeks and those with poor prognostic signs should start treatment with a DMARD with the aim of completely suppressing all clinical and laboratory evidence of inflammation.

Improving survival

For more than 50 years, RA has been known to be associated with premature mortality. In studies that have been large enough to explore cause-specific mortality, cardiovascular causes have accounted for most excess deaths. Originally, these cardiovascular deaths were thought to be directly related to rheumatoid heart disease, but it is now clear that they are the result of coronary heart disease and that patients with RA, just like those with diabetes, develop accelerated atherosclerosis.[12] Women with RA positive for rheumatoid factor are twice as likely to die from coronary heart disease in the first 10 years after they develop RA as age-and sex-matched controls from the general population. The risk of coronary heart disease is particularly marked in patients who are positive for rheumatoid factor. Atherosclerosis is increasingly recognised as an inflammatory condition, and many similarities exist between the histology of the inflamed rheumatoid joint and the histology of the atherosclerotic plaque. Within the general population, high sensitivity CRP is an independent predictor of cardiovascular disease. A similar trend is seen in patients with RA, in whom studies show that the risk of premature coronary death is related to the cumulative erythrocyte sedimentation rate or to baseline levels of CRP.

Rheumatoid arthritis is associated not only with excess cardiovascular mortality but also with excess cardiovascular morbidity. Studies have shown endothelial dysfunction, increased carotid intima medial thickness, and carotid plaques. The coronary heart disease in patients with RA often is silent – just as it is in patients with diabetes. Work from the Mayo Clinic showed that patients with RA have an increased prevalence of congestive heart failure and non-cardiac vascular events.

As already mentioned, RA is associated with an increased prevalence of smoking, and this without doubt plays a part in the aetiology of the accelerated atherosclerosis – as does dyslipidaemia. Patients with RA have reduced levels of total cholesterol and LDL cholesterol, which are influenced by the level of inflammation. The level of HDL cholesterol, however, is even further reduced, which leads to an adverse ratio of total cholesterol:HDL cholesterol. An interesting trial of atorvastatin in patients with RA showed an improvement not only in the lipid profile but also in activity of RA. Patients with RA thus might be expected to experience improved cardiovascular mortality if exposed to statins – not only through a reduction in their levels of cholesterol but also because of improved control of their disease.

☐ SUMMARY

The epidemiology and treatment options for patients with RA have changed quite significantly in the last 10 years. Real opportunities for primary and secondary prevention of the disease, as well as improved survival, are available.

REFERENCES

1   Symmons DP. Looking back: rheumatoid arthritis – aetiology, occurrence and mortality. *Rheumatology (Oxford)* 2005;44 (Suppl 4):iv14–7.

2   Gregersen PK, Silver J, Winchester RJ. The shared epitope hypothesis. An approach to understanding the molecular genetics of susceptibility to rheumatoid arthritis. *Arthritis Rheum* 1987;30:1205–13.

3   Hinks A, Barton A, John S *et al*. Association between the PTPN22 gene and rheumatoid arthritis and juvenile idiopathic arthritis in a UK population: further support that PTPN22 is an autoimmunity gene. *Arthritis Rheum* 2005;52:1694–9.

4   Arnett FC, Edworthy SM, Bloch DA *et al*. The American Rheumatism Association 1987 revised criteria for the classification of rheumatoid arthritis. *Arthritis Rheum* 1988;31:315–24.

5   Zendman AJ, van Venrooij WJ, Pruijn GJ. Use and significance of anti-CCP autoantibodies in rheumatoid arthritis. *Rheumatology (Oxford)* 2006;45:20–5.

6   Peterfy CG. New developments in imaging in rheumatoid arthritis. *Curr Opin Rheumatol* 2003;15:288–95.

7   Symmons DP. Epidemiology of rheumatoid arthritis: determinants of onset, persistence and outcome. *Best Pract Res Clin Rheumatol* 2002;16:707–22.

8   Klareskog L, Stolt P, Lundberg K *et al*. A new model for an etiology of rheumatoid arthritis: smoking may trigger HLA-DR (shared epitope)-restricted immune reactions to autoantigens modified by citrullination. *Arthritis Rheum* 2006;54:38–46.

9   Simon LS. The treatment of rheumatoid arthritis. *Best Pract Res Clin Rheumatol* 2004;18:507–38.

10 Feldmann M, Maini RN. Lasker Clinical Medical Research Award. TNF defined as a therapeutic target for rheumatoid arthritis and other autoimmune diseases. *Nat Med* 2003;9:1245–50.

11 Furst DE, Breedveld FC, Kalden JR *et al.* Updated consensus statement on biological agents, specifically tumour necrosis factor {alpha} (TNF{alpha}) blocking agents and interleukin-1 receptor antagonist (IL-1ra), for the treatment of rheumatic diseases, 2005. *Ann Rheum Dis* 2005;64 (Suppl 4):iv2–14.

12 Sattar N, McCarey DW, Capell H, McInnes IB. Explaining how 'high-grade' systemic inflammation accelerates vascular risk in rheumatoid arthritis. *Circulation* 2003;108:2957–63.

☐ RHEUMATOLOGY SELF ASSESSMENT QUESTIONS

Understanding osteoarthritis

1   Osteoarthritis is characterised pathologically by the following:
   (a) Osteochondral loose bodies
   (b) Marginal erosions and osteopenia
   (c) Diffuse loss of hyaline cartilage
   (d) Marginal osteophytes
   (e) An association with calcium crystal deposition

2   Risk factors for osteoarthritis of the knee include:
   (a) Obesity
   (b) Farming
   (c) Increased bone density
   (d) Male sex
   (e) Varus–valgus malalignment

3   The following are physiological associations of osteoarthritis of the knee:
   (a) Reduced knee proprioception
   (b) Increased tendency to fall
   (c) Repetitive knee bending while carrying loads
   (d) Quadriceps weakness
   (e) Increased sway when weight bearing

4   Pain and disability from OA of the knee can be improved in the long term by the following:
   (a) Avoidance of activity, especially weight-bearing activity
   (b) Weight loss if obese
   (c) Aerobic fitness training
   (d) Quadriceps strengthening exercises
   (e) Wearing shoes with raised heels

5   The following statements are true:
   (a) Osteoarthritis has appeared very recently in our evolutionary history
   (b) People with nodal osteoarthritis of the hands have an additional increased risk of osteoarthritis of the knee after meniscectomy
   (c) Most joints with structural OA are painful
   (d) Most people with nodal OA of the hand have a good long-term prognosis with respect to hand pain and function
   (e) Other animals, including dinosaurs, have been shown to develop OA

Developments in rheumatoid arthritis

1   Genetic susceptibility to RA is associated with:
   (a) HLA B27

   (b) HLA DR3

   (c) HLA DRB1 genes that bear the shared epitope

   (d) PTPN 22

   (e) TNFα receptor genes

2   With respect to anti-CCP antibodies:

   (a) They are more specific than rheumatoid factor in the diagnosis of RA

   (b) Testing for anti-CCP antibodies should replace testing for rheumatoid factor in patients with suspected RA

   (c) They are predictive of the development of extra-articular disease in RA

   (d) They are predictive of the development of erosions in RA

   (e) They are associated with smoking in patients with the shared epitope

3   Modification of the following lifestyle factors might be expected to reduce the incidence of RA:

   (a) Reduced alcohol consumption

   (b) Smoking cessation

   (c) Reduced consumption of citrus fruits

   (d) Reduced consumption of red meat

   (e) Weight reduction

4   Patients with RA have a reduced life expectancy:

   (a) Excess mortality is mainly attributable to gastrointestinal perforations and bleeds

   (b) Excess mortality is related to the cumulative burden of inflammatory disease

   (c) Excess cardiovascular mortality can be attributed to a high concentration of LDL cholesterol

   (d) Excess mortality is more marked in patients who are positive for rheumatoid factor

   (e) Baseline levels of C-reactive protein are a predictor of future cardiovascular events

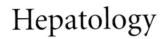

Hepatology

Intensive care for the liver

Julia Wendon

In the field of acute liver failure (ALF), the diagnostic groupings can be split into hyperacute, acute, and subacute liver failure. The aetiology remains broad, and although the most common cause worldwide is viral hepatitis (B), concern should be addressed in those in whom the diagnosis may be missed – particularly patients with ALF induced by drugs (for example, non-steroidal anti-inflammatory drugs and herbal remedies) and those with so-called seronegative disease (in whom all sought aetiologies are absent). Hyperacute and acute liver failure have a greater risk of cerebral oedema and cardiovascular failure but also a greater chance of spontaneous survival; conversely, patients with subacute liver failure have a lower risk of cerebral oedema and encephalopathy and the lowest chance of spontaneous survival.[1] In addition, subacute liver failure can be easily confused with chronic liver diseases associated with ascites and splenomegaly; this is especially important to remember when the aetiology is not clear, and the question 'Could this be acute liver failure and should transplantation be considered a possible option?' always should be asked.

☐ AETIOLOGY

Viral acute liver failure

Viral ALF is an uncommon complication of viral hepatitis that occurs in 0.2–4% of cases depending on the underlying aetiology. Hepatitis A rarely progresses to acute liver failure, however this risk rises with increasing age at time of exposure. Hepatitis B can cause ALF through a number of scenarios. The incidence of the delta virus seems to be decreasing, while vaccination and antiviral drugs should have some impact on the other mechanisms. Hepatitis C is rarely recognised as the sole cause of ALF.

Hepatitis E is common in parts of Asia and Africa, and the risk of developing ALF increases to more than 20% in pregnant women, being particularly high during the third trimester. Hepatitis E is also encountered in Europe and the United States and may account for up to 8% of cases that would previously have been described as seronegative hepatitis. Unusual causes of viral ALF include herpes simplex 1 and 2, herpesvirus 6, varicella zoster virus, Epstein-Barr virus, and cytomegalovirus.

Seronegative hepatitis is the most common presumed viral cause in some parts of the Western world. In the United Kingdom, it accounts for 56% of such cases. Middle-aged women are most frequently affected, and it occurs sporadically. The diagnosis is one of exclusion. Considerable uncertainty surrounds whether much, or all, of this category is the result of a viral infection.

Drug-related acute liver failure

Overdose of acetaminophen accounts for about 40% of cases of ALF in the United Kingdom and United States.[1] It is usually taken with suicidal or parasuicidal intent, but up to 8–30% of cases follow the therapeutic use of acetaminophen. Factors that increase susceptibility to acetaminophen toxicity include regular alcohol consumption, antiepileptic treatment (enzyme induction), and malnutrition. Acute liver failure develops in only 2–5% of those who take overdoses, and the mortality is highest at doses exceeding 48g. Staggered ingestion can make assessment a particular challenge.

Idiosyncratic drug reactions usually develop during the first exposure to the drug. The diagnosis is largely made on the basis of a temporal relation between exposure to the drug and the development of ALF. Estimates of the risk of developing ALF as a result of an idiosyncratic reaction range from 0.001% for non-steroidal anti-inflammatory drugs to 1% for the combination of isoniazid and rifampicin. Ecstasy (methylenedioxymethamphetamine (MDMA), a synthetic amphetamine) has been associated with a number of clinical syndromes ranging from rapidly progressive ALF associated with malignant hyperpyrexia to subacute liver failure.

Other aetiologies

Acute liver failure associated with pregnancy tends to occur during the third trimester. Three patterns are recognised, although a considerable degree of overlap exists:

- ☐ acute fatty liver of pregnancy – primagravids carrying a male fetus are most at risk

- ☐ HELLP (haemolysis, elevated liver enzymes, low platelets) syndrome

- ☐ ALF complicating pre-eclampsia or eclampsia.

In addition, a range of unusual causes of ALF exists. Wilson's disease may present as ALF, usually during the second decade of life. It is characterised clinically by a Coomb's negative haemolytic anaemia and demonstrable Kayser-Fleischer rings in most cases. Poisoning with *Amanita phalloides* (death cap mushroom) is most commonly seen in central Europe, South Africa, and the west coast of the United States. Severe diarrhoea, often with vomiting, is a typical feature and starts five or more hours after ingestion of the mushrooms. Liver failure develops 4–5 days later. Autoimmune liver disease may present as ALF, but is usually not responsive to treatment with corticosteroids. Budd-Chiari syndrome may present with ALF, and the diagnosis is suggested by hepatomegaly and confirmed by the demonstration of hepatic vein thrombosis. Malignancy infiltration, especially with lymphoma, is typically associated with hepatomegaly. Ischaemic hepatitis is increasingly being recognised as a cause of ALF, especially in older patients.

Paediatric causes include neonatal haemochromatosis, mitochondrial disorders, tyrosinaemia, galactosaemia, and fructose intolerance.

☐ CRITERIA FOR LIVER TRANSPLANTATION

Table 1 shows indications for consideration for liver transplantation; these represent the O'Grady criteria,[2] which seem to have withstood the test of time and remain sensitive and specific. Other criteria that seem equally robust are the Clichy criteria, which are based on the presence of encephalopathy, levels of factor VII, and age. More recently, criteria for paracetamol-induced acute liver failure have been suggested; these use blood levels of lactate (>3.5 mmol/l at more than 24 hours and with adequate volume therapy)[3] and a high level of phosphate on days 2–3.

Table 1 O'Grady criteria for consideration for liver transplantation in patients with acute liver failure.

Type of acute liver failure	Criteria
Acetaminophen induced	pH <7.3 (greater than 24 hours after ingestion and after full volume resuscitation) **or** all three of the following within a 24-hour timeframe: • INR >6.5 • Serum creatinine >300 µmol/l • Encephalopathy (grade 3 or above)

Non-acetaminophen induced	INR >6.5 **or** any three of the following:
	• Age <10 or >40 years
	• Aetiology:
	  – Non-A–E hepatitis
	  – Halothane hepatitis
	  – Drug reaction
	• Jaundice to encephalopathy >7 days
	• INR >3.5
	• Serum bilirubin >300 µmol/l

INR = international normalised ratio

☐ CLINICAL PRESENTATION AND MANAGEMENT

Acute liver failure is a multi-system disease with evidence of cardiovascular, respiratory, metabolic, haematological, abdominal, immunological, and neurological involvement. Coagulopathy and encephalopathy are essential for a diagnosis of acute liver failure, and the international normalised ratio imparts important prognostic information with respect to outcome. As such, coagulation parameters are not normally corrected (unlike in the setting of chronic liver disease). A small cohort of patients develop a syndrome of profound coagulopathy, with a high activated partial thromboplastin ratio (APTR), low levels of fibrinogen, and platelet dysfunction, which can result in significant bleeding; in this situation, replacement of factors is appropriate.

The metabolic disturbances are broad. Insulin resistance – both peripheral and hepatic – is common. Hyperlactataemia is frequently seen and is multifactorial in nature, relating to peripheral production and impaired hepatic clearance. Levels of lactate may be affected by volume status, and this should always be looked for and corrected in the first instance. Persistence of a high level of lactate is a poor prognostic feature and may be used as a guide to the need for transplantation in patients with acute liver failure. In patients with hyperacute and acute liver failure particularly, crystalloid depletion may result from vomiting, and this group might need normal saline in terms of fluid resuscitation. Nutritional status should always be considered, as patients in the subacute category are frequently poorly nourished. All patients with liver failure have been shown to have increased metabolic requirements, so aggressive enteral feeding should be undertaken early. Recent work has shown the safety of early use of a standard protein feed in patients with encephalopathy and acute-on-chronic liver disease: no differences were seen in mortality, positive nitrogen balance was maintained, and no increase was seen in the incidence of encephalopathy.[4]

A study by van de Berghe randomised 1,548 post-surgical critically ill patients to standard of care (glucose levels controlled at 10–11 mmol/l) or tight glucose control (insulin treatment aimed at achieving glucose levels of 4.4–6.1mmol/l). A significant mortality benefit was seen for the group with tight control of glucose levels; this effect was more pronounced in patients who remained in the intensive care unit for more than five days. In addition, this cohort of patients showed a lower incidence of hyperbilirubinaemia, decreased duration of ventilation, and reduced incidence of renal impairment, bacteraemia, and polyneuropathy. Subsequent work from this group suggested that glucose control might be very pertinent with respect to liver function. The authors also published the results of post-mortem biopsies of liver and muscle from 18 patients (matched for demographics, acute physiological disturbances, and interventions) in each of the treatment groups. In the standard-of-care group, 20–30% of the hepatocytes in 78% of the livers had abnormally large mitochondria, with disarrayed cristae and reduced electron density of the matrix. By comparison, the mitochondrial structure was normal in 91% of biopsies from patients who had been in the group that received tight control with insulin. No differences between the groups were seen with respect to skeletal muscle. When this tissue was examined further, a significant difference in complex 1, but no difference in complex 2, 3 or glyceraldehyde-3-phosphate dehydrogenase (GADPH), was noted. It thus was suggested that hyperglycaemia might result in impaired mitochondrial respiration and production of mitochondrial superoxide in reactive oxygen species. Indeed, glucose uptake in the liver is proportional to the level in blood, while uptake in the muscle is dictated by levels of glucose transporter 4. Tight glucose control thus might result in preservation of mitochondrial hepatocyte function. Although hypoglycaemia is always a concern in patients with liver disease, it is very rare in those who are being fed, and large numbers of patients will need treatment with insulin to maintain normal levels of glucose.

The development of hypotension in patients with liver failure is a poor prognostic sign. In adults, some 90% of patients who have acute or hyperacute liver failure and fulfil the criteria for liver transplantation may need norepinephrine support. Sadly, however, rapidly escalating levels of norepinephrine may preclude orthotopic liver transplant. It is difficult to determine exactly which mean arterial pressure should be aimed for, especially as patients with acute liver failure frequently do not autoregulate with respect to their cerebral haemodynamics. Clinical acumen is required in this context, along with assessment of end-organ function. These patients almost invariably have a high output state and initially may be fluid responsive. Subsequently, however, invasive haemodynamic monitoring is needed to ensure that fluid does result in an improvement in stroke volume and hence cardiac output. In order to ensure this in clinical practice, dynamic rather than static parameters of fluid status must be examined. In terms of invasive haemodynamic monitoring, the pivotal point must be the determination of fluid responsiveness and the monitoring of improvement in stroke volume index in response to a fluid challenge. This can be achieved with a variety of haemodynamic monitoring methods. Pressure monitoring in terms of central venous pressure or pulmonary artery flotation catheter to achieve pulmonary artery occlusion pressure, however, does not show good correlation with preload or indeed with fluid responsiveness. This may be further compounded by the development of intra-abdominal hypertension. Some measure of dynamic haemodynamic monitoring, such as can be achieved through stroke volume variation or pulse pressure variation, thus is needed.

In the literature in general intensive care, significant data suggest that epinephrine may be detrimental, resulting in increases in splanchnic consumption of oxygen and turnover of glucose. Phenylnephrine has been associated with decreased splanchnic blood flow and decreases in splanchnic oxygen consumption. Normally, norepinephrine is the first choice.

The type of fluid used for resuscitation remains an area of ongoing debate. The recent saline versus albumin fluid evaluation (SAFE) study did not show any clear-cut benefit for crystalloid or colloid in a general population of intensive care patients. A body of evidence suggests that 20% albumin may be beneficial in patients with acute-on-chronic liver disease with hepatorenal failure, but no significant evidence exists with respect to patients with acute liver failure.

Again in the literature in general intensive care, evidence suggests impaired response to synacthen (tetracosactide; a synthetic analogue of adrenocorticotrophic hormone (ACTH)) in patients with a critical illness. In an adult population of patients with acute hepatic necrosis, 57% of patients had an abnormal synacthen response, with hypotension associated with lower baseline and incremental values.[5] Similar observations have been seen in patients with chronic liver disease, with an increasing incidence of abnormal responses to synacthen with progression from Child-Pugh score A to Child-Pugh score C. Data in patients with chronic liver disease and sepsis also show a high incidence of abnormal response to ACTH, with increasing incidence with increasing Child-Pugh, model for end-stage liver disease (MELD), and sepsis-related organ failure assessment (SOFA) scores.[6] In a retrospective study by Harry *et al*, no difference in mortality was seen between patients treated with steroids and weaned off pressors compared to those not on steroids. This syndrome has also been reported by Marick *et al*, who again noticed a significant incidence of poor renal response after administration of 1 µg ACTH. No difference was seen in levels of albumin and creatinine between those with or without normal adrenal function, but a significant difference was seen in terms of high-density lipoprotein (HDL) cholesterol, which was significantly lower (8.2 mg/dl) in the group of poor responders compared with the normal responders (28.4 mg/dl). Overall, 75% of the pressor-dependent patients had impaired adrenal function; and in these, mortality was 26% in those treated with steroids and 46% in those who did not receive steroids.

Renal failure is common in patients with acute liver failure and is most frequently acute tubular necrosis rather than hepatorenal syndrome. Treatment relates to adequate volume repletion and blood pressure control, with removal of any potential precipitants. It should always be noted that urea will not provide an adequate reflection of renal function and that creatinine also may be a poor reflection, especially in patients with low muscle mass. The role of intra-abdominal pressure should be considered as a potential contributor to renal dysfunction – particularly in those with ascites. The nature of intra-abdominal hypertension is such that it will impact on the adequacy of venous return and contribute to impaired respiratory dysfunction. Pressure can be measured via the urinary catheter, and treatment options, such as drainage of a small volume of ascites, can then be considered.

Hypoxia is common in patients with acute liver failure and various aetiologies, and the precipitant of this hypoxia is often multi-factorial, relating to effusions, intra-abdominal hypertension with changes in thoraco-abdominal compliance, atelactasis, acute lung injury, acute respiratory distress syndrome (ARDS), and mismatches in pulmonary blood flow to the lungs (VQ mismatch). Chest X-rays frequently are unhelpful, and computed tomography may not be possible because of the risk of transporting hypoxic patients around the hospital. In this setting, invasive haemodynamic monitoring that allows measurement of extravascular lung water may allow delineation of optimal management profiles. In patients with chronic liver disease, consideration should always be given to hepatopulmonary syndrome, which can be diagnosed easily at the bedside with a bubble or contrast echocardiogram (contrast freely appearing in the left circulation at about three beats). Portopulmonary syndrome should be another diagnosis that is sought actively; it frequently contributes significantly to development of ascites and oedema. Optimal treatment is with liver transplantation, but case series suggest that agents such as sildenafil and nebulised epoprostenol may be beneficial.

Infection is common, and recent studies from Rolando *et al* showed that severe sepsis was associated with a 58% mortality and septic shock with a 98% mortality. Studies that examined selective gut decontamination showed decreased infection rates but no effect on mortality. The role of probiotic bacteria in this context requires examination.

Of note, increasing components of the systemic inflammatory response syndrome are associated with development of and deeper levels of encephalopathy. This relation is seen for inflammatory markers rather than infection per se. These findings have been noted by Rolando and Vaquero.[7,8] Encephalopathy is a significant component of acute liver failure, with cerebral oedema most prevalent in patients with hyperacute liver failure. A retrospective review of some 230 patients from King's Liver Unit showed an instance of clinical cerebral oedema in 24% of patients with hyperacute liver failure, 23% of those with ALF, and only 9% of those with subacute liver failure.

The relation between arterial ammonia and cerebral deaths has been shown by the Copenhagen group; a significant difference was seen between arterial levels of ammonia in patients who had cerebral herniation compared with those who survived or died from sepsis-related multiple organ failure. The cut-off point seemed to be 150 mmol/l.[9] This relation between levels of ammonia and outcome was also described recently by Bhatia *et al*. In addition, considerable variation is seen in measured levels of ammonia, depending on the site of sampling (venous versus arterial). Furthermore, patients with acute liver failure showed marked variations in cerebral blood flow and there seemed to be a loss of autoregulation with respect to pressure, although autoregulation is maintained with respect to changes in arterial levels of carbon dioxide.

Some work suggests that lowering body temperature restores autoregulation and also, with respect to pH, that partial pressure of ammonia correlates better with the level of encephalopathy than arterial levels of ammonia. One small study examined six patients with acute liver failure treated with terlipressin. This drug did not have any effect on mean arterial pressure but resulted in significant increases in cerebral blood flow and intracranial pressure – perhaps related to vasopressin receptors in the cerebral circulation. As such, terlipressin is best avoided in patients with acute liver failure.

Inflammatory markers, ammonia, systemic inflammatory response syndrome (SIRS) components, white cell count, and vasopressor requirements have been shown by Jalan *et al* to be associated with intracranial hypertension that requires treatment. The lowering of temperature has also been reported by Jalan in two publications that showed that cooling patients to 32–33°C resulted in a significant fall in intracranial pressure, lowered cerebral blood flow, and improved cerebral perfusion pressure, with decreases in arterial levels of ammonia and cerebral ammonia uptake.[10]

Animal models have suggested that hyponatraemia is associated with ammonia-induced brain oedema, and a prospective trial of hypernatraemia by Murphy *et al* shared a significant reduction in intracranial pressure in the treatment group with a decreased risk of needing treatment for intracranial pressure.[11]

Management of chronic liver disease and encephalopathy should ensure that all possible precipitants are sought and treated and that the airway is protected. Liver support systems have been examined in the fields of acute and acute-on-chronic liver failure. Molecular adsorbent recirculating system (MARS) therapy has been reported to be beneficial in regard to encephalopathy in abstract form and in relation to hepatorenal failure and management of acute-on-chronic liver disease in a small study. In respect of cardiovascular performance, some studies suggest improvement in blood pressure while others do not. Other non-cell-based liver support systems (Prometheus) are now being evaluated and seem to be efficacious with respect to clearance of parameters such as bile acids and bilirubin. Biological systems are more complex in their availability and application. The study of the bioartificial liver (BAL) system did not impact on outcome overall, although a benefit could be seen in subgroup analysis.

□ SUMMARY

The management of acute liver failure in adults needs a multidisciplinary approach with attention to detail and recognition that changes in physiology can occur rapidly and that transplantation will become a requirement in a cohort of patients. The aim of treatment should be to provide stability in an environment in which the liver can spontaneously regenerate. Patients for transplantation need to be optimally selected, but patients who will survive with orthotopic liver transplant must be chosen rather than those who will die without it. A decision to not proceed with liver transplant is fraught with difficulties, but the presence of fixed dilated pupils, rapidly escalating dose of norepinephrine with cyanosed peripheries, severe ARDS and multiple organ failure in older patients, and haemorrhagic pancreatitis would normally preclude progression to transplantation.

REFERENCES

1   O'Grady JG, Schalm SW, Williams R. Acute liver failure: redefining the syndromes. *Lancet* 1993;342:273–5.

2   O'Grady JG, Alexander GJ, Hayllar KM, Williams R. Early indicators of prognosis in fulminant hepatic failure. *Gastroenterology* 1989;97:439–45.

3   Bernal W, Donaldson N, Wyncoll D, Wendon J. Blood lactate as an early predictor of outcome in paracetamol-induced acute liver failure: a cohort study. *Lancet* 2002;359:558–63.

4   Cordoba J, Lopez-Hellin J, Planas M *et al.* Normal protein diet for episodic hepatic encephalopathy: results of a randomized study. *J Hepatol* 2004;41:38–43.

5   Harry R, Auzinger G, Wendon J. The clinical importance of adrenal insufficiency in acute hepatic dysfunction. *Hepatology* 2002;36:395–402.

6   Tsai MH, Peng YS, Chen YC *et al.* Adrenal insufficiency in patients with cirrhosis, severe sepsis and septic shock. *Hepatology* 2006;43:673–81.

7   Rolando N, Wade J, Davalos M *et al.* The systemic inflammatory response syndrome in acute liver failure. *Hepatology* 2000;32:734–9.

8   Vaquero J, Polson J, Chung C *et al.* Infection and the progression of hepatic encephalopathy in acute liver failure. *Gastroenterology* 2003;125:755–64.

9   Clemmesen JO, Larsen FS, Kondrup J *et al.* Cerebral herniation in patients with acute liver failure is correlated with arterial ammonia concentration. *Hepatology* 1999;29:648–53.

10 Jalan R, Olde Damink SW, Deutz NE, Hayes PC, Lee A. Moderate hypothermia in patients with acute liver failure and uncontrolled intracranial hypertension. *Gastroenterology* 2004;127:1338–46.

11 Murphy N, Auzinger G, Bernel W, Wendon J. The effect of hypertonic sodium chloride on intracranial pressure in patients with acute liver failure. *Hepatology* 2004;39:464–70.

Vascular liver disorders

Chundamannil E Eapen and Elwyn Elias

The major conduits of hepatic blood flow – the portal vein, hepatic artery (inflow channels), and hepatic veins (outflow channels) – are prone to a variety of disorders that vary widely in their clinical manifestations. This article summarises some of the recent advances in our understanding of disorders that affect the liver vasculature.

☐ VASCULAR OCCLUSION AS THE PRIMARY MECHANISM FOR PORTAL HYPERTENSION

Budd Chiari syndrome or hepatic venous outflow obstruction

Budd Chiari syndrome (BCS) consists of hepatic venous outflow obstruction and its manifestations, regardless of the cause and level of obstruction, from the small hepatic veins to the entrance of the right atrium. Intrahepatic sinusoidal obstruction syndrome, known as 'hepatic veno-occlusive disease' and most often seen in the context of recent bone-marrow transplantation and cardiac disorders, including constrictive pericarditis, thus are excluded.[1] The typical presentation is ascites, which is sometimes accompanied by pain over the liver. Diagnosis is achievable on careful evaluation of the hepatic veins with Doppler ultrasonography, although other methods including computed tomography and magnetic resonance imaging may give additional information. Liver biopsy may be diagnostic for hepatic venous outflow obstruction, but it is seldom essential other than when the hepatic veins visible on imaging are grossly normal and occlusion is within the smaller hepatic veins. The most sensitive diagnostic method involves hepatic venography via the transjugular route, which permits measurement of venous pressure gradients across stenotic lesions and at the same time provides access for attempts at venoplasty when hepatic veins are incompletely thrombosed.

Excellent medium-term outcomes with treatment by interventional radiology have been shown in patients with Budd-Chiari syndrome of all grades of disease severity, with an evolving change in approach from the traditional methods of portosystemic shunt surgery and liver transplantation to hepatic vein angioplasty and transjugular intrahepatic portosystemic shunt (TIPS).[2] When selecting a treatment approach with interventional radiology, it is useful to classify Budd-Chiari syndrome into two groups: discrete occlusion of proximal hepatic veins and diffuse occlusion of all hepatic veins. Discrete proximal stenoses in hepatic veins are amenable to angioplasty and occur in 41% of patients with Budd-Chiari syndrome.[2] In contrast, patients with diffuse occlusion of hepatic veins are amenable only to TIPS or surgical techniques.

The decision to treat a patient with Budd-Chiari syndrome depends on the presence or absence of symptoms, the presence of complications, and the type of hepatic venous outflow obstruction. Patients with discrete stenosis of proximal hepatic veins may be treated by angioplasty, even if the patient is asymptomatic, given the benefits of restoring physiologic hepatic venous outflow. On the other hand, in the presence of diffuse occlusion of hepatic veins that precludes angioplasty, only symptomatic patients are offered definitive treatment. Currently, TIPS is the preferred treatment in patients with diffuse occlusion of hepatic veins who present with ascites or variceal bleeding. It decompresses the portal circulation into the inferior vena cava (IVC) above the level at which it may be obstructed by an enlarged caudate lobe in patients with Budd-Chiari syndrome (Fig 1). This avoids a major pitfall, in which high pressure in the IVC below the caudate lobe may prevent effective hepatic decompression via mesocaval shunt surgery. In patients with diffuse occlusion of hepatic veins who present with hepatic encephalopathy, liver transplantation may be preferred.

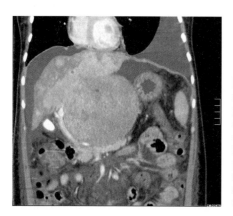

Fig 1 Selectively preserved venous outflow may lead to enlargement of the caudate lobe in patients with Budd-Chiari syndrome. When the caudate lobe compresses the inferior vena cava and a porto-caval shunt procedure is required, transjugular intrahepatic portosystemic shunts (TIPS) have the advantage over mesocaval shunts of decompressing the portal circulation into the supra-caudate portion of the inferior vena cava.

Haematological investigations have high success in revealing prothrombotic conditions such as Factor V Leiden (about 25%) and myeloproliferative disease. Such congenital and acquired disorders may interact within the same patient to produce Budd-Chiari syndrome a decade or more before myeloproliferative disease would otherwise become overt. Patients with Budd-Chiari syndrome are therefore likely to benefit from treatment with lifelong anticoagulation, even if an underlying prothrombotic state has not been identified.

Hepatic veno-occlusive disease (sinusoidal obstruction syndrome)

Hepatic veno-occlusive disease is typically the result of an inflammatory and fibrotic reaction that occludes the hepatic sinusoids. Although it was associated historically with a variety of toxic injuries (such as bush tea disease), nowadays it is encountered almost exclusively in the context of recent bone-marrow transplantation. The patient develops congestive hepatomegaly and ascites within days or weeks of engraftment. The pathogenesis involves a toxic drug injury to the sinusoidal endothelium and is more common with rapid metabolisers of cyclophosphamide and with pre-existent liver disease such as hepatitis C virus infection. It seems likely that depletion of hepatoprotective glutathione stores predisposes the endothelium to drug injury via toxic intermediate metabolites. As approximately 70% of patients with veno-occlusive disease recover spontaneously, initial treatment is primarily supportive with careful attention being given to sodium and water balance. Debibrotide, a polydeoxylribonucleotide with thrombolytic and antithrombotic properties but no systemic anticoagulant effect, has shown encouraging and sustainable responses in approximately 30% of patients who have been treated.

Portal vein thrombosis

With advances in imaging, acute portal vein thrombosis increasingly is being recognised. The aetiology and clinical presentation of portal vein thrombosis differs markedly between children, in whom it commonly occurs in countries in the developing world, and adults. Multiple local precipitating factors and underlying prothrombotic disorders are often present. The typical presentation is bleeding varices in a patient with palpable splenomegaly but no other indication of hepatic disease.

Portal biliopathy increasingly is recognised as a cause of cholestatic jaundice and choledocholithiasis.[3] Longstanding portal vein thrombosis is accompanied by cavernous transformation of the portal vein, many collaterals coursing within the wall of the bile duct with impingement on the lumen (Fig 2). Fibrotic stricture of the biliary system may follow, making resolution of jaundice uncertain despite surgical decompression of the varices by shunt surgery.

In patients with chronic portal vein thrombosis, evidence is accruing that anticoagulation is safe and effective in permitting recanalisation and preventing extension of thrombus. In a study of non-cirrhotic patients with chronic portal vein thrombosis followed for a median of 46 months, the incidence of thrombotic events was 5.5 per 100 patient years, while that of gastrointestinal bleeding was 12.5 per 100 patient years. The presence of an underlying prothrombotic state and the absence of anticoagulant treatment were independent predictors for thrombosis. In patients with an underlying prothrombotic state, the incidences of splanchnic venous infarction

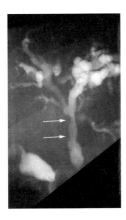

Fig 2 Scalloped indentation (arrowed) of the bile ducts as a result of compression from the portal vein is characteristic of portal biliopathy. Jaundice and intraductal gallstone formation may result.

were 0.82 and 5.2 per 100 patient years in periods with and without anticoagulation, respectively (p=0.01).[4] In a study of 251 cirrhotic patients listed for liver transplantation, all patients detected to have splanchnic vein thrombosis were treated with anticoagulation until they were transplanted. The proportion with partial or complete recanalisation of their portal vein at the time of transplantation was significantly higher in those who received anticoagulation (8/19) than in those who did not receive anticoagulation (0/10) (p=0.002). Survival was significantly shorter in those who had complete portal vein thrombosis at the time of surgery (p=0.04).[5]

Intrahepatic portal vein occlusion (non-cirrhotic portal hypertension)

Non-cirrhotic portal hypertension is caused by obliteration of intrahepatic portal vein radicles and presents as pre-sinusoidal portal hypertension initially and progressive liver failure much later. A variety of terms are used to describe this condition: nodular regenerative hyperplasia of liver (Fig 3), idiopathic portal hypertension, non-cirrhotic portal fibrosis, hepatoportal sclerosis, and incomplete septal cirrhosis. Vascular liver disorders are best named by describing the site of vascular occlusion, so 'intrahepatic portal vein occlusion' may become the preferred term to describe this condition.

Because of the difficulty in excluding cirrhosis on a needle biopsy specimen, diagnosis of non-cirrhotic portal hypertension has largely depended on wedge liver

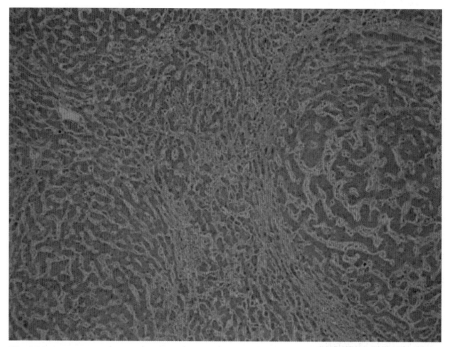

Fig 3 Nodular regenerative hyperplasia results from occlusion of some but not all of the peripheral portal vein branches. Hepatic lobules with intact portal vein supply enlarge, but those without portal vein inflow seem compressed. No fibrosis, as would be found in cirrhosis, is present.

biopsy samples taken at laparotomy or autopsy studies. In a study of 107 livers from patients with non-cirrhotic portal hypertension (wedge liver biopsy (n=92), autopsy (n=15)), portal fibrosis with associated obliterative lesions of small portal veins (<300 μm in diameter) was found in 100% of cases and irregular intimal thickening in medium and large portal veins (up to the third- or fourth-order branches of the right or left portal vein branches) in all livers from autopsies and frequently, but focally, in wedge biopsy livers.[6] With the move to use TIPS rather than abdominal surgery as portosystemic shunt treatment of portal hypertension, wedge liver biopsies are less frequently obtainable. To diagnose non-cirrhotic portal hypertension on a needle biopsy of the liver is a challenging task. Corrosion injection cast studies have shown that peripheral intrahepatic portal vein radicles are obliterated in patients with non-cirrhotic portal hypertension. Newer imaging techniques to study intrahepatic peripheral portal vein branches need to be evaluated as diagnostic tests for this condition.

Emerging evidence shows that gut-derived prothrombotic factors, such as immunoglobulin A cardiolipin antibody, may be driving the obliterative process in the intrahepatic portal vein radicles in this condition.[7] The role of anticoagulants in preventing progressive obliteration of intrahepatic portal vein radicles and secondary thrombosis of extrahepatic portal venous system in patients with non-cirrhotic portal hypertension (intrahepatic portal vein occlusion) needs to be evaluated.

☐ PULMONARY VASCULAR COMPLICATIONS OF PORTAL HYPERTENSION

Hepatopulmonary syndrome

The hepatopulmonary syndrome is characterised by dilatation of pulmonary capillaries to such an extent that oxygen is unable to diffuse adequately to prevent hypoxaemia. Diagnosis depends on the demonstration of right-to-left shunts by bubble echocardiography or 99-technetium macroaggregated albumin scintigraphy and the exclusion of all other causes of right-to-left shunts (Fig 4, overleaf). Patients show orthodeoxia, with marked reduction in arterial oxygen saturation when standing from a recumbent posture as a result of the effect of gravity, which increases perfusion of the lower lung fields, where capillary dilatation is maximal. Correction of hypoxaemia on breathing 100% oxygen, particularly when recumbent, is typical. No consistently effective medical treatment exists, but liver transplantation results in gradual resolution of the problem.[8]

Portopulmonary hypertension

Pulmonary hypertension occurs in up to 16% of patients with advanced liver disease, especially those assessed for or referred for liver transplantation.[8] The diagnosis of portopulmonary hypertension requires demonstration of increased pulmonary vascular resistance, thus excluding raised pressure caused solely by the hyperdynamic circulation frequently seen in patients with cirrhosis. The condition is reversible after liver transplantation, but, in view of the dangers of intraoperative right heart failure, many regard severe degrees of portopulmonary hypertension as a

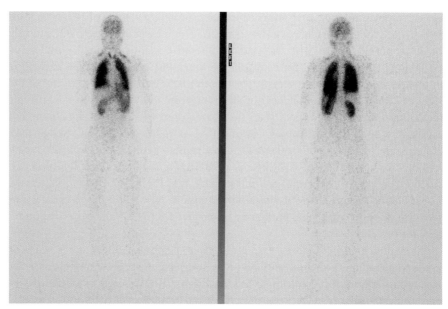

Fig 4 Intravenous injection of 99-technetium macroaggregated albumin (MAA) would normally provide images of the lungs in accordance with their perfusion pattern. In this patient with hepatopulmonary syndrome, some 50% (normal range 3–6%) of the MAA was not retained after passing through the dilated intrapulmonary capillaries.

contraindication to liver transplantation, hence the vital importance of making an early diagnosis.

☐ CONGENITAL AND HEREDITARY VASCULAR ANOMALIES

Patent ductus venosus

In the fetus, blood returning from the placenta largely bypasses the liver by flowing from the left branch of the portal vein through the ductus venosus into the inferior vena cava (Fig 5). Hypergalactosaemia detected on neonatal screening may be attributable to this. Persistent patency of the ductus venosus into adulthood has been associated with hepatic encephalopathy, large lesions of focal nodular hyperplasia in the liver, recurrent pedal oedema and fatigue, pulmonary hypertension, and right-sided heart failure.[9] Direct or magnetic resonance venography delineates the patent ductus venosus. Closure of patent ductus venosus using interventional radiology has been reported.

Hereditary haemorrhagic telangiectasia or Osler-Rendu-Weber disease

Hereditary haemorrhagic telangiectasia (HHT) is an autosomal dominant disorder characterised by mucocutaneous telangiectasia and arteriovenous malformations predominantly in the lungs (PAVM), brain (CAVM), and liver (HAVM). Liver involvement in HHT is reported in 8–31% of cases. A common hepatic artery

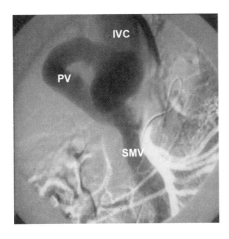

Fig 5 A patent ductus venosus has been shown after injection into the superior mesenteric artery. Blood flows through the superior mesenteric vein (SMV), portal vein (PV), and patent ductus directly into the inferior vena cava (IVC).

diameter of >7 mm and intrahepatic hypervascularisation have been identified as sonographic diagnostic criteria for liver involvement in HHT. Mutations in the genes encoding for endoglin (ENG) and activin receptor-like kinase 1 (ALK-1) lead to HHT-1 and HHT-2, respectively. Hepatic arteriovenous malformations have a higher frequency in women and are more frequent in HHT-2. Shunting from the hepatic artery to the hepatic veins is the predominant effect of liver involvement in HHT, although shunting between the hepatic artery and portal vein and between the portal vein and hepatic vein also occur. Hepatic involvement in HHT may produce symptoms as a result of high output cardiac failure, portal hypertension, or biliary disease.[10]

☐ BENIGN FOCAL VASCULAR LESIONS IN LIVER

Haemangioma

Haemangioma is the most common benign tumour in the liver and is usually detected as an incidental finding. The diagnosis is based on imaging characteristics, and follow up is generally not indicated. Extremely rarely, patients develop pain in association with rapid increase in size of an already large lesion, at which point resection may be considered.

Focal nodular hyperplasia

Focal nodular hyperplasia (FNH) is the second most common benign liver tumour after haemangioma. A central stellate scar (stalk) contains a large artery, unaccompanied by any portal vein radicle, from which blood flows to the periphery of the lesion. Diagnosis is made by demonstration of the central scar on imaging. Focal nodular hyperplasia may remain static or progress slowly with time and should be managed conservatively while reassuring the patient of its benign nature. The key in diagnosis is to differentiate between FNH and hepatic adenomas, which have a propensity for rupture and carry a low but significant risk of malignant transformation. Contrast-enhanced ultrasound and contrast-enhanced magnetic resonance imaging have been shown to improve accuracy in differentiating FNH from hepatic adenoma.

☐ VASCULAR MALIGNANCIES OF THE LIVER

Hepatic angiosarcoma

Angiosarcoma represents the malignant end of a spectrum of changes within sinusoidal endothelium of the liver that includes peliosis hepatis and sinusoidal dilatation. All three conditions can be related to vinyl chloride, arsenic, thorotrast, and anabolic steroids.

Polyvinyl chloride (PVC) is an important plastic resin for construction, pipes and tubing, sidings, and other uses. Exposure to vinyl chloride monomer during the early years of production resulted in an important sentinel health event: the recognition of an excess of a rare liver cancer, hepatic angiosarcoma, at facilities throughout the world. Vinyl chloride is a pluripotent carcinogen that is directed predominantly towards hepatic sinusoidal endothelial cells and secondly towards hepatic parenchymal cells.[11] Polymorphisms of cytochrome P450 CYP 2E1, glutathione S-transferase theta 1 (GSTT-1) and alcohol dehydrogenase-2 (ADH-2) may be a major reason for genetic susceptibility to vinyl chloride monomer-induced hepatic damage. The prognosis for patients with these tumours is very poor.

Hepatic epithelioid haemangioendothelioma

Hepatic epithelioid haemangioendotheliomas are rare, low-grade tumours with a more favourable prognosis than angiosarcomas. The malignant potential often remains unclear in the individual patient. Detection of endothelial markers (factor VIII antigen, lectins (Ulex europaeus agglutinin, UEA-I)) in the histochemistry of tumour cells is diagnostic. Surgical resection is considered the treatment of choice for resectable lesions. For unresectable liver lesions, liver transplantation is considered a reasonable option.

☐ NEWER IMAGING MODALITIES TO EVALUATE FOCAL LIVER LESIONS

With the advent of newer imaging techniques, it is increasingly possible to accurately differentiate focal liver lesions with non-invasive tests. Recent advances in contrast material-enhanced ultrasonography mainly include:

☐ development of low-acoustic-pressure (low-mechanical-index) harmonic software capable of obtaining real-time images without disrupting contrast material microbubbles

☐ commercialisation of new contrast media ('second-generation' contrast media) capable of producing intense echo signals in this low-mechanical-index setting.

With the use of low-mechanical-index continuous-mode contrast-enhanced ultrasound, the circulatory kinetic models of various focal liver lesions can be displayed dynamically. With its unique capacity to provide images in real time, low-mechanical-index contrast-enhanced ultrasound is the dynamic imaging modality of choice in the differential diagnosis of focal liver lesions.[12]

REFERENCES

1   Janssen HL, Garcia-Pagan JC, Elias E *et al*. Budd-Chiari syndrome: a review by an expert panel. *J Hepatol* 2003;38:364–71.

2   Eapen CE, Velissaris D, Heydtmann M *et al*. Favourable medium term outcome following hepatic vein re-canalisation and/or TIPS for Budd Chiari syndrome. *Gut* 2006;55: 878–84.

3   Chandra R, Kapoor D, Tharakan A, Chaudhary A, Sarin SK. Portal biliopathy. *J Gastroenterol Hepatol* 2001;16:1086–92.

4   Condat B, Pessione F, Hillaire S *et al*. Current outcome of portal vein thrombosis in adults: risk and benefit of anticoagulant therapy. *Gastroenterology* 2001;120:490–7.

5   Francoz C, Belghiti J, Vilgrain V *et al*. Splanchnic vein thrombosis in candidates for liver transplantation: usefulness of screening and anticoagulation. *Gut* 2005;54:691–7.

6   Nakanuma Y, Hoso M, Sasaki M *et al*. Histopathology of the liver in non-cirrhotic portal hypertension of unknown aetiology. *Histopathology* 1996;28:195–204.

7   Austin A, Campbell E, Lane P, Elias E. Nodular regenerative hyperplasia of the liver and coeliac disease: potential role of IgA anticardiolipin antibody. *Gut* 2004;53:1032–4.

8   Hoeper MM, Krowka MJ, Strassburg CP. Portopulmonary hypertension and hepato-pulmonary syndrome. *Lancet* 2004;363:1461–8.

9   Jacob S, Farr G, De Vun D, Takiff H, Mason A. Hepatic manifestations of familial patent ductus venosus in adults. *Gut* 1999;45:442–5.

10 Garcia-Tsao G, Korzenik JR, Young L *et al*. Liver disease in patients with hereditary hemorrhagic telangiectasia. *N Engl J Med* 2000;343:931–6.

11 Bolt HM. Vinyl chloride – a classical industrial toxicant of new interest. *Crit Rev Toxicol* 2005;35:307–23.

12 Catalano O, Nunziata A, Lobianco R, Siani A. Real-time harmonic contrast material-specific US of focal liver lesions. *Radiographics* 2005;25:333–49.

☐ HEPATOLOGY SELF ASSESSMENT QUESTIONS

Vascular liver disorders

1   In patients with Budd-Chiari syndrome, hepatic vein angioplasty is feasible in:
   (a) Those with discrete stenosis of proximal hepatic veins (10% of patients)
   (b) Those with diffuse occlusion of all hepatic veins (10% of patients)
   (c) Those with discrete stenosis of proximal hepatic veins (40% of patients)
   (d) Those with diffuse occlusion of all hepatic veins (40% of patients)
   (e) All patients, as long as expertise is available

2   The following interventional radiological treatment is advised for Budd-Chiari syndrome:
   (a) Hepatic vein angioplasty in symptomatic patients
   (b) Hepatic vein angioplasty in asymptomatic patients
   (c) TIPS in symptomatic patients
   (d) TIPS in asymptomatic patients
   (e) Thrombolysis as initial step in all patients

3   Regarding portal vein thrombosis:
   (a) Anticoagulation helps prevent extension of thrombus
   (b) Anticoagulation helps recanalisation of thrombus
   (c) Anticoagulation is contraindicated because of the risk of variceal bleed
   (d) Portal biliopathy can lead to bile duct stones
   (e) Detection of acute portal vein thrombosis is increasing

4   The site of vascular occlusion in patients with non-cirrhotic portal hypertension is:
   (a) Small (intrahepatic) hepatic vein branches
   (b) Hepatic sinusoids
   (c) Peripheral (intrahepatic) portal vein branches
   (d) Extrahepatic portal vein
   (e) Hepatic arterial branches

5   Regarding pulmonary vascular complications of portal hypertension:
   (a) Liver transplantation reverses portopulmonary hypertension
   (b) Severe portopulmonary hypertension is a contraindication for liver transplantation
   (c) Liver transplantation reverses hepatopulmonary syndrome
   (d) Hepatopulmonary syndrome is caused by pulmonary arterial vasoconstriction
   (e) Orthodeoxia is a feature of portopulmonary hypertension

Infectious diseases

Sepsis: new paradigms, novel therapies

Mervyn Singer

☐ INTRODUCTION

Incidence and impact of sepsis

Sepsis, the exaggerated systemic response to infection, is a major cause of mortality and morbidity. It was recently ranked the 10th greatest 'killer' overall in the US, which places it on a par with myocardial infarction. Unlike myocardial infarction, however, sepsis is on an inexorable rise. National data from the US indicate an annualised increase in the incidence of sepsis of 8.7% between 1979 and 2000 – from about 164,000 cases (82.7 per 100,000 population) to nearly 660,000 cases (240.4 per 100,000 population).[1] This predominantly is the result of larger numbers of complex surgical and medical interventions and the growing populations of elderly people and immunosuppressed patients. Sepsis also results in a huge economic burden – nearly $17 billion per annum in the US alone. In the UK, it is responsible for 25% of admissions to intensive care units (ICU).[2] Hospital mortality for such patients ranges from 25% to 60% depending on the severity of the condition. The major mode of death is through the development of multiple organ failure (MOF).

Definitions

Box 1 shows the definition of sepsis used to describe the severity of sepsis according to a consensus group.[3] This classification is still used widely and is augmented by other scoring systems to denote the severity of illness (such as the acute physiology and chronic health evaluation (APACHE) II score) and the degree of organ dysfunction (such as the sequential organ failure assessment (SOFA). This allows better delineation of the effect of sepsis on an individual patient and improves the ability to track disease progression and response to conventional or experimental treatments.

☐ A MULTI-SYSTEM RESPONSE

The focus of research, and thus the basis for the widely held perception of sepsis, has been its manifestation as an exaggerated systemic inflammatory response to infection. Reams of research publications have dissected microbial–host interactions and downstream signalling events, such as activation of transcription factors, which, in turn, encode for increased expression of a wide array of inflammatory mediators, adhesion molecules, and receptors. This knowledge, and the excitement generated by the discovery of yet another crucial pathway or mediator, has led to billions of dollars

Box 1 Classification of severity sepsis. Adapted from Bone *et al.*[3]

Systemic inflammatory response syndrome (SIRS)
Two or more of:
- Temperature >38°C or <36°C
- Heart rate >90 bpm
- Respiratory rate >20 breaths per minute or $PaCO_2$ <32 mmHg (4.3 kPa)
- White blood cells >12,000 cells/mm³, <4,000 /mm³, or >10% immature forms.

Sepsis
The systemic response to infection. Definition as for SIRS but as a result of infection.

Severe sepsis
Sepsis associated with organ dysfunction, hypoperfusion, or hypotension. These may include, but are not limited to, lactic acidosis, oliguria, or an acute alteration in mental status.

Septic shock
Sepsis with hypotension, despite adequate fluid resuscitation, plus presence of perfusion abnormalities.

Multi-organ dysfunction syndrome
Presence of altered organ function in an acutely ill patient such that homeostasis cannot be maintained without intervention. Multiple organ failure has not achieved worldwide uniformity of definition.

---

being thrown at immunomodulatory interventions. For the large part, these have proved futile or, in some cases, detrimental.[4]

The negative results of most of these immunomodulatory trials highlight the current paucity of our understanding of a phenomenally complex condition to which this short review will do scant credit. Until recently, little emphasis had been placed on attempting to understand how this systemic inflammation leads to organ dysfunction, how this inflammation resolves, and how the organs subsequently recover. Awareness also is increasing of the role of other systems, such as the microvascular, immune, hormonal, bioenergetic, metabolic, and coagulatory systems, especially as the degree of perturbation of each system has been associated independently with poor outcomes. We still have a poor grasp of the temporal relation and interactions between these different systems. For each of these systems, we now recognise an evolving process, with an initial upregulation in activity followed by depression. If the patient recovers, activity normalises or even overshoots. A striking example of this temporal change is in the immune response to sepsis. After early activation, subsequent downregulation will lead to immune suppression that, in the context of a heavily instrumented critically ill patient, will predispose to further bouts of infection, reactivation of the acute inflammatory response, and further aggravation of organ dysfunction. Crucially, we also have little realisation how most, if not all, of our current interventions (pharmacological and mechanical) impact upon these processes – whether positively or negatively.[5]

Genetic predispositions, which still are poorly defined, place the patient at higher risk of developing sepsis or subsequently succumbing to the illness, or both.[6] Numerous studies have highlighted a large variety of polymorphisms of genes that code for proinflammatory and other proteins as beneficial or detrimental. Unfortunately, we still are no closer to routine prospective identification of patients who are at risk, let alone modification of their phenotype or genotype. Likewise, understanding is limited about why pathogenic organisms are carried without problem by some patients but are catastrophic in others and why repeat episodes with similar microbes are seen rarely in otherwise healthy people.

Temporal evolution

The initial 'acute phase response' to the infectious insult consists of a rise in proinflammatory and immune activity – cellular and humoral – and an increase in 'fright, flight, and fight' hormones, such as the catecholamines and cortisol.[7] The increase in metabolic rate needed to serve this increased activity is matched by a rise in energy production, which is predominantly sourced as adenosine triphosphate (ATP) from the mitochondria. This constitutes a normal and appropriate defence strategy to the infecting organism; however, in some people, this is exaggerated greatly, such that even a relatively mild insult can produce an overwhelming systemic response. In such a situation, overactivation of coagulation pathways occurs.[8] Although this coagulopathy rarely translates into clinically apparent disseminated intravascular coagulation or histological evidence of microvascular thrombi, it will generate thrombin – a potent proinflammatory mediator – that further drives the inflammatory response.

At the vascular level, increased production of potent vasoactive substances (ranging from vasodilators such as nitric oxide and prostaglandin E1 to vasoconstrictors such as endothelin and thromboxane) will cause microvascular regional flow abnormalities, with areas of vasoconstriction and dilatation seen within the same organ bed. A high degree and persistence of microvascular abnormalities are poor prognostic signs.[9] Increased capillary leak results in increased extravasation of fluids into interstitial fluids, which potentially may act as a barrier to diffusion of oxygen and substrate to the cells and subsequent removal of waste products. A combination of capillary leak that leads to hypovolaemia and interstitital oedema, vasodilatation, and loss of vascular smooth muscle tone (mediated in part by overactivation of ATP-dependent potassium channels) may compromise organ perfusion. Paradoxically, despite this presumed lack of tissue oxygenation, cell death is not a feature of sepsis in most affected organs. Hotchkiss *et al* sought evidence to confirm their belief in the importance of necrotic and, in particular, apoptotic cell death by analysing biopsies taken from multiple organs in patients soon after death from MOF.[10] They acknowledged the virtual lack of histological damage in most of the organs examined, including the lungs, heart, liver, and kidneys. Only in rapidly dividing cells, such as epithelial cells from the gut, spleen cells, and lymphocytes, did they report an increase, albeit small, in the proportion of apoptotic cells.

A paradigm thus needs to be developed that can embrace dysfunctional organs with seemingly normal histology. A clue may be derived from the unexpected finding of high tissue oxygen tension (PO_2) in the bladder and gut mucosa of animal models and the thigh muscle of patients with sepsis. This tissue PO_2, which reflects the balance between local tissue oxygen supply and demand, decreases in patients with other states of shock, such as haemorrhage, heart failure, or hypoxaemia. Oxygen thus seems to be available at the cellular level but is underutilised. As >90% of the body's total consumption of oxygen is used by mitochondria towards generation of ATP by oxidative phosphorylation, this does implicate bioenergetic failure as an integral pathophysiological mechanism that underlies MOF.[11] Numerous studies – in laboratories and patients – consistently show mitochondrial dysfunction and damage with prolonged sepsis; the degree of this relates to poor outcome.[11,12] With insufficient energy to fuel metabolism, these processes must switch off, otherwise continuing energy consumption will decrease the tissue levels of ATP to below the threshold that triggers pathways for cell death. Kreymann and colleagues found that total body oxygen consumption and resting energy expenditure were high in patients with sepsis but decreased with progression of disease severity, such that patients in septic shock had levels equivalent to those in healthy people.[13] Only during the recovery phase was a rebound increase in energy expenditure seen (to 60% above normal).

The predominant absence of cell death thus does imply that switching off these processes successfully decreases metabolic activity, albeit at the expense of impaired organ functioning. This is clinically and biochemically manifest as 'organ failure'; however, it may actually represent a late-stage adaptive process of the body's attempts to cope with a prolonged bout of systemic inflammation.[7] Many analogies can be drawn across extreme conditions of nature, such as temperature excess or deficit, drought, and lack of oxygen that result in hibernation, estivation, and acclimatisation. Myocardial hibernation is an accepted phenomenon in patients with cardiac disorders: ongoing ischaemia results in decreased contractile function but eventual recovery after restoration of perfusion. Unlike cardiac arrest or major haemorrhage, in which the energy failure is abrupt and cell death may ensue, the more prolonged septic insult gives cells the time they need to adapt. This does provide survival advantage, as more hardy animals and patients who are resilient enough to withstand the infectious insult will recover their organ function and thus enhance their long-term prospects of survival and the ability to propagate future, hardier generations. The very low proportion of patients who require long-term dialysis after recovering from acute renal failure as a component of their multi-organ dysfunction syndrome is testament to this fact.

Alongside this bioenergetic–metabolic shutdown, evidence shows depressed inflammatory, immune, and hormonal activities; however, precise relations are not known. Even at the onset of inflammation, production of anti-inflammatory mediators, such as inteleukin (IL)-10 and IL-1 receptor antagonist, is increased. After an undefined period of a few days, the proinflammatory and anti-inflammatory balance shifts in favour of the anti-inflammatory response. Similar downregulation is seen in immune cells, with a shift in Th1:Th2 ratios in T-helper lymphocytes and a fall in monocyte human leucocyte antigen-DR (HLA-DR) expression. Recent data suggest that cellular immune downregulation may be related to energy failure. In the endocrine system, the profiling of most hormones alters considerably, and these changes independently prognosticate outcome. Clearly, whether these changes are causative or epiphenomenal needs to be established, but it is remarkable how many different hormones are affected by the septic process, including glucocorticoids, thyroid hormone, vasopressin, leptin, gut-derived hormones, prolactin, and the sex hormones. Downstream changes also occur, so circulating levels of hormones do not translate necessarily to normal bioactivity. Abnormalities have been described at or beyond the receptor for insulin (insulin resistance) and corticosteroids. Diurnal rhythms are lost, and the impact of therapeutic interventions should not be underestimated. For example, even low doses of dopamine have a marked effect on prolactin secretion, which, in turn, is an important modulator of inflammation. Importantly, cross-talk occurs between hormonal and bioenergetic pathways. For example, many of the actions of thyroid hormone are mediated through direct effects on mitochondrial respiration. Development of the low T3 syndrome, as is found commonly in sepsis, thus will have an inhibitory effect on ATP production, in addition to direct inhibition of the electron transport chain by nitric oxide and other reactive species and downregulation of mitochondrial gene expression.

Recovery processes

The hypothesis that organ failure is an adaptive, hibernation-like process yet has to be proved conclusively, although, conversely, no data at present undermine this concept of 'sleeping' organs. If the hypothesis is assumed to be valid, a 'switch' must be activated to restart these dormant downregulated pathways. Clearly, identification of this 'switch' will lead to a crucial therapeutic impact, as the acute inflammatory phase, at least by blood sampling, seems to have terminated within a few days, yet the ensuing organ failure can persist for weeks, during which time further episodes of infection and inflammation may supervene. More prompt recovery of these organs will decrease morbidity, reduce mortality, and significantly lessen hospital stays and the need for long-term social and medical support. If the central role of the mitochondrion is proved, processes that repair or renew mitochondria – mitochondrial biogenesis – could be accelerated. Knowledge in this field is expanding, with recognition that biogenesis can be stimulated by nitric oxide, leptin, and the transcriptional activator peroxisome proliferator-activated receptor gamma coactivator-1alpha (PGC-1) – all of which are affected by sepsis.

☐ NOVEL TREATMENTS

As stated earlier, most of the therapeutic efforts to date have been targeted at attenuating the inflammatory response, although with decidedly mixed outcomes. Only 'low-dose' corticosteroids (50 mg four times daily plus fludrocortisone) given to patients in septic shock who were not cortisol-responsive to stimulation of adrenocorticotrophic hormone and activated protein C given to patients with sepsis and APACHE II scores >24 have been shown in single multi-centre studies to reduce 28-day mortality significantly.[14,15] A single-centre study conducted in surgical patients admitted postoperatively to intensive care showed outcome benefit in the subgroup that received at least three days of a regimen of intensive insulin (plus nutritional) treatment and tight glycaemic control.[16] Although the study did not concentrate specifically on patients with concurrent sepsis, the greatest reduction in mortality involved deaths as a result of MOF with a proven septic focus. This advantage recently was reproduced by the same group in a medical population of patients in ICU. The mechanism(s) of benefit remain uncertain, although mitochondrial protection, improvement of dyslipidaemia, and anti-inflammatory effects all may contribute.

Notwithstanding the relatively low success rate of preceding trials, numerous strategies have been developed that target different aspects of the septic process. Many are still at the laboratory stage, although promising results in rodents, pigs, and other mammals is certainly no guarantee of success in clinical trials. Some of these novel approaches are highlighted below. This is not intended as a comprehensive listing of all putative treatments but rather aims to give a flavour as to the directions in which treatment is (or could be) heading.

Bacterial–host interactions

Blocking Toll receptors may decrease the ability of bacteria to initiate an inflammatory response. In a mouse model, survival was increased from 0% to >60% with an antagonistic Toll-like receptor (TLR)-2 antibody.

Modulation of inflammatory response

Activation of Toll factor stimulates pathways that lead to eventual activation of the nuclear transcription factor NF-κB. This leads to increased expression of numerous proinflammatory mediators, including cytokines and inducible nitric oxide synthase. Various inhibitors of NF-κB (such as parthenolide, PC-SPES, and isohelenin) all have shown benefit in rodent models of sepsis.

After many false dawns regarding inhibitors of proinflammatory cytokines, attention has shifted towards blocking late-onset cytokines, notably high mobility group box-1 (HMGB-1) protein. Mortality in a murine endotoxin model was reduced significantly, even when given 18 hours after endotoxin. The clinical relevance of this protein is shown by its markedly higher levels in patients who did not survive sepsis compared with eventual survivors (83.7 ng/ml *v* 25.2 ng/ml).

Immune modulation

Recognition that immunosuppression is a frequent finding in patients with prolonged sepsis has encouraged investigation of treatments that reduce lymphocyte apoptosis (such as caspase-3 inhibitors) or stimulate the immune response. Alas, early and encouraging studies with interferon γ in patients whose monocytes had low HLA-DR expression have not been followed up by larger randomised studies.

Hormonal modulation

Other than the intensive insulin regimen and low dose corticosteroid approaches described earlier, other types of hormonal supplementation have been examined. For example, leptin – an adipocyte-derived hormone that has numerous roles including satiety, immunomodulatory, reproductive energy regulation, and mitochondrial biogenesis – has been administered to a fasted rat model of sepsis, improving survival outcomes from 0% to 35%. In patients, plasma levels of leptin were significantly higher in patients who survived sepsis, while fasting is an important means of depleting leptin levels. A multi-centre study in Canada is examining the benefits of vasopressin supplementation in patients with septic shock, as plasma levels of this hormone have been found to be inappropriately 'normal' in such patients.

Bioenergetic modulation

If decreased production of energy secondary to mitochondrial dysfunction is central to the pathogenesis of organ failure, a number of strategies could be applied that protect the mitochondria (for example, boosting levels of mitochondrial anti-oxidants such as glutathione or manganese superoxide dismutase), modulate substrate (such as bypassing inhibition at Complex I with succinate), or stimulating recovery or regeneration of new mitochondria.

REFERENCES

1   Martin GS, Mannino DM, Eaton S, Moss M. The epidemiology of sepsis in the United States from 1979 through 2000. *N Engl J Med* 2003;348:1546–54.

2   Padkin A, Goldfrad C, Brady AR *et al.* Epidemiology of severe sepsis occurring in the first 24 hrs in intensive care units in England, Wales, and Northern Ireland. *Crit Care Med* 2003;31:2332–8.

3   Bone RC, Balk RA, Cerra FB *et al.* Definitions for sepsis and organ failure and guidelines for the use of innovative therapies in sepsis. The ACCP/SCCM Consensus Conference Committee. American College of Chest Physicians/Society of Critical Care Medicine. *Chest* 1992;101:1644–55.

4   Natanson C, Esposito CJ, Banks SM. The sirens' songs of confirmatory sepsis trials: selection bias and sampling error. *Crit Care Med* 1998;26:1927–31.

5   Singer M, Glynne P. Treating critical illness: the importance of first doing no harm. *PLoS Med* 2005;2:e167.

6   Angus DC, Burgner D, Wunderink R *et al.* The PIRO concept: P is for predisposition. *Crit Care* 2003;7:248–51.

7   Singer M, De Santis V, Vitale D, Jeffcoate W. Multiorgan failure is an adaptive, endocrine-mediated, metabolic response to overwhelming systemic inflammation. *Lancet* 2004;364:545–8.

8   Levi M, Keller TT, van Gorp E, ten Cate H. Infection and inflammation and the coagulation system. *Cardiovasc Res* 2003;60:26–39.

9   Sakr Y, Dubois MJ, De Backer D, Creteur J, Vincent JL. Persistent microcirculatory alterations are associated with organ failure and death in patients with septic shock. *Crit Care Med* 2004;32:1825–31.

10 Hotchkiss RS, Swanson PE, Freeman BD *et al.* Apoptotic cell death in patients with sepsis, shock, and multiple organ dysfunction. *Crit Care Med* 1999;27:1230–51.

11 Brealey D, Brand M, Hargreaves I *et al.* Association between mitochondrial dysfunction and severity and outcome of septic shock. *Lancet* 2002;360:219–23.

12   Singer M, Brealey D. Mitochondrial dysfunction in sepsis. In: Brown GC, Nicholls DG, Cooper CE, eds. *Mitochondria and cell death. Biochemical Society Symposium 1999; 66.* London: Portland Press:149–66.

13   Kreymann G, Grosser S, Buggisch P *et al.* Oxygen consumption and resting metabolic rate in sepsis, sepsis syndrome, and septic shock. *Crit Care Med* 1993;21:1012–9.

14   Annane D, Sebille V, Charpentier C *et al.* Effect of treatment with low doses of hydrocortisone and fludrocortisone on mortality in patients with septic shock. *JAMA* 2002;288:862–71.

15   Bernard GR, Vincent JL, Laterre PF. Efficacy and safety of recombinant human activated protein C for severe sepsis. *N Engl J Med* 2001;344:699–709.

16   van den Berghe G, Wouters P, Weekers F *et al* Intensive insulin therapy in the critically ill patients. *N Engl J Med* 2001;345:1359–67.

☐ INFECTIOUS DISEASES SELF ASSESSMENT QUESTIONS

Sepsis: new paradigms, novel therapies

1 Sepsis:
   (a) Is a major cause of morbidity and mortality
   (b) Is increasing in incidence worldwide
   (c) Constitutes the systemic inflammatory response to infection
   (d) Has well-defined genetic predispositions
   (e) Has seen marked improvements in outcomes in the past decade

2 Sepsis:
   (a) Causes simultaneous release of proinflammatory and anti-inflammatory mediators
   (b) Induces activation of multiple non-inflammatory pathways
   (c) Induces later downregulation of the same pathways
   (d) Induces multiple organ failure in most affected patients

3 Paradoxical findings in sepsis include:
   (a) Minimal cell death in most affected organs
   (b) Normal microcirculation
   (c) Elevated tissue oxygen tensions
   (d) Recovery of failed organs within days to weeks
   (e) Immunosuppression

4 Mechanisms involved in the development of organ failure include:
   (a) Mitochondrial dysfunction
   (b) Activation of coagulation
   (c) Metabolic shutdown
   (d) Hyperthyroidism
   (e) Excess nitric oxide production

Croonian Lecture

Understanding hypoxia signalling in cells – a new therapeutic opportunity?

Peter J Ratcliffe

Effective delivery of oxygen to metabolising tissues is a central physiological challenge for all large multicellular organisms. In man, the pulmonary, cardiac, vascular, and erythropoietic systems all contribute to the formidable task of ensuring appropriate delivery of oxygen to the body's approximately 10^{14} respiring cells, and very precise coordination of growth and physiological function is needed to avoid metabolic compromise or the risk of toxicity from excessive oxygenation.

The first major steps in the understanding of oxygen delivery by these systems can be traced to the times of the benefactor of this lecture, Thomas Croone, in the mid-17th century. The description of the blood circulation by William Harvey in *De motu cordis et sanguinis in animalibus* (1628) left an open question as to its purpose. Harvey's landmark deduction was based, in part, from the observation that rates of blood flow were much higher than previously supposed – and inconceivable without recirculation. Hence the focus of attention after this discovery was on the purpose of this rapid movement of the blood. Richard Lower (1631–91) working in Oxford with Robert Hooke (1635–1702) noted that while the blood leaving the heart for the lungs was blue, the blood returning from the lungs to the heart was red. Lower mixed blood with air in a glass vessel and noted the same colour change, concluding that 'nitrous spirit of the air, vital to life, is mixed with the blood during transit through the lungs.' It was to be another 100 years before the work of Priestley, Scheele and Lavoisier defined the essential 'spirit of the air' as oxygen and Lavoisier correctly described the chemistry of combustion, concluding that biological energy metabolism was essentially the same process. A further 100 years passed before the early environmental physiologists gained the first insights into the control mechanisms that respond to altered oxygen availability. In the late 19th century, a correlation between life at altitude and increased haemoglobin content of the blood was noted by Paul Bert,[1] but it was Mabel Fitzgerald (a colleague of JS Haldane on the expedition of 1911 to Pike's Peak, Colorado, to study breathing responses at altitude) who first clearly described the sensitivity of this response, illustrating that relatively minor reductions in barometric pressure at modest altitude were associated with a discernable elevation of haemocrit.[2] These observations were the first of many that ultimately defined the extremely sensitive control of red blood cell production in response to changes in blood oxygen availability. Although studies at this time also suggested the operation of a circulating factor in the regulation of red cell production,[3] hormonal control by erythropoietin was finally proved beyond doubt by Erslev's classic plasma transfer experiments in the early 1950s.[4]

Circulating levels of erythropoietin can be increased several 100-fold within hours of hypoxic stimulation. The response cannot be induced by metabolic poisoning with mitochondrial inhibitors, but it can be induced by transition metals, such as cobaltous ions, and iron chelators – distinctive properties that suggested the operation of a specific oxygen-sensing process and formed the point of entry for recent molecular analyses of oxygen sensitive signal pathways (reviewed in Jelkmann[5]). Two advances in the mid-1980s greatly facilitated this approach: molecular cloning of the erythropoietin gene and the development of tissue culture models for studying regulation by oxygen.

Unexpectedly, early studies of erythropoietin gene regulation revealed that the oxygen sensitive signal pathways that underlie erythropoietin regulation operate in essentially all mammalian cells irrespective of their relevance to erythropoietin production and that they regulate many other genes.[6] Central to the response is a series of closely related transcription factors, termed hypoxia-inducible factors (HIFs), that induce a very extensive transcriptional cascade – directly or indirectly controlling the expression of hundreds of genes in any given cell type. Hypoxia-inducible factor transcriptional targets are now recognised to play a key role in enhanced angiogenesis, as well as enhanced erythropoiesis, vasomotor regulation, matrix metabolism, cell proliferation and survival decisions, energy metabolism, and many other cellular and systemic responses to hypoxia (Fig 1) (for review, see Semenza[7]). The recent elucidation of pathways that regulate HIF, as novel signalling systems mediated by post-translational protein hydroxylation, has provided some of the first molecular biochemical insights into the complex task of maintaining physiological oxygen homeostasis (for review see Schofield[8]). Given the prevalence of ischaemic and hypoxic pathology in human disease, these insights have also generated considerable interest as a potential basis for drug design. This lecture will outline the biological perspective of the new findings and consider the challenge of therapeutic translation.

☐ THE HIF HYDROXYLASE SYSTEM

Hypoxia-inducible factor is an α/β heterodimer of basic-helix-loop-helix proteins that binds DNA sequences within the hypoxia response elements (HRE) at the loci of target genes.[9] Both HIF-α and HIF-β subunits exist as a series of isoforms encoded by distinct genetic loci. The HIF-β subunits are constitutive nuclear proteins, whereas HIF-α subunits are inducible by hypoxia. The proteolytic stability of HIF-α and its transcriptional activity are regulated by distinct mechanisms that have the oxygen-dependent hydroxylation of specific amino acid residues in common. Hydroxylation at two prolyl residues (Pro 402 and Pro 564 in human HIF-1α) mediates interactions with the von Hippel-Lindau E3 ubiquitin ligase complex that targets HIF-α to the ubiquitin-proteasome pathway for proteolytic destruction.[10,11] These hydroxylations are catalysed by a series of three closely related HIF prolyl hydroxylases, termed prolyl hydroxylase domain (PHD) 1–3.[12] In a

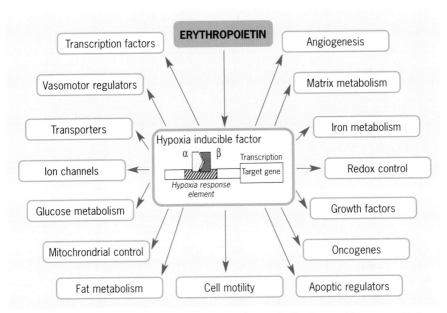

Fig 1 The hypoxia-inducible factor (HIF) transcriptional cascade directly regulates genes with key functions in a broad range of processes. The complex binds in a sequence-specific manner to control elements in DNA, termed hypoxia-response elements, at target gene loci.

second hydroxylation-dependent control, β-hydroxylation of an asparaginyl residue in the C-terminal activation domain of HIF-α (Asn 803 in human HIF-1α) is catalysed by a HIF asparaginyl hydroxylase termed factor inhibiting HIF (FIH).[13–15] Hydroxylation at this site blocks interaction of the HIF-α C-terminal activation domain with the transcriptional coactivators p300/CBP (Fig 2). The HIF hydroxylases are all iron (II)- and 2-oxoglutarate-dependent dioxygenases that have an absolute requirement for molecular oxygen. In hypoxia, therefore, hydroxylation of both the prolyl residues and the asparaginyl residue is reduced, which allows HIF-α to escape von Hippel-Lindau (VHL) ubiquitin ligase complex-mediated proteolysis, to recruit coactivators, and to activate the transcription of hypoxia-inducible genes. The enzymatic process splits dioxygen, with one oxygen atom creating the hydroxylated amino acid and the other oxidising 2-oxoglutarate to succinate with the release of carbon dioxide (Fig 3). Iron (II) at the catalytic centre is loosely bound by a 2-histidine-1-carboxylate coordination motif and may be displaced or substituted by other metals, such as cobalt (II), with loss of catalytic activity, which accounts for the classic properties of activation of HIF, and induction of hypoxia-responsive genes such as erythropoietin, by cobaltous ions and iron chelators (for review see Schofield[8] and Kaelin[16]).

The 2-oxoglutarate dioxygenase superfamily is widely represented across both prokaryotes and eukaryotes, but to date it is unclear whether the HIF hydroxylases have evolved unique catalytic features or are relatively ordinary 2-oxoglutarate-dependent oxygenases that simply use their absolute requirement for molecular oxygen in a signalling role. The evolutionary origin of the oxygen-sensing function

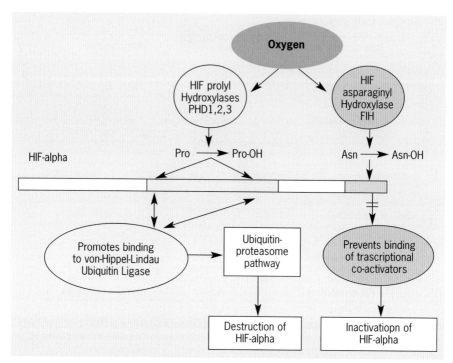

Fig 2 Dual regulation of hypoxia-inducible factor (HIF)-α subunits by oxygen-dependent prolyl (Pro) and asparaginyl (Asn) hydroxylation.

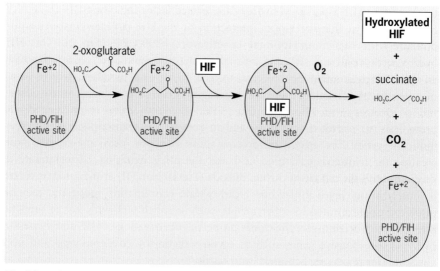

Fig 3 Reaction catalysed by the hypoxia-inducible factor (HIF) prolyl hydroxylase (PHD) enzymes and the HIF asparaginyl hydroxylase (FIH). On the basis of precedent for other enzymes of this type, molecular oxygen is postulated to bind the catalytic centre after ordered binding of the cosubstrate, 2-oxoglutarate, and the prime substrate, HIF. In a radical reaction at the catalytic iron centre, molecular oxygen is split, with one atom incorporated into the hydroxylated amino acid residue and the other into the oxidative decarboxylation of 2-oxoglutarate.

of 2-oxoglutarate oxygenases in higher animals is also unclear. Members of the 2-oxoglutarate oxygenase family and related enzymes oxidise both small- and large-molecule substrates and are involved in diverse biological functions. None of these processes point clearly to an ancestral oxygen-sensing mechanism, however, and in lower organisms, such as bacteria and yeast, other types of enzyme have been implicated in this role. Although strikingly conserved across nematode worms, insects, and vertebrates, both HIF and the HIF hydroxylases are apparently confined to higher eukaryotes – perhaps suggesting that the system developed in response to the challenge of oxygen homeostasis in multicellular animals.

☐ BIOLOGICAL CONTROL OF HIF HYDROXYLASE ACTIVITY

Given the very broad range of processes that manifest regulation by the HIF hydroxylase system and their operation in cells that operate at substantially different oxygen tension within the intact organism, an important challenge now is to understand how the biochemical process of oxygen-dependent protein hydroxylation can generate the flexibility necessary for a role in physiological oxygen homeostasis.

In vitro assays of enzyme kinetics indicate that the apparent K_m (concentration of substrate that gives half-maximal activity) for oxygen for the HIF hydroxylases is well above the physiological range, with reported values of 230–250 µM for the PHDs and about 100 µM for FIH.[12,17,18] Important caveats to these analyses exist, however, such as the use of relatively short peptides rather than native HIF-α polypeptides and the necessary use of unphysiological reaction conditions in the *in vitro* assays. Nevertheless, it seems likely that concentrations of oxygen in tissues, believed to be in the range of 10–30 µM, will essentially always be below the K_m for oxygen of the HIF hydroxylases and thus limiting for enzyme activity over the entire physiological range. For oxygen-sensitive operation of the system, it is also important that the overall cellular capacity for HIF hydroxylation is such that, within the physiological range, hydroxylation is rate limiting for HIF degradation or inactivation (Fig 4). Evidence that is indeed the case is provided by observations that modest changes in enzyme activity achieved genetically by overexpression or small interfering RNA (siRNA)-mediated suppression of individual hydroxylase enzymes have clear effects on levels of HIF-α levels and HIF transcriptional target gene expression. In this respect, it is also interesting that the PHD enzymes exhibit marked inducible and cell-type specific patterns of expression. In particular, PHD2 and PHD3 are markedly inducible by hypoxia by mechanisms that include transcriptional activation by HIF itself. Increases in enzyme abundance will increase the rate of HIF hydroxylation at any given oxygen tension. Increased levels of hydroxylase in hypoxic cells (or reduced levels in well-oxygenated cells) thus may serve a 'range-extending' function that matches hydroxylation capacity to that required for regulation of HIF over a wider range of oxygen concentrations.

Interestingly, emerging data suggest that HIF hydroxylase activity might also be controlled at a number of other levels in addition to the level of oxygen, potentially providing flexibility for directing physiological responses to hypoxia (see Fig 4) (for review, see Schofield[8] and Kaelin[16]). In this respect, a number of properties of the

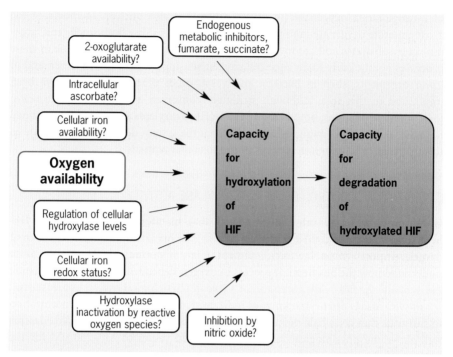

Fig 4 Actual and potential regulatory inputs to the hypoxia-inducible factor (HIF) hydroxylases. These processes are postulated to serve to enable flexible operation of the system in physiological oxygen homeostasis. Note that cellular capacity for hydroxylation of HIF must be in a similar range to cellular capacity for degradation of hydroxyated HIF for optimum oxygen sensitivity of the pathway.

HIF hydroxylases, including their relatively complex cosubstrate and cofactor requirements, are intriguing.

Use of the citric acid cycle intermediate 2-oxoglutarate as cosubstrate, and the action of other citric acid cycle intermediates such as fumarate and succinate as competitive inhibitors of 2-oxoglutarate binding, in *in vitro* assays of dioxygenase activity raises the interesting possibility of dual control by oxygen and energy metabolism. Whether and under what circumstances these metabolites reach critical levels for modulation of hydroxylase activity in cells, however, is unclear. Intriguingly, however, genetic defects in succinate dehydrogenase and fumarate hydratase (enzymes of the citric acid cycle) have been associated with tumours that manifest enhanced angiogenesis or activation of HIF, or both, possibly arising from suppression of hydroxylase activity by accumulation of succinate or fumarate.[19,20]

Another property that may contribute to control is dependence on iron (II) and ascorbate. As noted above, iron binding by the 2-histidine-1-carboxylate motif at the catalytic centre is relatively labile and the HIF hydroxylases are readily inhibited by iron chelators, which explains the activation of HIF transcription by such agents. Ascorbate is another cofactor that is needed for the full catalytic activity of many 2-oxoglutarate-dependent dioxygenases, including the HIF hydroxylases. The precise mechanism of action is unclear, although in the case of one group of enzymes

– the procollagen prolyl hydroxylases – ascorbate seems to be used in reduction of the catalytic iron centre after uncoupled cycles that generate an inactive oxidised iron centre. Whether physiological changes in cellular iron (II) availability or ascorbate affect HIF hydroxylase activity *in vivo* is unclear. Addition of iron or ascorbate to tissue culture medium, however, readily suppresses the accumulation of unhydroxylated HIF-α that is frequently observed in rapidly growing, but apparently well-oxygenated, cultures of tumour cells. This indicates that, at least under these conditions, availability of these cofactors does indeed become limiting. It will now be of interest to determine whether similar mechanisms contribute to HIF activation and excessive angiogenesis observed in native cancer growth.

Other possibilities supported by evidence in cultured cells are that HIF hydroxylase activity may be inhibited by nitric oxide or inactivation of the catalytic iron centre by oxygen radicals, which potentially links the pathway to other signalling systems. Again, the challenge now is to determine to what extent such processes operate physiologically, particularly in the intact organism.

☐ THERAPEUTIC DEVELOPMENT

The role of the HIF transcriptional cascade in many adaptive and potentially protective physiological responses to hypoxia has suggested that pharmacological augmentation of HIF activation might be used in the treatment of hypoxic or ischaemic conditions. The enzymatic basis of HIF regulation, together with the requirement of the HIF hydroxylases for cosubstrates such as 2-oxoglutarate, provides a typical system for drug targeting through development of competitive 2-oxoglutarate analogues or more complex inhibitors. Indeed, such an approach has previously been taken in attempts to develop procollagen prolyl hydroxylase inhibitors that might limit tissue fibrosis. Some of the prolyl hydroxylase inhibitors developed in this way also inhibit HIF hydroxylases and clearly activate HIF target genes. Relative specificity for HIF versus procollagen prolyl hydroxylases is observed for certain compounds, however, which supports the feasibility of selective inhibition.

Analysis of the action of HIF hydroxylase inhibitors and other means of HIF activation in models of anaemia and ischaemic vascular diseases has suggested efficacy in a number of situations. Therapeutic development, however, still presents a number of challenges. Bioinformatic predictions made possible by genome-sequencing projects suggest the existence of an extensive family of 2-oxoglutarate oxygenases, with up to 40 or so predicted members encoded by the human genome.[21] Such insights provide the means to identify and limit potential unwanted 'off-target' effects from relatively unselective 2-oxoglutarate analogues. Nevertheless, to achieve and prove specificity for PHD enzymes against a range of 2-oxoglutarate oxygenases with known and unknown functions remains a challenging task. The pleotrophic nature of the HIF transcriptional response also creates both opportunity and challenge. This is well illustrated by considering the role of HIF in promoting two processes that might be of medical benefit – erythropoiesis and angiogenesis. In each case, activation of HIF can promote an effective response, and in each case efficacy is most probably based on the ability of HIF activation to regulate a range of targets in the relevant pathway. In angiogenesis, therefore, the aim of pharmacological HIF activation would be to augment the physiological activation of angiogenesis by hypoxia. The HIF pathway modulates the expression of not only a range of key angiogenic growth factors such as vascular endotheial growth factor (VEGF) but also growth factors receptors and molecules that play ancillary roles in the angiogenic process, such as matrix metalloproteinases (for review, see Pugh[22]). This coordinated response will likely induce more effective angiogenesis than treatment with any one factor. For instance, short-term exposure to the growth factor VEGF is associated with the growth of leaky vessels that may be unwanted in the treatment of ischaemic tissue. In contrast, transgenic expression of a stabilised HIF-1α gene in the skin of mice promotes the growth of new vessels that show little leakage.[23] Activation of HIF thus may offer advantages over treatment with recombinant VEGF.

In anaemia, the efficacy and safety of recombinant erythropoietin sets a high barrier for any new treatment. However, additional functions of the HIF system, such as induction of other haematopietic growth factors or receptors and alterations in iron metabolism that support efficient erythropoiesis, likely may enable treatment of conditions that are currently partly or completely refractory to erythropoietin. The pleotrophic effects of HIF activation thus may be of benefit in each of these conditions. Promotion of angiogenesis, however, is likely to be undesirable in a treatment aimed at promoting erythropoiesis and vice versa.

Current insights into the HIF hydroxylase system gained through biochemical analysis and observation in tissue culture system would suggest that separation of these effects might be difficult to achieve. Observations in intact organisms, however, provide a different perspective. Despite the pleotrophic effects of HIF activation in tissue culture, the well-studied effects of systemic hypoxia at altitude are largely confined to effects on erythropoiesis and respiration. Although hypoxic induction of angiogenesis is clearly observed in injured and neoplastic tissue, the normal circulation in the intact organism seems much less responsive. The reasons for this paradox remain unclear. It seems likely that additional levels of control serve to limit the expression and action of HIF target gene products in the cells of the intact organism, but the mechanisms are not well understood. Further insights into these processes are important but can most likely be obtained only in the intact organism.

Thus, just as the switch of experimental effort into tissue culture systems provided the impetus for molecular analysis of the cellular response to hypoxia, it is now clear that effective therapeutic translation will require a refocus on studies in the intact organism and, wherever possible, man. Further molecular analysis will be important in guiding these studies and in revealing potential risks of unwanted effects. Nevertheless, as with other potential drug targets, it is important that insights into the massive complexity of physiological pathways that are now possible through molecular and genomic analyses are used to assist, rather than outface, safe therapeutic development.

□ ACKNOWLEDGEMENTS

I am grateful to the members of my own laboratory and my colleague Christopher Schofield's laboratory for their many contributions to this work and for support from Wellcome Trust, Medical Research Council, Cancer Research UK, Kidney Research UK, and British Heart Foundation.

REFERENCES

1   Bert P. Sur la richesse en hémoglobine du sang des animaux vivant sur les hauts lieux. *Comptes Rendu Academie Science Paris* 1882;94:805–7.

2   Fitzgerald ML. VIII. The changes in the breathing and the blood at various high altitudes. *Philos Trans R Soc Lond B Biol Sci* 1913:351–71.

3   Carnot P, Deflandre C. Sur l'activité hémopoïétique du sérum au cours de la régénération du sang. *C R Acad Sci Paris* 1906;143:384–6.

4   Erslev AJ. Humoral regulation of red cell production. *Blood* 1953;8:349–57.

5   Jelkmann W. Erythropoietin: structure, control of production, and function. *Physiol Rev* 1992;72:449–89.

6   Maxwell PH, Pugh CW, Ratcliffe PJ. Inducible operation of the erythropoietin 3' enhancer in multiple cell lines: evidence for a widespread oxygen-sensing mechanism. *Proc Natl Acad Sci USA* 1993;90:2423–7.

7   Semenza GL. HIF-1 and human disease: one highly involved factor. *Genes Dev* 2000;14:1983–91.

8   Schofield CJ, Ratcliffe PJ. Oxygen sensing by HIF hydroxylases. *Nat Rev Mol Cell Biol* 2004;5:343–54.

9   Wang GL, Jiang B-H, Rue EA, Semenza GL. Hypoxia-inducible factor 1 is a basic-helix-loop-helix-PAS heterodimer regulated by cellular O2 tension. *Proc Natl Acad Sci USA* 1995;92:5510–4.

10   Ivan M, Kondo K, Yang H, Kim W, Valiando J, Ohh M, et al. HIFalpha targeted for VHL-mediated destruction by proline hydroxylation: implications for O_2 sensing. *Science* 2001;292:464–8.

11   Jaakkola P, Mole DR, Tian YM *et al.* Targeting of HIF-alpha to the von Hippel-Lindau ubiquitylation complex by O_2-regulated prolyl hydroxylation. *Science* 2001;292:468–72.

12   Epstein ACR, Gleadle JM, McNeill LA *et al.* *C. elegans* EGL-9 and mammalian homologues define a family of dioxygenases that regulate HIF by prolyl hydroxylation. *Cell* 2001;107:43–54.

13   Lando D, Peet DJ, Whelan DA, Gorman JJ, Whitelaw ML. Asparagine hydroxylation of the HIF transactivation domain: a hypoxic switch. *Science* 2002;295:858–61.

14   Lando D, Peet DJ, Gorman JJ *et al.* FIH-1 is an asparaginyl hydroxylase enzyme that regulates the transcriptional activity of hypoxia-inducible factor. *Genes Dev* 2002;16:1466–71.

15   Hewitson KS, McNeill LA, Riordan MV *et al.* Hypoxia-inducible factor (HIF) asparagine hydroxylase is identical to factor inhibiting HIF (FIH) and is related to the cupin structural family. *J Biol Chem* 2002;277:26351–5.

16   Kaelin WG. Proline hydroxylation and gene expression. *Annu Rev Biochem* 2005;74:115–28.

17   Hirsila M, Koivunen P, Gunzler V, Kivirikko KI, Myllharju J. Characterization of the human prolyl 4-hydroxylases that modify the hypoxia-inducible factor. *J Biol Chem* 2003;278:30772–80.

18   Koivunen P, Hirsila M, Gunzler V, Kivirikko KI, Myllharju J. Catalytic properties of the asparaginyl hydroxylase (FIH) in the oxygen sensing pathway are distinct from those of its prolyl-4-hydroxylases. *J Biol Chem* 2003;279:9899–904.

19   Selak MA, Armour SM, MacKenzie ED *et al.* Succinate links TCA cycle dysfunction to oncogenesis by inhibiting HIF-alpha prolyl hydroxylase. *Cancer Cell* 2005;7:77–85.

20   Isaacs JS, Jung YJ, Mole DR *et al.* HIF overexpression correlates with biallelic loss of fumarate hydratase in renal cancer: novel role of fumarate in regulation of HIF stability. *Cancer Cell* 2005;8:143–53.

21   Elkins JM, Hewitson KS, McNeill LA *et al.* Structure of factor-inhibiting hypoxia-inducible factor (HIF) reveals mechanism of oxidative modification of HIF-1 alpha. *J Biol Chem* 2003;278:1802–6.

22   Pugh CW, Ratcliffe PJ. Regulation of angiogenesis by hypoxia: role of the HIF system. *Nat Med* 2003;9:677–84.

23   Elson DA, Thurston G, Huang LE *et al.* Induction of hypervascularity without leakage or inflammation in transgenic mice overexpressing hypoxia-inducible factor-1alpha. *Genes Dev* 2001;15:2520–32.

Linacre Lecture

Attacking the disease spiral in chronic obstructive pulmonary disease

Michael I Polkey and John Moxham

☐ INTRODUCTION

Chronic obstructive pulmonary disease (COPD) is the most common respiratory cause of mortality and morbidity in adults in the UK. Although the condition is initially a pulmonary one, data exist to support the concept that factors associated with COPD, including immobility, gives rise to secondary effects, including a quadriceps myopathy, which in turn cause anaerobic metabolism at low work rates. This, through bicarbonate buffering, leads to CO_2 retention which, because of constraints imposed by pulmonary mechanics, cause acidosis and dyspnoea. Various therapeutic strategies to reverse this spiral may be employed including pulmonary rehabilitation, quadriceps strength training and surgical or bronchoscopic lung volume reduction.

Chronic obstructive pulmonary disease (COPD) is a common and serious problem. It is currently the fourth leading cause of chronic morbidity and mortality in the USA and is predicted to rank fifth in the worldwide burden of disease by 2020.[1] COPD is one of the few major chronic diseases that continues to increase in both prevalence and mortality rate. With the exception of smoking cessation,[2] no intervention has been shown to reduce progression of the condition. Despite maximal medical therapy with inhaled steroids and bronchodilators, people with COPD are frequently symptomatic and may be admitted with acute exacerbation. As a consequence, every physician practising general internal medicine will regularly encounter patients with advanced COPD.

Although COPD is initially a pulmonary disease, two arguments exist to support the notion that a wholly pulmonary disease is not a useful construct when considering patients with advanced COPD. First, the cardinal index of airflow obstruction, the volume expired in the first second of a forced expiration (FEV_1), is a very poor guide to symptoms[3] and a relatively weak guide to mortality.[4] Second, correction of the pulmonary abnormality by double lung transplantation fails to restore exercise performance to normal.[5]

From this basis, we have developed the concept of a disease spiral that seems to better suit the clinical path of patients with COPD. It is important to emphasise that, as with many medical ideas, the concept is merely a resynthesis of previously described ideas, but it has nevertheless been helpful in generating hypotheses for ongoing studies. The overall schema is shown in Fig 1.

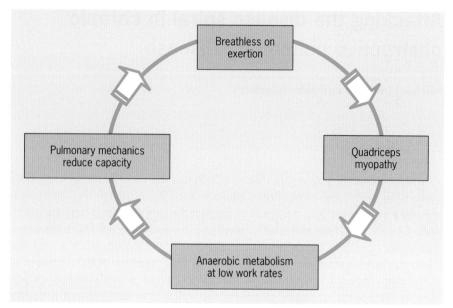

Fig 1 Disease spiral in chronic obstructive pulmonary disease (COPD).

☐ DOES EVIDENCE EXIST TO SUPPORT THE DISEASE SPIRAL?

Breathless on exertion

Most physicians accept that patients with COPD experience dyspnoea on exertion. However, in a landmark paper, Killian and co-workers identified that a surprisingly high number of patients with COPD also experience symptoms of leg fatigue (see later).[6] We revisited this problem and took the opportunity to study both cycle and treadmill-walking exercise.[7] We found that during a walking task, the majority (about 75%) of patients stopped walking because of dyspnoea alone, although a minority placed leg fatigue as an equal or more important cause of exercise limitation. For cycle exercise, the proportion of patients citing breathlessness alone as the cause of exercise limitation was diminished.

Quadriceps myopathy

It is reasonably well accepted that patients with COPD have quadriceps wasting and weakness.[8] At a microscopic level, the changes associated with COPD are characterised by a loss of fatigue-resistant type I fibres and of oxidative enzymes[9,10] without differences in capillarity or mitochondria.[11] Interestingly, type II fibres seem to have reduced mechanical efficiency and consequently reduced power output for a given level of oxygen uptake. The importance of quadriceps involvement in COPD is demonstrated by its association with increased use of healthcare resources[12] and by the fact that, independently of FEV_1, reduced quadriceps cross-sectional area is associated with a poorer prognosis (Fig 2).[13]

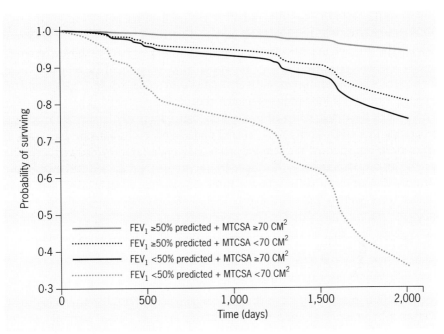

Fig 2 Risk of death in chronic obstructive pulmonary disease (COPD) stratified according to the volume expired in the first second of a forced expiration (FEV_1) and quadriceps bulk assessed as mid-thigh cross-sectional area (MTCSA) assessed using computed tomography (CT). If FEV_1 is less than 50% predicted, then muscle wasting wields a more marked effect. Reproduced from Marquis *et al* with permission of the American Thoracic Society.[13]

The origin of quadriceps weakness in COPD remains a matter of considerable controversy; for a more detailed review, see Couillard and Prefaut.[14] The simplest hypothesis, and that used in the disease spiral, is that weakness arises as a result of immobility induced by the breathlessness. However, the picture is complicated by the clinical observation that quadriceps weakness may also complicate steroid administration, although this seems a less important problem in stable patients at the doses used in a conventional steroid trial.[15] The picture is also clouded by the link between COPD and cachexia. Cachexia is certainly associated with a poor prognosis in COPD,[16,17] but quadriceps weakness may occur in patients without nutritional depletion and this, therefore, cannot account entirely for quadriceps weakness. That disuse is a necessary condition for weakness is supported strongly by the finding that in patients with quadriceps muscle weakness, the strength of the diaphragm, adductor pollicus[18] and abdominal muscles[19] is normal; the relevance of these muscles is that they are continuously active, even in patients with the most severe disease. The presence of cofactors with immobility is not excluded by these data. In normal life,[20] and especially during acute exacerbation, people with COPD have substantially reduced physical activity. It is well known that muscle strength is lost rapidly during disuse,[21] and it is inevitable that quadriceps strength was shown recently to exhibit a significant reduction during admission for acute exacerbation of COPD.[22] Spruit *et al* hypothesised a role for the cytokine interleukin 8 (IL-8) for muscle weakness in this context, and other groups have separately suggested a role for tumour necrosis factor alpha (TNF-α)[23] and interleukin 6 (IL-6).[24] Other factors may also be relevant, in particular gene polymorphisms: we have established recently that, independent of lung function, the type II polymorphism of the gene that codes for angiotensin-converting enzyme is associated with reduced quadriceps strength in patients with COPD but not in age-matched controls.[25]

Recently, data have emerged to confirm that quadriceps fatigue is symptom-generating in COPD. Thirty-two patients underwent a constant-rate exercise test; magnetic stimulation of the femoral nerve was undertaken before and after the test.[26] This measurement was developed by our group[27] and is a sensitive test for the identification of quadriceps fatigue.[7] Of the 32 patients, 22 developed quadriceps fatigue; these patients had more glycolytic enzymes and fewer capillaries than non-fatiguers. Importantly, patients who developed fatigue had higher leg-symptom scores, suggesting that fatigue is associated directly with symptom generation.

Anaerobic metabolism at low work rates

The reduction in oxidative enzymes results in patients with COPD producing lactic acid as a by-product of anaerobic metabolism at much lower rates of exercise compared with age-matched controls.[10] Lactic acid is buffered by bicarbonate to produce carbon dioxide (CO_2) and water. The lungs can normally excrete CO_2, but this is not the case in patients with COPD, who have flow limitation. One would therefore predict that such patients would retain CO_2 during whole-body exercise. When we tested this hypothesis in patients with a mean FEV_1 of 24% predicted, we found this to be the case, with a mean rise of $Pa\,CO_2$ during constant-rate treadmill exercise from 5.38 kPa to 6.32 kPa and a fall in pH from 7.41 to 7.36.[28]

Pulmonary mechanics reduce capacity

Breathlessness may arise for several reasons. The proposition that pulmonary mechanics limit exercise in COPD is not synonymous with the start of our spiral, patients becoming breathless on exertion. The observation that flow limitation was present in COPD is longstanding,[29,30] but it has become apparent that increasing lung volumes during exercise – dynamic hyperinflation – contribute to symptom generation in COPD[31] and a reduction in dynamic hyperinflation can reduce dyspnoea in the absence of changes in FEV_1.[32,33] Dynamic hyperinflation can be measured easily using the inspiratory capacity measurement technique (Fig 3) and should form part of future intervention studies.

☐ ARE THERE TREATMENT OPPORTUNITIES IN THE SPIRAL?

Preventing development of myopathy

Pulmonary rehabilitation is an established treatment option[34] endorsed by the National Institute of Health and Clinical Excellence (NICE), which believes that 'Pulmonary rehabilitation should be made available to all appropriate patients with

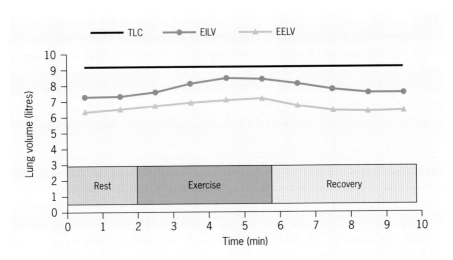

Fig 3 Example of dynamic hyperinflation induced by exercise in a patient with chronic obstructive pulmonary disease (COPD) in our laboratory. EELV = end expiratory lung volume; EILV = end inspiratory lung volume; TLC = total lung capacity.

COPD' (www.nice.org.uk/pdf/CG012_niceguideline.pdf). It is clear that in patients with mild disease, high-intensity pulmonary rehabilitation can elicit a true training benefit[35] and pulmonary rehabilitation can increase the oxidative enzyme content of skeletal muscle.[36]

If skeletal muscle were to develop weakness in a stepwise manner around exacerbations, as proposed by Spruit *et al*,[22] then logically it would be appropriate to target pulmonary rehabilitation around the time of exacerbation. This was done in a study by Man and coworkers, in which patients admitted with acute exacerbation were randomised at discharge to receive usual care or, in addition, to receive pulmonary rehabilitation.[37] The intervention group had a significant reduction in visits to accident and emergency departments at 3 months (10% *v* 43%, p=0.01) and greater improvement in shuttle walking distance (+90 m *v* −25 m, p=0.002). Although this approach seems promising, it is unknown whether over a longer period early pulmonary rehabilitation confers a greater advantage than standard pulmonary rehabilitation and, if so, whether this benefit is conferred by improvements in muscle strength.

Train the quadriceps muscle

As noted above, in patients with mild to moderate disease, it is possible to train the quadriceps muscle using pulmonary rehabilitation. However, the same approach does not work in patients with more severe COPD, as they are unable to reach a sufficiently high work intensity.[38] An alternative approach is to train the quadriceps muscle in isolation using percutaneous electrical stimulation. Two studies have trialled this approach,[39,40] but although significant benefits have been claimed from these studies the method has not yet moved into general use. One problem is that it is hard to design an appropriate placebo, since the recipient is aware of the electrical stimuli. Therefore, in our own approach to this problem, we have opted to train only one leg and to use the other leg as a control and to assess response in terms of muscle-biopsy appearances and the twitch tension elicited by magnetic stimulation of the femoral nerve,[27] since these measures are independent of patient effort. Studies are ongoing and we plan to report in early 2007.

Reduce the impact of anaerobic metabolism

High-intensity exercise in COPD gives rise to acidosis and hypercapnia. Intuitively, approaches to rehabilitation that allow the patient to exercise with reduced minute ventilation could allow the patient to cope better with hypercapnia. Little detailed work has been done in this regard, although it has been established that very-high-intensity supplemental oxygen reduces dynamic hyperinflation,[41] and this approach is in use by some groups.

An obvious option is to use non-invasive ventilation (NIV) to assist exercise in pulmonary rehabilitation. NIV is an established therapy in the care of patients admitted with acute exacerbations of COPD.[42,43] When used acutely during exercise in COPD, NIV reduces respiratory muscle work[44,45] and attenuates exercise-induced lactataemia. Based on these findings, we hypothesised that NIV given during a PR programme could allow patients to reach a higher level of exercise and therefore achieve a true physiological training benefit. We tested this hypothesis in a prospective randomised controlled study in 19 patients with severe COPD.[46] The patients receiving NIV during exercise were able to achieve a higher level of exercise and, when studied during a constant-rate exercise test without NIV after the programme, such patients had a 30% reduction in blood lactate compared with patients who had exercised without NIV (Fig 4). This difference showed a trend towards statistical significance (p=0.09), and a larger multicentre study to assess the place of NIV in pulmonary rehabilitation is required. Two other studies have addressed this question: one showed benefit[47] and one did not.[48] The only clear factor that explains the difference is that our study and that of Costes *et al*[47] enrolled patients with more severe disease compared with Bianchi *et al*,[48] and it seems reasonable that this adjunctive therapy would be most helpful in patients with more severe disease.

Improving pulmonary mechanics

It has become clear that a variety of drugs may improve pulmonary mechanics in the absence of a clear improvement in FEV_1, including beta$_2$ agonists,[49] tiotropium[50] and low-density gas mixtures.[51]

Lung transplantation, either single or double, may provide a considerable improvement in lung function,[52] but this is not a therapeutic option for most patients because of the shortage of donor organs and because the mortality of the procedure (15% at 1 year, 50% at 5 years) is unattractive to patients with all but the most severe disease.

Lung-volume reduction surgery (LVRS) was revived in the mid 1990s,[53] and

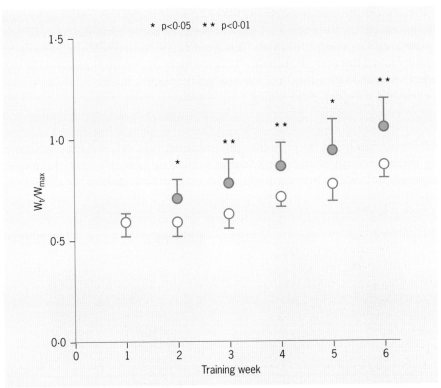

Fig 4 Mean work rates achieved each week in people with chronic obstructive pulmonary disease (COPD) undergoing pulmonary rehabilitation (PR) with (closed symbols) and without (open symbols) the benefit of non-invasive ventilation (NIV). Data from Hawkins *et al* (2002), reproduced with permission of the BMJ Publishing Group.[46]

randomised controlled studies have established that the procedure can improve exercise performance and mortality in patients with heterogeneous upper-zone bullous emphysema.[54,55] Unfortunately, there are several drawbacks to LVRS. First, the surgery is beneficial only in patients with upper-lobe bullous disease, who constitute at most 25% of patients with emphysema. Second, the mortality rate of approximately 5% is unattractive to many patients. Third, in order to minimise mortality, most groups, including our own, set minimum fitness criteria for patients being considered for LVRS of a shuttle walk distance of more than 150 m and a carbon monoxide gas transfer (TL_{CO}) greater than 30% predicted. In practice, this means that many patients prepared to consider the operation fail on safety criteria. Finally, even in the best hands, improvement does not occur in about 25% of patients, and no good method of identifying non-responders preoperatively has been found.

It has become a matter of interest to find a less invasive method of achieving lung-volume reduction. Two main approaches have been advocated. One is to create an extra-pulmonary pathway to allow additional drainage of air from the lung. Ex vivo this approach is satisfactory,[56] but no in vivo data are yet in the public domain. An alternative concept is to place a one-way valve in the airway, which prevents air entering the subtended lobe but allows air to exit. The theory is that the subtended lobe will then collapse, causing volume reduction. This certainly can work (Fig 5); importantly, in series reported from our[57,58] and other[59–61] institutions, it seems to be free of major side effects. As with LVRS, a beneficial response is not universal, but the valves can at least be removed if desired. Physiological analysis indicates that improvement in walking distance can be explained almost entirely by a reduction in dynamic hyperinflation and improved ventilation/perfusion matching.[58] Current thinking is that the best choice of treatment (extra-pulmonary bypass versus endobronchial blocker) may be influenced by the presence or absence of collateral ventilation (desirable with the former approach, not with the latter), and this can be conveniently assessed at bronchoscopy.[62]

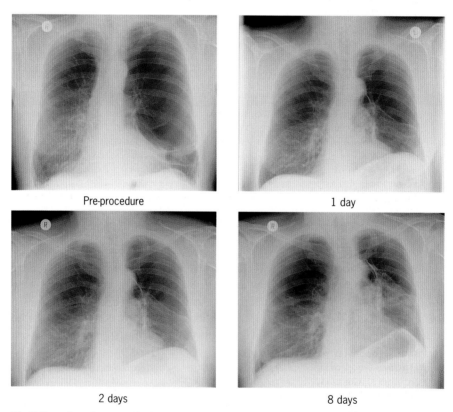

| Pre-procedure | 1 day |
| 2 days | 8 days |

Fig 5 Examples of consecutive X-rays from a responder to bronchoscopic lung volume reduction.

☐ CONCLUSION

COPD is not simply a pulmonary disease, and consideration of the disease spiral may allow for additional treatment and research opportunities that may be of considerable benefit to patients.

CONFLICT OF INTEREST

Dr Polkey has received research funding from Emphasys Medical.

CITATION

This chapter has been published in *Clinical Medicine* Vol 6 No 2 March/April 2006 pp190–6. Please cite only from the journal.

REFERENCES

1 Pauwels RA, Buist AS, Calverley PM, Jenkins CR, Hurd SS. Global Strategy for the Diagnosis, Management, and Prevention of Chronic Obstructive Pulmonary Disease. NHLBI/WHO global initiative for chronic obstructive lung disease (GOLD) workshop summary. *Am J Respir Crit Care Med* 2001;163:1256–76.

2 Fletcher C, Peto R. The natural history of chronic airflow obstruction. *BMJ* 1977;1:1645–8.

3 Jones PW. Health status measurement in chronic obstructive pulmonary disease. *Thorax* 2001;56:880–87.

4 Celli BR, Cote CG, Marin JM, Casanova C *et al*. The body–mass index, airflow obstruction, dyspnea, and exercise capacity index in chronic obstructive pulmonary disease. *N Engl J Med* 2004;350:1005–12.

5 Williams TJ, Patterson GA, McClean PA, Zamel N, Maurer JR. Maximal exercise testing in single and double lung transplant recipients. *Am Rev Respir Dis* 1992;145:101–5.

6 Killian KJ, Leblanc P, Martin DH, Summers E *et al*. Exercise capacity and ventilatory, circulatory, and symptom limitation in patients with chronic airflow limitation. *Am Rev Respir Dis* 1992;146:935–40.

7 Man WD, Soliman MG, Gearing J, Radford SG *et al*. Symptoms and quadriceps fatigability after walking and cycling in chronic obstructive pulmonary disease. *Am J Respir Crit Care Med* 2003;168:562–7.

8 Bernard S, LeBlanc P, Whittom F, Carrier G *et al*. Peripheral muscle weakness in patients with chronic obstructive pulmonary disease. *Am J Respir Crit Care Med* 1998;158:629–34.

9 Jakobsson P, Jorfeldt L, Brundin A. Skeletal muscle metabolites and fibre types in patients with advanced chronic obstructive pulmonary disease, with and without chronic respiratory failure. *Eur Respir J* 1990;3:192–6.

10 Maltais F, Simard AA, Simard C, Jobin J *et al*. Oxidative capacity of the skeletal muscle and lactic acid kinetics during exercise in normal subjects and in patients with COPD. *Am J Respir Crit Care Med* 1996;153:288–93.

11 Richardson RS, Leek BT, Gavin TP, Haseler LJ *et al*. Reduced mechanical efficiency in chronic obstructive pulmonary disease but normal peak VO2 with small muscle mass exercise. *Am J Respir Crit Care Med* 2004;169:89–96.

12 Decramer M, Gosselink R, Troosters T, Verschueren M, Evers G. Muscle weakness is related to utilization of health care resources in COPD patients. *Eur Respir J* 1997;10:417–23.

13 Marquis K, Debigare R, Lacasse Y, LeBlanc P *et al*. Midthigh muscle cross-sectional area is a better predictor of mortality than body mass index in patients with chronic obstructive pulmonary disease. *Am J Respir Crit Care Med* 2002;166:809–13.

14 Couillard A, Prefaut C. From muscle disuse to myopathy in COPD: potential contribution of oxidative stress. *Eur Respir J* 2005;26:703–19.

15 Hopkinson NS, Man WD, Dayer MJ, Ross ET *et al*. Acute effect of oral steroids on muscle function in chronic obstructive pulmonary disease. *Eur Respir J* 2004;24:137–42.

16 Chailleux E, Laaban JP, Veale D. Prognostic value of nutritional depletion in patients with COPD treated by long-term oxygen therapy: data from the ANTADIR observatory. *Chest* 2003;123:1460–66.

17 Schols AM, Slangen J, Volovics L, Wouters EF. Weight loss is a reversible factor in the prognosis of chronic obstructive pulmonary disease. *Am J Respir Crit Care Med* 1998;157(6 Pt 1):1791–7.

18 Man WD, Soliman MG, Nikoletou D, Harris ML *et al.* Non-volitional assessment of skeletal muscle strength in patients with chronic obstructive pulmonary disease. *Thorax* 2003;58:665–9.

19 Man WD, Hopkinson NS, Harraf F, Nikoletou D *et al.* Abdominal muscle and quadriceps strength in chronic obstructive pulmonary disease. *Thorax* 2005;60:718–22.

20 Pitta F, Troosters T, Spruit MA, Probst VS *et al.* Characteristics of physical activities in daily life in chronic obstructive pulmonary disease. *Am J Respir Crit Care Med* 2005;171:972–7.

21 Harris ML, Polkey MI, Bath PM, Moxham J. Quadriceps muscle weakness following acute hemiplegic stroke. *Clin Rehabil* 2001;15:274–81.

22 Spruit MA, Gosselink R, Troosters T, Kasran A *et al.* Muscle force during an acute exacerbation in hospitalised patients with COPD and its relationship with CXCL8 and IGF-I. *Thorax* 2003;58:752–6.

23 Creutzberg EC, Schols AM, Weling-Scheepers CA, Buurman WA, Wouters EF. Characterization of nonresponse to high caloric oral nutritional therapy in depleted patients with chronic obstructive pulmonary disease. *Am J Respir Crit Care Med* 2000;161(3 Pt 1): 745–52.

24 Debigare R, Marquis K, Cote CH, Tremblay RR *et al.* Catabolic/anabolic balance and muscle wasting in patients with COPD. *Chest* 2003;124:83–9.

25 Hopkinson NS, Nickol AH, Payne J, Hawe E *et al.* Angiotensin converting enzyme genotype and strength in chronic obstructive pulmonary disease. *Am J Respir Crit Care Med* 2004;170:395–9.

26 Saey D, Michaud A, Couillard A, Cote CH *et al.* Contractile fatigue, muscle morphometry, and blood lactate in chronic obstructive pulmonary disease. *Am J Respir Crit Care Med* 2005;171:1109–15.

27 Polkey MI, Kyroussis D, Hamnegard C-H, Mills GH *et al.* Quadriceps strength and fatigue assessed by magnetic stimulation of the femoral nerve in man. *Muscle Nerve* 1996;19:549–55.

28 Polkey MI, Hawkins P, Kyroussis D, Ellum SG *et al.* Inspiratory pressure support prolongs exercise induced lactataemia in severe COPD. *Thorax* 2000;55:547–9.

29 Dayman H. Mechanics of breathing in health and emphysema. *J Clin Invest* 1951;30:1175–90.

30 Christie RV. The elastic properties of the emphysematous lung and their clinical significance. *J Clin Invest* 1934;13:295–319.

31 O'Donnell DE, Revill SM, Webb KA. Dynamic hyperinflation and exercise intolerance in chronic obstructive pulmonary disease. *Am J Respir Crit Care Med* 2001;164:770–77.

32 Man WD, Mustfa N, Nikoletou D, Kaul S *et al.* Effect of salmeterol on respiratory muscle activity during exercise in poorly reversible COPD. *Thorax* 2004;59:471–6.

33 Hadcroft J, Calverley PM. Alternative methods for assessing bronchodilator reversibility in chronic obstructive pulmonary disease. *Thorax* 2001;56:713–20.

34 Griffiths TL, Burr ML, Campbell IA, Lewis-Jenkins V *et al.* Results at 1 year of outpatient multidisciplinary pulmonary rehabilitation: a randomised controlled trial. *Lancet* 2000;355:362–8.

35 Casaburi R, Patessio A, Ioli F, Zanaboni S *et al.* Reductions in exercise lactic acidosis and ventilation as a result of exercise training in patients with obstructive lung disease. *Am Rev Respir Dis* 1991;143:9–18.

36 Maltais F, LeBlanc P, Simard C, Jobin J *et al.* Skeletal muscle adaptation to endurance training in patients with chronic obstructive pulmonary disease. *Am J Respir Crit Care Med* 1996;154 (2 Pt 1):442–7.

37 Man WD, Polkey MI, Donaldson N, Gray BJ, Moxham J. Community pulmonary rehabilitation after hospitalisation for acute exacerbations of chronic obstructive pulmonary disease: randomised controlled study. *BMJ* 2004;329:1209.

38 Casaburi R, Porszasz J, Burns MR, Carithers ER *et al.* Physiologic benefits of exercise training in rehabilitation of patients with severe chronic obstructive pulmonary disease. *Am J Respir Crit Care Med* 1997;155:1541–51.

39   Neder JA, Sword D, Ward SA, Mackay E *et al.* Home based neuromuscular electrical stimulation as a new rehabilitative strategy for severely disabled patients with chronic obstructive pulmonary disease (COPD). *Thorax* 2002;57:333–7.

40   Bourjeily-Habr G, Rochester CL, Palermo F, Snyder P, Mohsenin V. Randomised controlled trial of transcutaneous electrical muscle stimulation of the lower extremities in patients with chronic obstructive pulmonary disease. *Thorax* 2002;57:1045–9.

41   Somfay A, Porszasz J, Lee SM, Casaburi R. Dose—response effect of oxygen on hyperinflation and exercise endurance in non-hypoxemic COPD patients. *Eur Respir J* 2001;18:77–84.

42   Plant PK, Owen JL, Elliott MW. Early use of non-invasive ventilation for acute exacerbations of chronic obstructive pulmonary disease on general respiratory wards: a multicentre randomised controlled trial. *Lancet* 2000;355:1931–5.

43   Bott J, Carroll MP, Conway JH, Keilty SEJ *et al.* Randomised controlled trial of nasal ventilation in acute respiratory failure due to chronic obstructive airways disease. *Lancet* 1993;341:1555–7.

44   Polkey MI, Kyroussis D, Mills GH, Hamnegard C-H *et al.* Inspiratory pressure support reduces slowing of inspiratory muscle relaxation rate during exhaustive treadmill walking in severe COPD. *Am J Respir Crit Care Med* 1996;154:1146–50.

45   Kyroussis D, Polkey MI, Hamnegard CH, Mills GH *et al.* Respiratory muscle activity in patients with COPD walking to exhaustion with and without pressure support. *Eur Respir J* 2000;15:649–55.

46   Hawkins P, Johnson LC, Nikoletou D, Hamnegard CH *et al.* Proportional assist ventilation as an aid to exercise training in severe chronic obstructive pulmonary disease. *Thorax* 2002;57:853–9.

47   Costes F, Agresti A, Court-Fortune I, Roche F *et al.* Noninvasive ventilation during exercise training improves exercise tolerance in patients with chronic obstructive pulmonary disease. *J Cardiopulm Rehabil* 2003;23:307–13.

48   Bianchi L, Foglio K, Pagani M, Vitacca M *et al.* Effects of proportional assist ventilation on exercise tolerance in COPD patients with chronic hypercapnia. *Eur Respir J* 1998;11:422–7.

49   O'Donnell DE, Voduc N, Fitzpatrick M, Webb KA. Effect of salmeterol on the ventilatory response to exercise in chronic obstructive pulmonary disease. *Eur Respir J* 2004;24:86–94.

50   Celli B, ZuWallack R, Wang S, Kesten S. Improvement in resting inspiratory capacity and hyperinflation with tiotropium in COPD patients with increased static lung volumes. *Chest* 2003;124:1743–8.

51   Palange P, Valli G, Onorati P, Antonucci R *et al.* Effect of heliox on lung dynamic hyperinflation, dyspnea, and exercise endurance capacity in COPD patients. *J Appl Physiol* 2004;97:1637–42.

52   Martinez FJ, Orens JB, Whyte RI, Graf L *et al.* Lung mechanics and dyspnea after lung transplantation for chronic airflow obstruction. *Am J Respir Crit Care Med* 1996;153:1536–43.

53   Cooper J, Patterson G, Sundaresan R, Trulock E *et al.* Results of 150 consecutive bilateral lung volume reduction procedures in patients with severe emphysema. *J Thorac Cardiovasc Surg* 1996;112:1319–30.

54   Geddes D, Davies M, Koyama H, Hansell D *et al.* Effect of lung-volume-reduction surgery in patients with severe emphysema. *N Engl J Med* 2000;343:239–45.

55   Fishman A, Martinez F, Naunheim K, Piantadosi *et al.* A randomized trial comparing lung-volume-reduction surgery with medical therapy for severe emphysema. *N Engl J Med* 2003; 348:2059–73.

56   Lausberg HF, Chino K, Patterson GA, Meyers BF *et al.* Bronchial fenestration improves expiratory flow in emphysematous human lungs. *Ann Thorac Surg* 2003;75:393–8.

57   Toma TP, Hopkinson N, Hillier J, Hansell DM *et al.* Bronchoscopic volume reduction with valve implants in patients with severe emphysema. *Lancet* 2003;361:931–3.

58   Hopkinson NS, Toma TP, Hansell DM, Goldstraw P *et al.* Effect of bronchoscopic lung volume reduction on dynamic hyperinflation and exercise in emphysema. *Am J Respir Crit Care Med* 2005;171:453–60.

59   Snell G, Holsworth L, Borrill ZL, Thomson KR *et al.* The potential for bronchoscopic lung volume reduction using bronchial prostheses. *Chest* 2003;124:1073–80.

60   Yim AP, Hwong TM, Lee TW, Li WW *et al.* Early results of endoscopic lung volume reduction for emphysema. *J Thorac Cardiovasc Surg* 2004;127:1564–73.

61   Venuta F, de Giacomo T, Rendina EA, Ciccone AM *et al.* Bronchoscopic lung-volume reduction with one-way valves in patients with heterogeneous emphysema. *Ann Thorac Surg* 2005;79:411–7.

62   Morrell NW, Wignall BK, Biggs T, Seed WA. Collateral ventilation and gas exchange in emphysema. *Am J Respir Crit Care Med* 1994;150:635–41.

The
William Withering Lecture

William Withering's legacy – for the good of the patient

Alasdair Breckenridge

☐ INTRODUCTION

The lessons that the physician William Withering learned from his studies of digitalis are still relevant today. This paper highlights four of these lessons and updates them using the tools of clinical pharmacology and pharmacoepidemiology. First, Withering learned that failure to prepare digitalis from the foxglove in a standard manner resulted in a product with unpredictable clinical effects. Preparation of medicines from plants since then has not followed similar good practice and medicines have often not been granted marketing authorisation because of variability in their quality. Second, differences in the response to digitalis were noted by Withering, but he had little idea of their basis. Clinical pharmacology has shown that for drugs such as digitalis differences are caused by variability both in receptor sensitivity and in drug disposition. Third, the dose-response characteristics of digitalis were well known to Withering. Modern techniques of measuring response, such as the use of biomarkers, have made such studies easier, although clinical observations remain the gold standard. Fourth, Withering documented many of the adverse effects of digitalis. The use of various modern databases has facilitated the analysis of clinical toxicology and thus of risk-benefit profiles.

William Withering was born in Wellington, Shropshire in 1741 and died in 1799 of pulmonary tuberculosis. He was a true polymath, being not only a physician of national repute, but also an expert botanist and a mineralogist, with both a genus of plants and a mineral named after him. But he is best known for his work on digitalis; his book, *An account of the foxglove and some of its medical uses*, was published in 1785 and is, by any standards, a remarkable work.[1]

It has been said that if digitalis were to come before a medicines regulatory committee today, it would be refused a licence. This can be disputed, for as a former Withering Lecturer, Michael Rawlins, said of Withering's book:

> *Its contents would do justice to an Expert Report accompanying a Product Licence application to the drug regulatory authority of any state in the European Union.*[2]

In his book, Withering describes how he:

- ☐ collected and prepared the leaves of the purple foxglove (*Digitalis purpurea*) to obtain a product of reasonable consistency

- ☐ demonstrated that some individuals were more responsive to digitalis than others

- ☐ investigated the dose-response characteristics of digitalis, with respect to both slowing the heart rate and inducing a diuresis

- ☐ identified most of the adverse effects of digitalis and their relation to dose, and how toxicity could be minimised by dose reduction.

Withering's impressive understanding of his newly discovered drug serves as a model for much of today's therapeutics, and it is no exaggeration to describe him as the father of clinical pharmacology.

This paper will take each of the lessons that Withering learned from studying digitalis and show how it has influenced modern clinical pharmacology and thus the regulation of medicines. The paper draws extensively on the writings of Jeffrey Aronson on Withering and digitalis.[3]

☐ LESSON 1: MEDICINES FROM PLANTS – VARIATIONS IN BIOAVAILABILITY

The production of medicines from plants has a long and variable history that is bedevilled by problems of impurities and poor standardisation, which makes Withering's efforts of over 200 years ago all the more remarkable:

> I was well aware of the uncertainty which must attend on the exhibition of the root of a biennial plant and therefore continued to use the leaves. These I found to vary much at different seasons of the year, but I found that if gathered at one time of year, namely when it was in its flowering state and carefully dried, the dose could be determined as exactly as any other medicine. The more I saw of the great powers of this plant, the more it seemed necessary to bring the doses to the greatest degree of accuracy.[1]

Unfortunately, not all these lessons have been learned and remembered. Over the past 10 years, one of the most contentious areas of therapeutics has been the drug treatment of depression with tricyclic antidepressants and selective serotonin reuptake inhibitors (SSRIs). Concerned about the adverse effects of these drugs, many depressed subjects have had recourse to herbal antidepressants, in particular St John's wort (SJW). SJW is widely used as an antidepressant in Germany, where more SJW than fluoxetine (Prozac) is sold for the treatment of depression, and in 1998 the sales value of SJW in Europe was $6 billion.

The herbal preparation consists of the dried flower tops or other parts of SJW, which are usually harvested shortly before or during the flowering season. However, the concentrations of the main active principle of SJW, hypericin, varies as much as 10-fold in different formulations, depending on which part of the plant is used, variations in growth conditions, and the time of year that it is gathered.[4]

SJW has pharmacological effects by virtue of its actions on the neurotransmitters serotonin, noradrenaline, and dopamine. However, SJW has important properties other than its antidepressant action, namely the ability to interact with other medications taken at the same time. It inhibits and then induces the metabolism of several important isozymes of CYP450. Thus, marked changes in the levels of such commonly used medicines as cyclosporin, warfarin, and constituents of oral contraceptive have been well documented in patients starting SJW.[4] SJW also induces the activity of the transporter p-glycoprotein, which is involved in the disposition of digoxin.

Several applications have been made to medicine licensing authorities to market preparations of SJW for the treatment of depression but all have failed – one reason being the variability in the content of active principle in the various batches.

A second modern example of variations in bioavailability concerns digoxin.[5] In 1969, Burroughs Wellcome, one of the main manufacturers of digoxin, decided to improve the formulation of their proprietary brand of digoxin, Lanoxin. The amount of digoxin in the tablet remained unchanged, but several of the excipients in the tablet were altered. The clinical importance of these changes went undetected for some time and it was only due to skilful detective work that the reason was unearthed for a lack of response to Lanoxin in some patients. Four-fold variability in the bioavailability of different batches of Lanoxin was eventually found, causing great variability in plasma digoxin levels in patients due to the differing rates of digoxin release from tablets in the stomach and intestine. In 1975, British pharmacopoeia standards for digoxin were published to prevent a repeat of this problem.

☐ LESSON 2: INTERINDIVIDUAL VARIATION IN RESPONSE TO DIGOXIN

Withering was aware that not all patients responded in the same beneficial way to digitalis administration. He knew little, of course, of how digoxin exerted its therapeutic effects and even less of its disposition within the body.

Today, one of the basic tenets of clinical pharmacology is that:

drug + receptor → drug-receptor complex → pharmacological effect

Variability in response to digoxin can therefore depend on variation in the sensitivity of the receptor on which digoxin acts, ie in its pharmacodynamics, or on variation in its disposition within the body, ie in its pharmacokinetics.

Pharmacodynamics

Four levels of action can be described:

1 At the *molecular level* there is strong evidence that digitalis inhibits the ubiquitous magnesium-dependent membrane-bound enzyme Na^+/K^+-ATPase and thus alters the intracellular disposition of Na^+, K^+ and indirectly Ca^{2+}.

2 At the *cellular level*, this results in an increased rate of contractility of cardiac muscle fibres (although this is not so in acute myocardial infarction or cor pulmonale, for reasons that are not entirely clear).

3 At the *whole heart level*, this results in an increase in cardiac output. In hypertrophic obstructive cardiomyopathy, however, due to the outflow obstruction, this increase may result in a worsening of the clinical situation rather than an improvement.

4 At the *whole body level*, the beneficial effects of digitalis manifest as alleviation of the symptoms and signs of heart failure.[3]

Marked variability in each of these stages has been documented.

Pharmacokinetics

Advances in our understanding of the pharmacokinetics of digitalis have been even more profound, and central to this is an appreciation of the role of the transporter protein p-glycoprotein.

Transporter proteins are key determinants of drug transport across cell membranes of the intestine, pancreas, liver hepatocytes, kidney and blood-brain barrier, where they are expressed in the apical portion of epithelial cells. These proteins influence both the influx and efflux of drugs across membranes. Much is now known of the molecular structure of these proteins, of their genetic control, and of the gene families that encode individual members. Genetic polymorphisms in several transporter proteins have been documented and their clinical relevance explored.[6]

The transporter protein p-glycoprotein is expressed in the apical segment of the epithelial cells of the jejunum, colon, proximal convoluted tubules of the kidney, biliary canaliculi of hepatocytes, and brain capillaries. P-glycoprotein acts as an efflux pump for many drugs, including digoxin, at these various sites. Over-expression of p-glycoprotein is associated with multidrug resistance (MDR) to many anticancer drugs as it removes these drugs from the intestine to the gut lumen. Thus, p-glycoprotein is also known as the MDR transporter.

With respect to digoxin, p-glycoprotein is an efflux transporter in the gut and at the blood-brain barrier, but less so within the kidney. In MDR knockout mice, ie mice that do not express p-glycoprotein activity, administration of digoxin results in a 30-fold increase in brain digoxin levels and a four-fold increase in digoxin plasma levels compared to control mice.[6]

In man, Greiner *et al* showed a significant correlation between the plasma area under the curve (AUC) of administered digoxin and the expression of p-glycoprotein in jejunal biopsies.[7] Further, when these subjects were given the inducing agent rifampicin and jejunal biopsies were taken before and after its administration, three- to four-fold increases in p-glycoprotein activity were found and the correlation between the plasma AUC of administered digoxin and p-glycoprotein activity was maintained (Fig 1).

Thus, the genetics of p-glycoprotein and the effects of other drugs that induce or inhibit p-glycoprotein activity are central to our understanding of the pharmaco-kinetics and thus the interindividual variability of the response to digoxin.

☐ LESSON 3: DOSE-RESPONSE CHARACTERISTICS OF DIGITALIS

The two main issues that Withering grappled with were the indications for digitalis administration and the appropriate dose. It is worth remembering that while Withering found that digitalis was remarkably effective in treating cases of dropsy, and that in doing so, he noted a slowing of the heart, the diagnoses, let alone the pathophysiology, of heart failure and atrial fibrillation were beyond the understanding of 18th century physicians.

Fig 2 shows Aronson's estimation of the efficacy of digitalis in the 162 cases of dropsy treated by Withering.[3] Withering encountered considerable toxicity, but

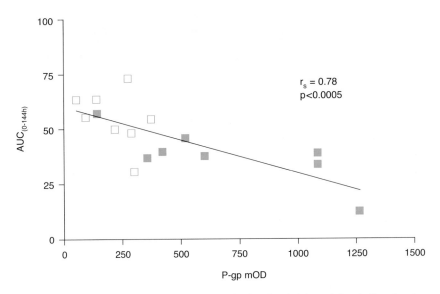

Fig 1 Correlation between area under the curve (AUC) of orally administered digoxin (1 mg) and expression of p-glycoprotein (n=16) measured by Western blot. Open squares = without rifampicin; filled squares = with rifampicin (600 mg). Reproduced from Greiner *et al* with permission of American Society for Clinical Investigation.[7]

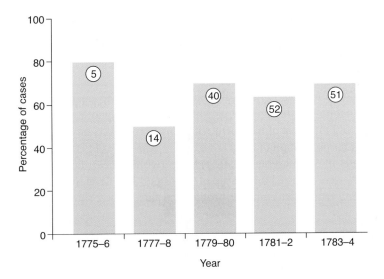

Fig 2 Percentage rates of therapeutic efficacy achieved by Withering with the foxglove, classified by year of use. The numbers in each bar refer to the number of cases treated during the relevant years. Reproduced from Aronson with permission of Oxford University Press.[3]

Aronson's estimation also show that as Withering became more adept at selecting dosage regimens, the incidence of adverse effects decreased.

The debate continues even today as to the appropriate dose of digitalis, and whether its dose-response characteristics in heart failure and atrial fibrillation are similar. The main problem is how to measure its efficacy; atrial fibrillation poses fewer problems than heart failure. While the gold standard for assessment of the therapeutic efficacy of a drug remains, changes in mortality or in quality-of-life measurements, such as improvement in disease-related symptoms or in activity or need for hospitalisation, require long and large studies of new drugs or in dose finding.

Thus, there is great interest in the use of surrogate measurements (reliable endpoint substitutes (physical signs or laboratory measurements), which should correlate with the frequency and intensity of the disease endpoint both as an epidemiological marker and as a therapeutic response) and biomarkers (laboratory measurements used as a surrogate measurement) in therapeutic drug evaluation.[8] The ideal marker should be biologically plausible, be detectable in most subjects at all stages of the disease, change towards normal when an effective agent is given, predict the ultimate clinical response in patients taking the drug, and discriminate between patients who will do well and those who will not.

Many biomarkers for heart failure have been proposed over the years; one of the more interesting and potentially valuable is B-type natriuretic peptide (BNP). BNP is released from ventricular myocytes, augments urine volume and sodium excretion, and inhibits the sympathetic nervous system and the renin angiotensin system. It has also been used as a possible treatment for heart failure.[9]

Two studies illustrate the potential usefulness of BNP measurements in situations with which Withering would have been familiar. First, the BNP for Acute Shortness of Breath Evaluation (BASEL) study investigated 452 patients presenting to the emergency room of a medical centre:[10] 225 patients were assigned to a diagnostic strategy involving measurement of BNP, while 227 were assessed in the standard manner. A plasma BNP concentration of >100 pg/ml was used as a discriminator for the diagnosis of heart failure from shortness of breath due to other causes. When used with other clinical information, rapid measurement of BNP in the emergency room improved the evaluation and treatment of patients with acute dyspnoea, reducing the time to discharge and total cost of treatment with no adverse effects on mortality or rate of subsequent hospitalisation (Table 1).

Second, a subset of 3,346 asymptomatic patients (without heart failure) in the Framingham study were followed for a mean of 5.2 years.[11] BNP level was measured at the first screening visit to determine its prognostic value. Table 2 shows that each

Table 1 B-type natriuretic peptide (BNP) for evaluation of acute shortness of breath.[10]

	BNP group	Standard group	p
Hospitalised (%)	75	85	0.008
Requiring intensive care (%)	15	24	0.01
Median time to discharge (days)	8.0	11.0	0.001
Cost of treatment ($)	5,410	7,264	0.006
30-day mortality (%)	10	12	0.45

Table 2 Prognostic value of B-type natriuretic peptide (BNP) measurement at first clinic visit in 3,346 persons without heart failure, followed for mean of 5.2 years.[11]

1 SD increment in BNP associated with:	p
27% increased risk of death	0.009
28% increased risk of first cardiovascular event	0.03
77% increased risk of heat failure	<0.001
66% increased risk of atrial fibrillation	<0.001
53% increased risk of stroke	0.002

incremental increase in BNP level correlates significantly with both mortality and cardiovascular morbidity. Interestingly, excess risk was apparent at BNP levels well below current thresholds for the diagnosis of heart failure.

BNP levels taken in isolation, however, must be interpreted with caution. Whether data such as that obtained by Wang et al[11] help in clinical management was questioned in a leading article published alongside the original article:

> *Looking at BNP in isolation may be akin to seeing smoke trailing out of the window of a house without having any notion of what is on fire, where that fire is, or how it can best be extinguished.*[9]

☐ LESSON 4: ADVERSE REACTIONS TO DIGITALIS

As Withering gained more experience with the use of digitalis, he noted fewer adverse effects.[1] Whether or not this related to different dosage regimens is more problematical, but we do know that over the years he experimented with different preparations of digitalis which probably had varying degrees of bioavailability.

The issue of the risk-benefit balance of digitalis is very much alive today. I have argued that the use of biomarkers such as BNP might be useful in documenting the benefit of digitalis. Are there equivalent tools to help our understanding of safety issues? The safety of medicines still depends very much on careful clinical observation and documentation, combined with biomarkers of toxicity. What has changed over the years is the sophistication of the way we study adverse reactions.

It is widely appreciated that when a medicine is granted a marketing authorisation, the understanding of its overall safety profile is very incomplete, relying on what can be extrapolated from animal pharmacology and from the limited clinical trial evidence that is available at that time. An appreciation of the safety profile of a new medicine can only be gained after it is marketed, and tools are required to capture this information. These tools are spontaneous adverse reaction reports, clinical databases, and clinical studies, both observational and experimental.

So, Withering's first port of call today if he were interested in the clinical toxicology of digitalis would be to access the reports of adverse reactions reported to a regulatory authority such as the Medicines and Healthcare products Regulatory Agency. Since 1963, when the UK Yellow Card database was set up, until the end of 2005, some 628 reports of adverse reactions to digoxin (104 cardiac and 94 gastrointestinal) were reported, 36 of which have been fatal (14 cardiac and 3 gastrointestinal). It might be considered that this is a remarkably small number, but it is known that all such spontaneous reporting systems suffer from under reporting, that such schemes have great difficulty in distinguishing adverse drug reactions from similar common symptoms that occur frequently in the population, and that for old drugs such as digitalis, prescribers are asked only to report severe and unusual reactions. In this respect, it is interesting that 20 cases of reproductive and breast disorder, including gynaecomastia, and 28 cases of eye disorders, mainly perturbation of colour vision, have been reported on Yellow Cards.

Further investigation of the adverse events following digitalis therapy could be carried out using the General Practice Research Data Base (GPRD) which contains some four million ongoing clinical records.

To study the cardiac side effects, however, it would be necessary to mount a clinical study, either an observational study (cohort or case-control) or a controlled clinical trial, since this is the best way of distinguishing adverse drug effects from similar events that are commonly seen in the community. Cardiovascular toxicity following therapy with rofecoxib (Vioxx) has recently been defined in a clinical trial;[12] spontaneous reports failed to document this toxicity.

□ CONCLUSION

The subtitle of this article is 'for the good of the patient'. By going back to the lessons that William Withering taught us over 200 years ago, and putting them in a modern context, this paper attempts to fulfil his legacy.

ACKNOWLEDGEMENTS

I am grateful to Jeffrey Aronson, Iain Chalmers and Trevor Jones for their helpful advice in the preparation of this paper.

CITATION

This chapter has been published in *Clinical Medicine* Vol 6 No 4 July/August 2006 pp393–7. Please cite only from the journal.

REFERENCES

1 Withering W. *An account of the foxglove and some of its medical uses.* London: CGJ and J Robinson, 1785.

2 Rawlins M. Pharmacovigilance: paradise lost, regained or postponed? *J R Coll Physicians* 1995;29:41–9.

3 Aronson JK. *An account of the foxglove and its medical uses 1785–1985.* Oxford: Oxford University Press, 1985.

4 Henderson L, Yue QY, Berqvist C *et al.* St. John's wort: drug interactions and clinical outcomes. *Br J Clin Pharmacol* 2002;54:349–56.

5 Munro-Faure AD, Fowle ASE, Fox J *et al.* Recognition of variable bioavailability as an international problem: a review of earlier studies. *Postgrad Med J* 1974;50(Suppl 6):14–8.

6   Mizuno N, Niwa T, Yotsumoto Y *et al*. Impact of drug transporter studies on drug discovery and development. *Pharmacol Rev* 2003;55: 425–61.

7   Greiner B, Eichelbaum M, Fritz P, *et al*. The role of intestinal P-glycoprotein in the interaction between digoxin and rifampicin. *J Clin Invest* 1999;104:147–53.

8   Jortani SA, Prabhu SD, Valdes R. Strategies for developing biomarkers for heart failure. *Clin Chem* 2004;50:265–78.

9   Mark DB, Felker GM. B-type natriuretic peptide-a biomarker for all seasons? *N Engl J Med* 2004;350:718–20.

10 Mueller C, Scholer A, Laule-Kilian K *et al*. Use of B-type natriuretic peptide in the evaluation and management of acute dyspnoea. *N Engl J Med* 2004;350:647–54.

11 Wang TJ, Larson MG, Levy D *et al*. Plasma natriuretic peptide levels and the risk of cardiovascular events and death. *N Engl J Med* 2004;350:655–63.

12 Bresalier RS, Sandler RS, Quan H *et al*. Cardiovascular events associated with rofecoxib in a colorectal adenoma chemoprevention trial. *N Engl J Med* 2005;352:1092–102.

Answers to self assessment questions

☐ RESPIRATORY

Management of acute respiratory distress syndrome

1a True	2a False	3a False	4a False
b True	b True	b True	b False
c False	c False	c False	c False
d True	d False	d True	d False
e False	e False	e True	e False

Improving outcomes in lung cancer

1a True	2a False	3a False	4a True
b True	b True	b True	b True
c False	c True	c False	c True
d False	d False	d True	d False
e True	e False	e True	e True

☐ CARDIOVASCULAR

Of stents and stem cells – advances in the management of ST elevation myocardial infarction

1a True	2a False	3a True	4a False
b True	b False	b False	b False
c True	c True	c True	c True
d False	d False	d False	d True
e True	e False	e True	e False

Angina pectoris: second wind, warm up and walk through

1a False	2a True	3a True
b True	b False	b True
c True	c True	c True
d False	d False	d True
e False	e True	e True

Minimally invasive valve replacement

1a True	2a True	3a True	4a True
b False	b True	b True	b False
c False	c False	c False	c False
d True	d False	d True	d True
e True	e True	e False	e True

Hypertension: lessons from the eponymous syndromes

1a True	2a True	3a True
b False	b False	b True
c False	c False	c True
d True	d False	d True
e True	e False	e False

☐ GASTROENTEROLOGY

Recent progress in inflammatory bowel disease: from bench to bedside

1a True	2a False
b True	b False
c False	c True
d False	d False
e False	e False

Progress in understanding and managing functional gastrointestinal disorders

1a False	2a False	3a False
b True	b False	b True
c False	c False	c True
d True	d True	d False
e True	e False	e True

Neuroendocrine tumours of the gastrointestinal tract and pancreas

1a True	2a False	3a True
b True	b True	b True
c True	c True	c False
d False	d True	d False
e False	e False	e True

Biomedical review – inflammation and cancer

1a False	2a False	3a True
b True	b True	b False
c False	c False	c False
d True	d True	d True
e True	e True	e True

□ NEUROLOGY

Stroke: advances in acute treatment and secondary prevention

1a False	2a True	3a False
b True	b False	b True
c False	c False	c True
d False	d True	d True
e False	e True	e False

Mitochondrial disorders – more common than you thought?

1a False	2a True	3a False
b False	b False	b False
c True	c True	c True
d True	d True	d True
e False	e True	e True

□ REHABILITATION

Rehabilitation following neurological injury

1a True	2a True	3a False	4a True	5a False
b False	b True	b False	b False	b True
c False	c True	c False	c False	c False
d True	d False	d True	d False	d False
e True	e False	e True	e True	e True

□ DERMATOLOGY

Pigmentation and sunburn

1a False	2a False	3a False
b True	b False	b True
c True	c False	c False
d True	d False	d True
e False	e True	e False

□ DIABETES/ENDOCRINOLOGY

Understanding glucocorticoids

1a True	2a False	3a True
b True	b False	b True
c False	c False	c False
d False	d True	d True
e False	e False	e False

Cushing's syndrome

1a	False	2a	True	3a	False
b	True	b	True	b	False
c	True	c	False	c	False
d	False	d	False	d	False
e	True	e	False	e	False

☐ GERIATRICS

Advances in Parkinson's disease

1a	True	2a	False	3a	True	4a	False	5a	False
b	True	b	False	b	False	b	False	b	True
c	True	c	False	c	True	c	True	c	True
d	True	d	False	d	False	d	True	d	True
e	False	e	True	e	True	e	True	e	True

☐ NEPHROLOGY

IgA nephropathy and Henoch-Schönlein purpura

1a	False	2a	True	3a	True	4a	False
b	False	b	False	b	False	b	False
c	True	c	True	c	True	c	True
d	True	d	False	d	False	d	False
e	True	e	True	e	True	e	True

Haemolytic uraemic syndrome

1a	False	2a	True	3a	True	4a	False
b	False	b	False	b	True	b	False
c	False	c	True	c	True	c	True
d	True	d	False	d	False	d	True
e	True	e	True	e	True	e	False

☐ RHEUMATOLOGY

Understanding osteoarthritis

1a	True	2a	True	3a	True	4a	False	5a	False
b	False	b	False	b	True	b	True	b	True
c	False	c	True	c	True	c	True	c	False
d	True	d	False	d	True	d	True	d	True
e	True	e	True	e	True	e	False	e	True

Developments in rheumatoid arthritis

1a False	2a True	3a False	4a False
b False	b False	b True	b True
c True	c False	c False	c False
d True	d True	d True	d True
e False	e True	e True	e True

☐ HEPATOLOGY

Vascular liver disorders

1a False	2a True	3a True	4a False	5a True
b False	b True	b True	b False	b True
c True	c True	c False	c True	c True
d False	d False	d True	d False	d False
e False	e False	e True	e False	e False

☐ INFECTIOUS DISEASES

Sepsis: new paradigms, novel therapies

1a True	2a True	3a True	4a True
b True	b True	b False	b True
c True	c True	c True	c True
d False	d False	d True	d False
e False		e True	e True